This book is dedicated to all the gluten-free people who have ever been less than impressed with the total at the bottom of their supermarket receipts.

BECKY EXCELL

BUDGET GLUTEN FREE

OVER 100 EASY AND AFFORDABLE
RECIPES FOR EVERY DAY

Photography by Hannah Hughes

Quadrille

AIR FRYER FAVOURITES 62

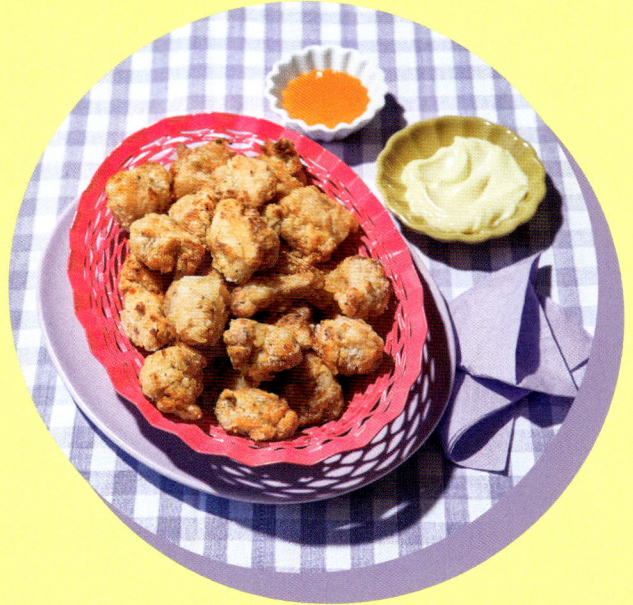

LUNCH + ON-THE-GO 32

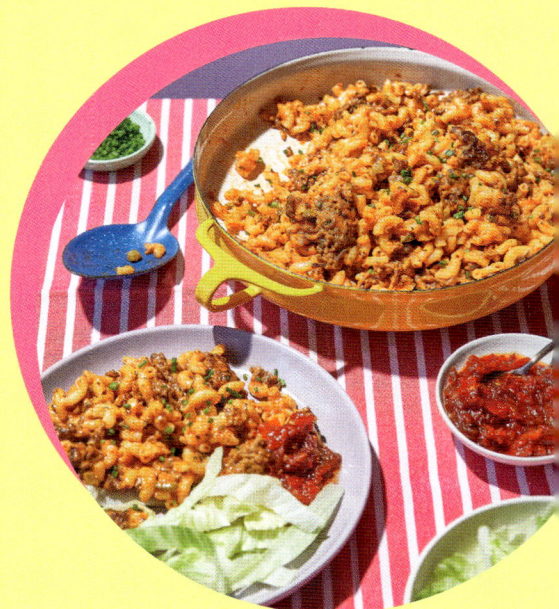

SAVVY STREET FOOD 84

BIG BATCH SLOW
COOKING 170

SPEEDY SUPPERS
120

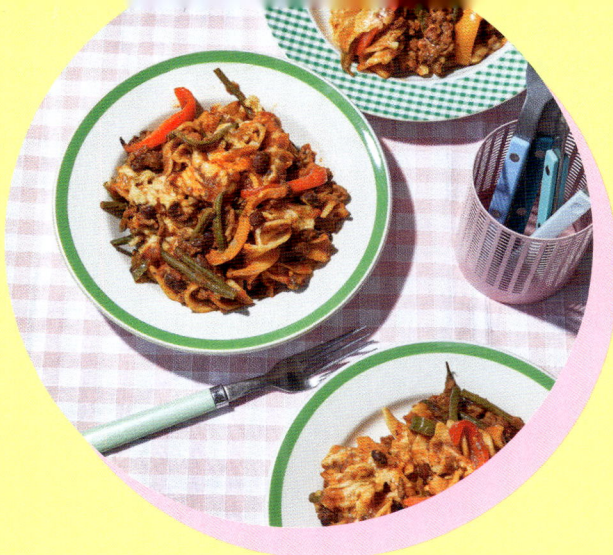

BARGAIN
BAKES 204

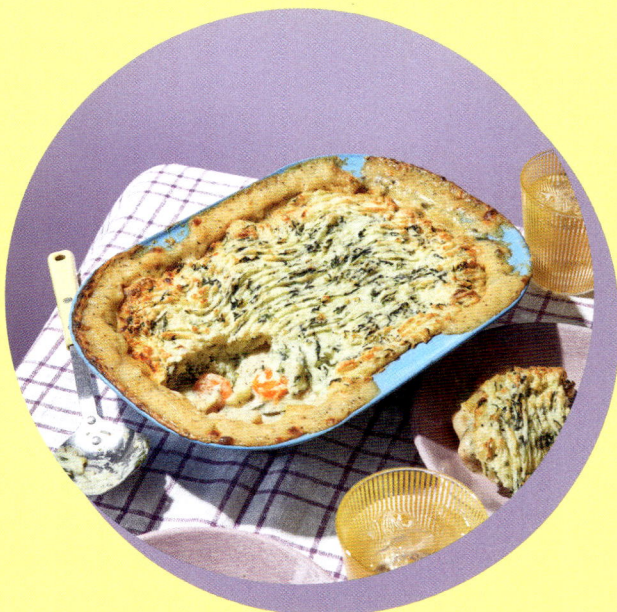

LOW-COST
COMFORT FOOD 140

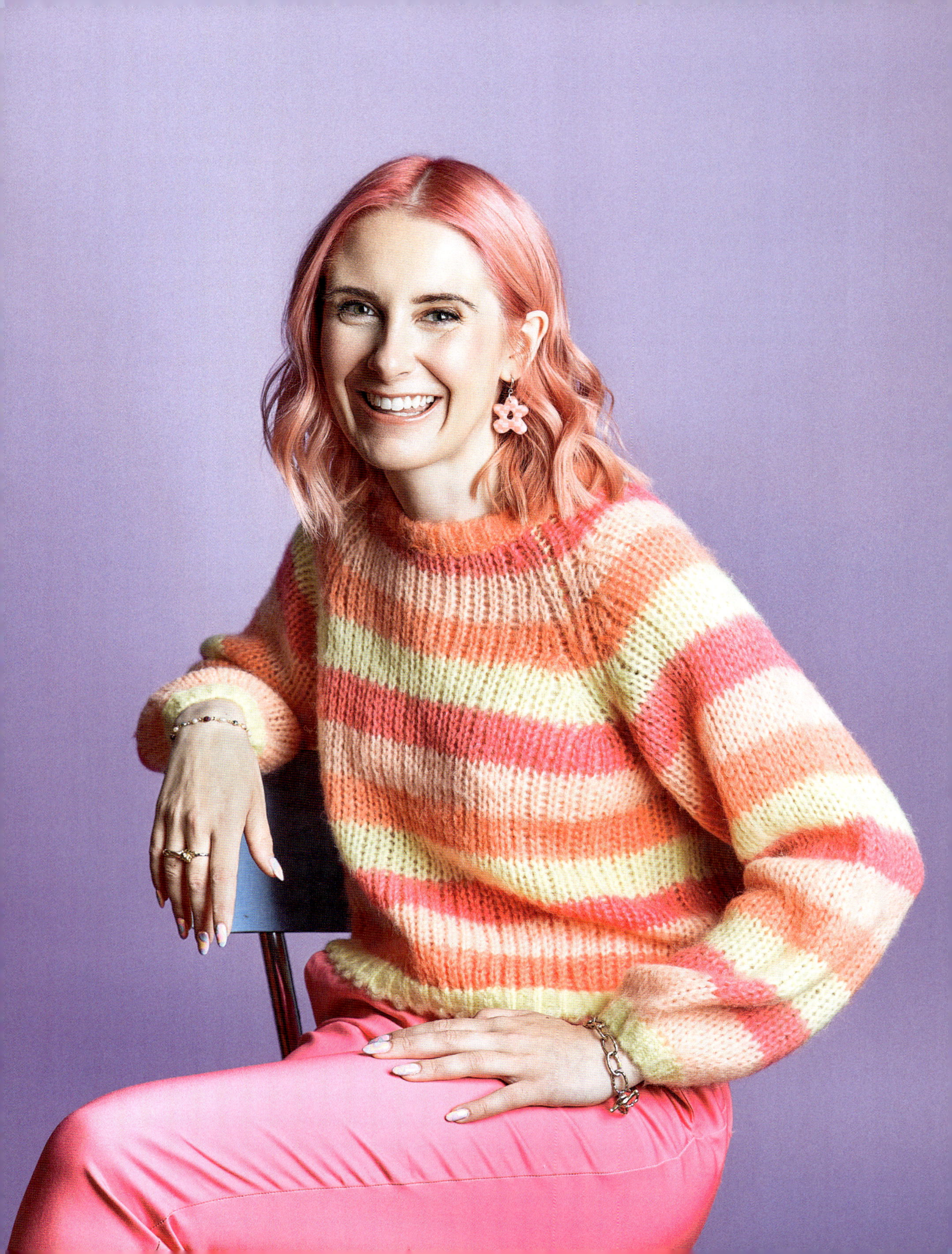

INTRODUCTION

Whether you've been on a gluten-free diet for one day or several decades, you'll very likely already know how expensive gluten-free products and ingredients can be. Whenever I tell friends and family that the price of a supermarket loaf of gluten-free bread can be up to seven times more expensive than a 'normal' loaf of bread, I'm always met with a look of pure shock. Yes, that's right, some people spend their disposable income on holidays of a lifetime, but I spend mine on making a sandwich.

But that gluten-free premium doesn't end at bread: other everyday essentials like flour, cereals and pasta are often twice as expensive as their gluten-containing counterparts, with other non-negotiable key ingredients being no exception. Imagine if I was to add up all those extra costs I've spent over my sixteen years of being on a gluten-free diet... I shudder to think of how much extra I've spent in total, which is exactly why I've never added it up! But what's the solution? Abstain from them entirely and live in a world where we all eat soup (without bread!) for every meal? And if we're not doing that, then how on earth could this book possibly make any real impact or difference to your supermarket receipts?

Well, against all odds, this book *can* make a difference. I've shared all the know-how and tricks behind my own budget-friendly cooking and baking philosophy that I've learned throughout my sixteen years on a gluten-free diet, across 100+ delicious recipes that nobody would ever know were gluten-free or budget-friendly. Not only will you quickly be able to make savings that will more than cover the cost of this book, you'll crucially learn how to offset the dreaded 'gluten-free tax' that's inevitably applied to most gluten-free products and ingredients. Using this book won't mean spending hours in the kitchen either, it actually encourages quite the opposite – time is money, after all!

My hit-and-miss experience with budget-friendly recipes over the years made me certain on one thing when I first began to write this book: I needed this book's definition of a 'budget-friendly recipe' to be as clear and concise as possible. This book had to deliver a clear promise on what my personal 'rules' are so you aren't left wondering why I've included these particular recipes; and that's exactly what I did (see page 8) before I even wrote a single recipe. That way, not only will you be able to understand exactly what's been hard-wired into each recipe and how they take cost very seriously, you'll also be able to apply my philosophy outside of these 100+ recipes.

But what about the big gluten-free elephant in the room? How does being gluten free factor into all of this if we're *not* going to be abstaining from the use of costlier gluten-free products entirely? Well, perhaps the best part of my budget cooking and baking philosophy is that I developed it entirely with being gluten free in mind. Don't thank me – I didn't have much choice! My entire approach to creating budget-friendly recipes developed as a way to counterbalance the increased cost of using essential gluten-free products. When I realized it was working so well that I was often spending even less money than before I was gluten free, I was absolutely set on writing this book and sharing it with the gluten-free community. By making savings to this degree, not only was I still able to include necessary gluten-free products in my recipes, the savings also allowed me to afford other eye-wateringly expensive essentials like gluten-free bread.

I hope it also goes without saying that a huge part of my budget cooking and baking philosophy is the notion that the end product of a budget-friendly gluten-free recipe need not look, taste or be any less than magnificent. After all, I'm a firm believer that all gluten-free food should be affordable, accessible and downright delicious and, not surprisingly, so is this book.

If you have total unyielding trust in me and just want to get started, taking a deep dive into my approach over the next few pages is absolutely not mandatory. After all, my own personal approach is hard-wired into every recipe in this book anyway! However, if you ever do have questions as to why a recipe uses a particular ingredient or instructs a particular cooking method, remember that you'll always find the answer laid out somewhere in my definition of budget-friendly cooking and baking on page 8. One caveat to that: you'll probably want to swing by the savvy shopping tips over on page 12, because knowing how to source affordable ingredients is probably more integral to budget cooking and baking than the actual recipes themselves!

So if you're tired of looking at your supermarket receipt and wondering if you accidentally scanned fifteen extra products at the self-service checkout, I can assure you that you've picked the right book! I hope it brings you a lifetime of savings, a savviness that supermarkets wish you didn't have, and endless plates of gluten-free food that'll quickly become family favourites while restoring a deserved sense of normality.

ABOUT ME

Hello, I'm Becky! I'm a gluten-free food writer, #1 *Sunday Times* best-selling author with now well over 1 million of you following me across social media. You might even have seen me on TV (politely) correcting common misconceptions surrounding Coeliac disease and gluten-free food in general. Now, if you told me I'd be writing all of the above in my *seventh* cookbook when I first started a gluten-free diet sixteen years ago... I probably wouldn't have believed you!

Back then, I was still just an eighteen-year-old student who had only recently started her first year of university studying law. I'd just moved 250 miles to Manchester from the small town I grew up in (and from my boyfriend, Mark) to live with seven new flatmates in student halls. One of the first unexpected challenges I faced there was learning how to shop, cook and live on a shoestring budget, all while possessing very basic cooking skills. Yet just as I was beginning to get to grips with things, there was a far greater challenge to come...

Every single time I went out to eat with my flatmates (we had vouchers for a local pizza place) I would almost immediately feel unwell. Not only did I feel bloated – along with many other unpleasant gut symptoms that I won't go into right now – but I was totally exhausted and I had no idea why. So I continued eating out (mostly so I didn't feel left out!) and, as a result, I felt like I was about to explode! To cut a long story short, I eventually went to the doctor and he recommended I remove gluten from my diet,* which did improve how I felt.

With gluten-loaded pizza taken away from me and a sudden reliance on far costlier gluten-free products (of which there weren't many!), my weekly food budget instantly became ten times harder to manage. Not forgetting that I had absolutely zero support, information or resources in navigating a gluten-free diet on a tight budget. And here's me thinking that all I'd have to worry about in my first year of university were my grades! That's not even mentioning the dizzying implications of living alongside seven other people; cross-contamination was an absolute nightmare.

Needless to say, having to get to grips with a gluten-free diet couldn't have come at a worse time. After struggling for months, I eventually dropped out entirely and went back home (in shame!). Though the reasons I decided to call it a day weren't solely due to the additional stresses of being gluten-free on a tight budget (I didn't enjoy studying law, I missed Mark, I didn't really feel like I fitted in... I could go on!) there's

no doubt that it absolutely didn't help. When I should have been in the library reading books, instead I often found myself in supermarkets reading ingredient lists and assessing prices!

Maybe if I wasn't constantly preoccupied with feeling unwell, feeling awkward around food in social situations, being hypervigilant about cross-contamination or persistently stressing about what I could both eat and afford, perhaps this story would have had a happier ending? I certainly would have been able to focus on my studies and social life a lot more.

You'll be pleased to know that I eventually did go back to university and conquer the initial trials and tribulations of surviving being gluten-free on a tight budget. And even though I didn't realize it at the time, that experience became the foundation of my approach to budget cooking and baking forevermore; an approach that would be further tried, tested, honed and sharpened throughout my adult years.

Ever since then, I've always wanted to write the book that I sorely needed when I first started a gluten-free diet all those years ago; one that would have allowed me to quickly get back to worrying about my aims and ambitions, not about what was for dinner. Yet it dawned on me that if I wrote that book, I would also be writing one that many gluten-free people likely also need *right now* when the costs of being gluten-free are higher than ever.

So I decided to sit down and condense everything I know about budget cooking and baking on a gluten-free diet. I put everything that I've learned, from 100% tried and true real life experience, into 100+ recipes and a series of easy-to-understand practically minded guides. That way, whether this book is absolutely vital to quickly restoring a sense of normality to your life, or you just want to decrease the cost of your weekly shop, you're free to embrace it as much as desired.

Being gluten free isn't a choice and I firmly believe that every person has a right to exciting, accessible, nourishing meals (and the odd sweet treat!) regardless of their dietary requirements or budget. So unsurprisingly, this book reflects that belief too!

Of course, don't forget to check out my blog (www.glutenfreecuppatea.co.uk) and my social media channels (@beckyexcell) for tons more budget-friendly recipes, with no doubt many more to come in the future.

Let's get saving!

Becky x

* It wasn't until a while later that I found out I should have been tested for Coeliac disease before giving up gluten. Testing for Coeliac disease when you haven't regularly been eating gluten won't provide an accurate result – so this is a quick reminder to anyone who has any symptoms (and there are plenty more than I've mentioned) to not remove gluten from your diet until you have been properly tested! Check the website of your country's Coeliac society for more information about the diagnosis of Coeliac disease.

MY DEFINITION OF 'BUDGET-FRIENDLY' COOKING + BAKING

So in the spirit of total transparency (and I also think you'll learn more from these recipes if you understand the thinking behind them), this section outlines my personal philosophy, rules and approach when creating budget-friendly, gluten-free recipes.

It can sometimes be difficult to just look at a recipe that claims to be 'budget-friendly' and reverse engineer exactly why it's been labelled this way. So, in this section, I thought it would make sense to clearly define my own personal budget-cooking philosophy so you never have to wonder why any of the recipes that are in this book are here. Plus, I strongly feel that these are the types of things that every home cook or baker should know so that you're empowered to make any recipe as budget-friendly as you need it to be.

Of course, reading this entire section is by no means mandatory, because each of these 'pillars' of my philosophy is built into each and every recipe – be it within the ingredients I call for you to use, a particular way of performing a certain task or strongly within the underlying context of any given chapter. However, here are my nine pillars I consider to be incredibly important in budget cooking and baking:

1. SAVVY SHOPPING

Believe me when I say this: it all starts here! Yep, budget cooking and baking starts way before you ever start heating your pan, oven, slow cooker or air fryer. After all, if you take a budget recipe and make it using the most expensive ingredients known to man, there won't be a budget-friendly meal waiting for you at the end of it all, will there? Knowing how to source products for the best price is a cornerstone of any form of budget cooking and baking.

While I could crudely sum it up as 'go to the supermarket and buy the cheapest items, then use them in the recipes in this book', in reality it isn't always that easy, especially on a gluten-free diet. That's why I've created a detailed guide on savvy supermarket shopping on page 12, complete with the ins and outs of sourcing everything you need for the best prices, without the process turning into a new, unwanted pastime.

The ability to source all the ingredients you need at the cheapest prices can make such a difference to the cost of each meal that savvy supermarket shopping alone can instantly slim your weekly food shop receipts. So for that reason, I highly recommend you ensure you're doing it already using the tips on page 12, because when combined with the other pillars here, you can really start to significantly save and offset the cost of using dedicated gluten-free products and ingredients.

2. USE GLUTEN-FREE PRODUCTS ONLY WHEN NECESSARY OR UNAVOIDABLE + MAKE USE OF AFFORDABLE, NATURALLY GLUTEN-FREE ALTERNATIVES WHENEVER YOU CAN

What does using a gluten-free product 'only when necessary' actually mean? Well, essentially, if you fancy a pasta dish, you're going to need gluten-free pasta, regardless of its cost! And in that sense, when the use of a costlier gluten-free product is absolutely essential to the dish, that's totally fine; that's where other pillars of my budget cooking philosophy can come into play to offset the cost of using them. This is exactly why I say there's no need to permanently abstain from using gluten-free products, as you can always offset their costs elsewhere! The same applies to when gluten-free soy sauce is an integral part of a dish – yes, removing it would mean a cheaper overall cost, but it would also likely mean a bland meal that nobody really enjoys. In both of the above scenarios, both ingredients are essential. After all, we already have so much taken away from us from the day we embark on a gluten-free diet, so why should we have to take away gluten-free products too?

But though this book makes use of gluten-free products and ingredients when absolutely necessary, it also partly endeavours to introduce exciting naturally gluten-free recipes into the mix too – those based around rice, for example – which can further offset the days where you do use costlier gluten-free products and ingredients. In fact, the entire lunch chapter was written as an alternative to using gluten-free bread – an essential ingredient for a sandwich, but why should a sandwich be essential for lunch every day? With that chapter in your back pocket, it certainly doesn't need to be!

And lastly, how could the use of a gluten-free product ever possibly be avoidable? Well, this part pertains to only using gluten-free products when there's no other way around it – which there often can be! Take my Ouma's Tangy Beef Babotie for example (page 152), a delicious South African casserole that's traditionally made with a slice of white bread soaked in milk. Instead of using a costly slice of gluten-free bread, I managed to adapt the recipe to achieve the same result without it. You're definitely not expected to work this all out yourself, because I've already done this part for you – though you might never realize it! However, this has always been a key part of my approach to creating budget-friendly recipes, and absolutely should be a part of yours when using recipes outside of this book.

3. SMART SWAPS

To me, smart swaps are those that replace noticeably costly ingredients with super-cost-effective ones that perform the exact same job – and for once we're not exclusively talking about gluten-free products. Budget-friendly recipes I've tried online in the past are often quite happy to use small amounts of expensive ingredients; that's because the cost of a small amount is relatively low, making the recipe still seem affordable and appealing.

A common example of this would be a budget recipe calling for 20g (¾oz) of an expensive ingredient like Parmesan. I always think: well, yes, the cost of that isn't a lot by itself (especially when you divide it per person) but what about the cost of the other 180g (6½oz) I've now got sitting in the fridge?! And let's not forget that the average block of Parmesan costs the same as the most expensive loaf of gluten-free bread.

So to combat that, I've simply swapped common expensive ingredients out entirely, usually for affordable ones that I already have in the fridge anyway. Following this particular example, I simply swap out Parmesan for mature Cheddar, which currently costs less than half the price despite fulfilling a similar role. Again, in the recipes in this book, these types of swaps have already been done for you and following them will no doubt result in noticeable savings.

By making smart swaps, all that's likely to vary is a subtle difference in flavour, yet in a dish or bake with several other ingredients, that flavour difference matters less. Just like with the next pillar of budget cooking and baking philosophy, it could be very easy to see these swaps negatively. But the aim is to swap costlier ingredients for better-value ones that always still pull their weight in terms of flavour, taste and texture. Otherwise I wouldn't swap them!

4. SMART BULKING

If cutting open a chicken pie only to find two chunks of chicken has taught us anything, it's that scrimping on costlier ingredients and bulking them out with cheaper ingredients isn't always the answer. We need to be smarter about it. That's why I make the distinction between 'smart bulking' and what I guess can only be considered 'dumb bulking'.

So, what is smart bulking? Think of some of your favourite Chinese takeaway dishes (which generally excel at 'smart bulking') – how many of your favourite dishes feature beansprouts, carrots, peppers, big chunks of onion, bamboo shoots etc.? And do you mind that they're there or do you just appreciate the dish as a whole? All of these ingredients are considerably cheaper than meat or fish, yet they add a different texture, flavour, visual appeal and extra nutrition to the finished dish. They make it a well-rounded, exciting plate so it's not just 'protein and sauce' – a pleasing balance of protein to veg that no one even notices and simply makes the dish go further. It allows the cost of each meal per person to be incredibly low while still churning out delicious, balanced and nutritious meals. If done right, you won't even notice or care!

5. BUDGET COOKING KNOW-HOW

I know this sounds vague, but in reality, lots of you might possess varying degrees of this knowledge already. This know-how centres on little tips and tricks surrounding the process of preparing, cooking or baking food that either:

- Make ingredients go further
- Taste better at little extra cost
- Economize the use of costlier essential ingredients
- Make use of small appliances with cheaper running costs
- Or maybe even use leftovers to reduce the amount of food that ends up going to waste

Take something as simple as using vegetable oil in a spray bottle, for example: in the past I would use anything from 1–2 tablespoons of vegetable oil to grease my pan. However, when greasing with a rapid succession of sprays of oil (anywhere from 5–10 sprays depending on the size of my pot), I found that I was actually using less than 1 millilitre. That's the type of cost difference that very quickly adds up!

You'll find this sort of mystical 'know-how' seared into every recipe in this book and, simply by using them, you'll soon begin to spot all of my sneaky tricks!

6. REPEATED USE OF THE SAME INGREDIENTS

While I own a veritable arsenal of spices, canned ingredients, jars of flavour-enhancing pastes, pickled veg, different naturally gluten-free flours and starches (I could go on), this book never assumes that you do. Why? Because buying six different spices to use for one recipe that you seldom use again doesn't sound very budget-friendly, does it? So in this book, I've tried to keep them as close to the list opposite as possible, which I deem to be the absolute essentials for not only this book, but cooking and baking in general! You can read more about why I've opted to use these particular spices over on page 24.

Budget store-cupboard essentials:

- Mild curry powder
- Smoked paprika
- Dried mixed herbs
- Chinese five spice
- Salt and black pepper (sometimes coarsely ground black pepper, but it's not a huge deal if you use regular)
- Jarred jalapeños (though dried chilli flakes work well too; each 10g/¼oz of jarred jalapeños is usually equivalent to 1 teaspoon of dried mild chilli flakes)
- Honey (the runny kind – nothing fancy!)
- Ginger paste and garlic paste (garlic paste is always optional as I can't personally tolerate it and I know all these meals taste perfectly fine without it!)

Baking essentials:

- Gluten-free plain (all-purpose) flour
- Gluten-free self-raising flour
- Xanthan gum
- Gluten-free baking powder
- Bicarbonate of soda (baking soda)

The exact same notion applies to many other ingredients throughout this book too. For example, for 95% of the recipes in this book I use mature Cheddar cheese when required. I also often use tomato purée (paste) for thickening sauces and stews. The list goes on, over on page 22.

Not only does using repeated ingredients ensure you'll actually finish them, instead of them hibernating in your cupboard or fridge until they expire (which is essentially money going to waste!), but it also has a convenient side effect of just making cooking feel infinitely easier and simpler.

7. MAKE USE OF LOW-RUNNING-COST APPLIANCES WHERE POSSIBLE

As I mentioned in my last book, *Gluten Free Air Fryer*, an air fryer can actually be up to five times cheaper to run than a conventional fan oven. Slow cookers are also not only one of the cheapest small appliances to buy, but they can also be up to four times cheaper than running the oven.

If you have a modern induction hob, these can cost even less to run than slow cookers (and tend to cook the food faster, meaning it doesn't need to be on as long). And who could forget the microwave? Its running costs are comparable to an air fryer as it only heats the food in it and not the air around it.

So with all that in mind, it would be crazy not to use these small appliances as much as possible, wouldn't it? That's why you'll find lots of air fryer methods throughout this book, as well as an entire chapter dedicated to slow cooking, whether that be in a literal slow cooker, or just in a big pot on the hob.

But all of this doesn't mean that you should steer clear of your oven at all costs and instead rush out and buy all of the above small appliances if you don't have them already. It's just to give you as many options as possible in case you have these small appliances already or were considering getting one anyway. Also, take a recipe like my Yorkshire pudding wraps (page 103): with the variety of things that need cooking all at once and in the quantity required, only an oven is large enough to cook it all at once, making it the most cost-efficient way to do so. If you were to air fry each individual element separately or in small batches, the air fryer would be on so long that you might as well just use the oven!

8. COOK A LARGER QUANTITY OF FOOD WHEN YOU DO COOK (+ UNDERSTAND HOW TO FREEZE/DEFROST IT) SO YOU ACTUALLY END UP COOKING FROM SCRATCH LESS OFTEN.

With the running costs of appliances in mind, the concept of batch cooking (cooking more food than you need right now and freezing it for future meals) becomes even more appealing! Not only will it mean you're firing up your cooking appliances less often, but you'll also be washing up less and, as a bonus, will spend infinitely less time in the kitchen.

That's why I wrote an entire chapter dedicated to making 'too much' food in the Big Batch Slow Cooking chapter. Of course, it wouldn't be much good if I didn't tell you how to freeze those intentional leftovers and then bring them back to life when dinner next rolls around – that's why you'll find all the freezing and defrosting info you'll need for those recipes and more on page 28.

Having these homemade ready meals to hand brings back a convenience to being gluten free that I had long forgotten was possible! And, of course, when you haven't got anything planned for dinner and a costly last-minute takeaway or ready meal might otherwise be on the cards, at least you've got the option of a delicious home-cooked meal that can be defrosted and on plates ASAP so you can actually make a proper choice instead of feeling forced. Remember: your freezer is your friend and it'll actually cost less to run if it's well used; a fuller freezer takes less energy to keep cold!

9. YOU DON'T HAVE TO BE VEGETARIAN OR VEGAN TO ENJOY MEAT-FREE MEALS.

What more can I say? Of course, this doesn't mean that half of the entire book is now suddenly vegetarian! But there's no denying that meat-free dinners are some of the most cost-effective meals around and that by introducing them to your meal plans even once a week they will certainly make a noticeable difference. That's why you'll find some of our favourite veggie meals that I'm absolutely confident couldn't be improved by randomly adding meat to them!

The meat-free meals in this book shouldn't necessarily be thought of as 'eating a vegetarian meal', in the same way you wouldn't eat a cheese sandwich and call it a 'vegetarian sandwich'. They're just meals that either happen to not have meat or simply don't need meat at all! And I feel that notion needs to be fully embraced when you're taking being gluten free on a budget seriously; after all, if you're eating meat every day for dinner, introducing a few meat-free meals to your meal plans every now and then gives you so much room for making significant savings. Savings that can quickly offset the cost of using gluten-free products when you do need to use them!

SAVVY SUPERMARKET SHOPPING TIPS

Without a doubt, the successful use of the recipes in this book and achieving the ultimate goal of slimming your supermarket receipts starts here. After all, what use is a budget recipe if you use the costliest ingredients the world has to offer? That's why this section exists – to give you practical tips and advice on sourcing ingredients for the best prices.

For years, when asked for my biggest money-saving tips on a gluten-free diet, I've imparted this wisdom: shop outside of free-from and gluten-free aisles where possible, limiting the products you buy there to absolute essentials. Assuming that you've got your head around being able to identify safe, gluten-free products without needing to rely on a big, bold 'gluten-free label' (see step 1 on page 17 if not), these tips focus on how to source the best-value products to use with the recipes in this book that are largely *outside* of conventional gluten-free aisles.

As I know some of you share my same, short attention span, the headlines for each tip contain exactly what you need to know. However, a little extra explanation doesn't ever really hurt, does it? So you'll find exactly what I mean, as well as the practical implications behind it, below each tip.

1. LEARN TO RECOGNIZE SUPERMARKET OWN-BRAND 'ESSENTIALS' RANGES THAT ARE EVEN CHEAPER THAN THEIR OWN-BRAND PRODUCTS.

Though these ranges *should* be easily identifiable by looking out for their obvious branding, often they aren't that easy to spot. In some supermarkets, their 'essentials' range will conveniently all fall under the same brand name with consistent, recognizable packaging. Yet in others, products in this range might have similar labels, but all under completely random, fictitious brand names and, rather unhelpfully, in all different colours. Do note that supermarket own-brand 'essentials' products are distinctly separate from even supermarket own-brand products – the 'essentials' range will be even cheaper than the latter and is created purely to price-match budget supermarkets!

To help you get off to a good start so that you know what you're looking for, here's a list of all the super value products that most definitely exist in all supermarkets under their 'essentials' range and are crucial for achieving the lowest cost-per-portion when making the recipes in this book. You'll find these specific products in both budget supermarkets and conventional supermarkets in their own budget-supermarket-style packaging:

- Canned chopped tomatoes and tomato purée (paste)
- Canned chickpeas, lentils and beans
- Long-grain rice
- Most cuts of chicken, beef and pork, including bacon
- Large bags of fresh vegetables
- Bags of frozen vegetables, especially including mushrooms, broccoli, cauliflower, mixed (bell) peppers, peas, sweetcorn, mixed frozen veg
- Frozen white fish fillets (specifically!)

A counterpoint to this tip might sound something like this: 'Yes, these products are cheap, but isn't that because they're poor quality?' But in fact, with all of the above products being wholefoods and simple ingredients, there's little room for them to be any less in quality than any 'big brand' product; for example, a chickpea is a chickpea and rice is rice! So please remember to occasionally re-evaluate whether your loyalty to the brands you buy is truly earned.

With that being said, part of shopping savvy will always involve dodging 'big brand' products wherever you can and feel comfortable doing so. There are always big savings at stake whenever big brands are involved!

2. CONSIDER + COMPARE THE COST OF INGREDIENTS BY THE PRICE PER GRAM OR KILOGRAM (OZ OR POUND).

I'm 99.9% sure that if the price of all supermarket products were displayed purely by their cost per weight, the nation's shopping habits would be very different. Supermarkets know that we will often buy the cheapest product on the shelf,

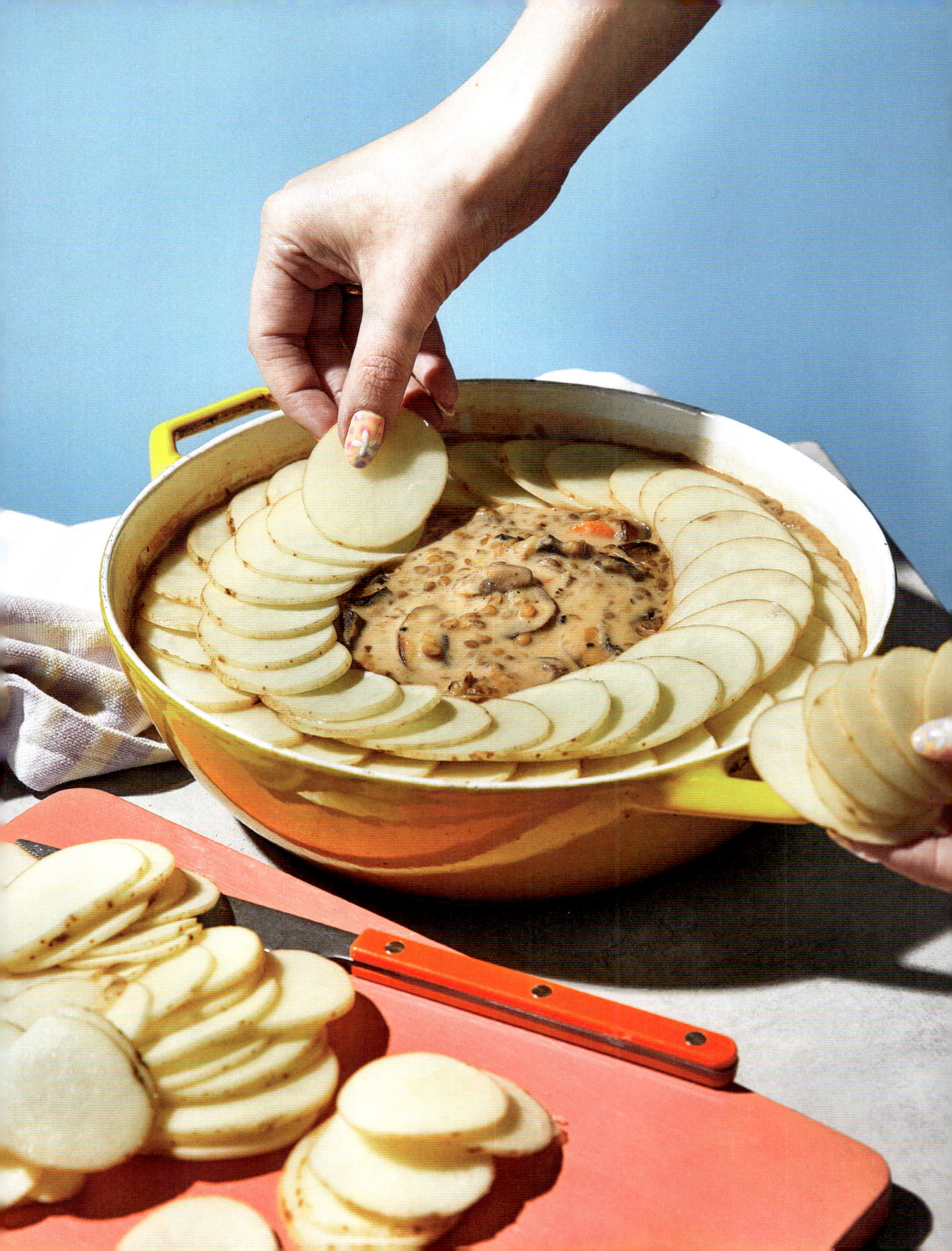

so some products are strategically portioned and priced to make you feel like you're getting good value, when in reality the pricing actually favours their own pockets.

Here's a real life example: which is cheaper? A 25g packet of cashew nuts for 60p or 300g pack for £3? Well, I phrased it to be a bit of a trick question, because of course, the 25g packet is literally cheaper! But let's take a look at their cost per weight: these prices make the 60p packet a whopping £24 per kilogram, whereas the £3 packet is £10 per kilogram. So while the smaller packet is cheaper, it's 2.4 times worse value for money. So paying attention to the price by weight will instantly help you to identify which product is truly the best value, not just the cheapest.

This information is often in small type underneath on the price label in the supermarket, just below the actual price of the product. Looking for this information never fails to truly answer the question, 'which of these products is actually cheaper?' and that's why you should always pay close attention to it.

3. BE AWARE OF THE INEVITABLE HIGH COST THAT COMES WITH CONVENIENCE.

Convenience products most definitely earn their place in any kitchen, and on a gluten-free diet (which inevitably involves more cooking and baking from scratch) their appeal only heightens. However, if you're in the habit of buying some of these products, there's a massive opportunity to save a noticeable amount on the total cost of your annual food shop, and again further offset the increased cost of being on a gluten-free diet.

Take this real-life example, which puts the previous tip into action. At the time of writing, the cheapest packet of 250g *microwavable* rice is 45p and the cheapest 1kg bag of *dried* rice is 55p – a difference of just 10p. This can easily make it feel like buying the microwavable rice is a worthwhile choice or at the very least, not *too much worse* value than buying the dried rice and cooking it yourself, right? In reality, if we consider the price per kilogram of both products, the microwavable rice is over 3 times more expensive if both were sold in equal weights. However, there's one thing we haven't yet considered that's about to make this comparison a whole

lot worse, which is that the 250g packet of microwavable rice is already cooked! That means that the water absorbed from the process of cooking it has been factored into its weight. So, how much would the 1kg bag of dried rice weigh if it were also cooked? Well, dried rice actually weighs around three times more when it's cooked! So with that in mind, if we now make the price comparison based on both products being cooked, you're now looking at 250g of microwavable rice versus a whopping 3kg of cooked dried rice. Yes, that's right, you'd get 2.75kg more rice for 10p extra simply by cooking it yourself. It's literally the difference between one packet of microwavable rice that serves 1–2 people, versus having enough rice to feed around 26 people.

To put that into perspective, if you bought 4 packets of microwavable rice per week for a year, you'd end up spending £93.85 on 208 packets (that's a lot of plastic packaging too!). If you bought the equivalent of dried rice and cooked it yourself, you'd spend £9.50 across a year for the exact same amount of cooked rice (around 17 bags of dried rice). I'll just give you a moment to let that sink in. That difference translates to a lot of loaves of even the most expensive gluten-free bread, in case you were wondering! This comparison could be even worse too as it was based on the cheapest available packet of microwavable rice – big brand equivalents cost almost twice as much for even less quantity!

Of course, the lesson this example teaches us is that convenience can be quite sneakily costly! Since this example can be a considerable saving per year, you won't be surprised to find an incredibly hands-off method to cook dried rice on the hob over in my chicken zinger ricebox recipe (page 88) or in the microwave in my microwave sweet and sour recipe (page 128) – yes, it takes longer than 2 minutes, but all you do is add rice and boiling water, cover it and come back when it's done! It's a simple habit change of putting on the rice just before you start cooking, instead of microwaving packets at the very end before serving.

I don't mean to launch a tirade against microwavable rice, as it definitely has its uses, but it's just such a great way to save a considerable amount of money that I had to give it as an example here.

4. LIMIT FREE-FROM AISLE PURCHASES TO ESSENTIAL ITEMS ONLY + ALWAYS REMEMBER TO SHOP AROUND.

While the free-from or gluten-free aisle should most definitely be your friend, watch out for products with free-from branding that are simply just 'normal' items with a high price mark-up: jars of tomato pasta sauce, lasagne white sauce, carbonara sauce, etc. are the usual main suspects – their 'normal' equivalents over in the other aisles shouldn't contain gluten to start with! Watch out for free-from cake mixes too, as they still require you to add eggs and butter, so all you're essentially buying is pre-weighed gluten-free self-raising flour and sugar (and maybe cocoa powder) at up to seven times the price of a bag of supermarket own-brand gluten-free flour.

One more crucial thing to highlight is that the prices of gluten-free and free-from products most definitely vary from store to store, as well as the range and variety of products. For example, at the time of writing, the price of gluten-free pasta is notably cheaper in two of the UK's major supermarkets than it is in others. Fortunately, shopping around for the cheapest prices no longer means you need to schedule a road trip of every local supermarket in existence – a quick check online will immediately yield a full catalogue of any given supermarket's range, complete with prices. Not surprisingly, the supermarket with the cheapest gluten-free flour, bread and dried pasta is where I often do my weekly shop now!

I also highly recommend using supermarket own-brand gluten-free flour blends (plain/all-purpose and self-raising) for the recipes in this book where possible. Not all supermarkets sell their own-brand flour blends, but when they do, they can be almost half the price of name-brand gluten-free flour blends, and they work exceptionally well too.

5. WHEN POSSIBLE, BUY INGREDIENTS IN LARGE QUANTITIES

I'm sure you might have noticed that buying cooking ingredients in more realistic quantities often means that you're effectively paying more per kilogram for the pleasure of receiving less. In most cases, this tip especially applies to those larger bags of vegetables (such as carrots and potatoes) or the biggest packets of meat (chicken breasts, thighs and beef mince) – all of these will yield quite a considerable saving when bought in a larger quantity if you pay attention to the price per gram or ounce. However, using up large quantities of ingredients before they spoil can be tough if you haven't planned on what you're going to be using them for!

Of course, a little meal planning always helps to ensure you can still take advantage of the lower price of bulk buying, but to make life easier I've written an entire chapter in this book that was made for quickly using up larger quantities of ingredients – Big Batch Slow Cooking. Usually, larger quantities of meat will come in 1kg (2lb 3oz) packs so I've ensured that these particular recipes will use 500g (lb 2oz) for example, so you can completely use up that full amount across two cooking sessions. Of course, this means that if you're a small household, you'll inevitably have leftovers – which is exactly why I've included instructions on how to store, freeze and defrost them, so absolutely nothing goes to waste. Think of it as creating your own pre-prepared ready meals at absolutely no extra cost, time investment or effort – you can thank me (and yourself) for the extra zero-effort meals later!

6. LOOK OUT FOR REDUCED OR CLEARANCE ITEMS.

Nothing beats the feeling of finding a product or ingredient that's heavily discounted, and it can make such a big difference to the final balance on your supermarket receipt. Having repeated success in finding reduced products can obviously vary, but it is possible to increase your success rate in hunting down those elusive yellow-ticket items.

For example, there are often lots of local supermarkets (from small convenience stores to medium-sized supermarkets) dotted around, that always kindly stock all the gluten-free essentials you need for a gluten-free diet. However, as products like gluten-free bread often don't have the best shelf-life in the world, and it's not necessarily an item that sells in large quantities everywhere, smaller stores are often great places to check for reduced gluten-free bread. Of course, when buying gluten-free bread that's been reduced, the best idea is to freeze it immediately. Slices can easily be toasted, or if you don't want to make sandwiches from toast, simply pop it into the air fryer at 160°C (320°F) for a few minutes to end up with warm bread as though it was freshly baked.

However, don't forget to check the 'regular' bread clearance section in larger supermarkets, as that's where they'll put the reduced gluten-free bread too. You're also far more likely to find reduced general cooking ingredients in larger supermarkets. Due to the sporadic nature that you might find, or fail to find, reduced products, their use across this book isn't assumed in each recipe's 'budget-friendly factor' – so consider it a bonus if you find any! Oh and while we're making this comparison, remember that larger supermarkets will have cheaper prices, more deals and a greater selection of budget-friendly products than smaller stores.

7. HEAD TO BUDGET SUPERMARKETS FOR WHOLEFOODS + SPICES.

Ever since the explosion of budget supermarkets, their lack of gluten-free essentials such as bread, pasta, cereal and flour has been a sticking point for most of us. While I'd love to shop there every week, their limited considerations of gluten-free eaters can mean I then have to end up going to two supermarkets just to get everything I need. In some countries, well-known budget supermarket chains have a brilliant range of gluten-free products, so if that's the case for you, then absolutely take advantage of it!

Despite this, you can still make the most of their excellent prices when it comes to meat, fish, vegetables (fresh and frozen) as well as spices, herbs and dairy products. After all, these form a huge part of cooking-from-scratch and budget-friendly cooking in general! However, if budget supermarkets aren't conveniently located for you or a double supermarket trip is simply out of the question, then the next tip might help…

8. LOOK ABOVE + BELOW EYE LEVEL OR 'GRAB LEVEL' WHEN SHOPPING IN SUPERMARKETS – THAT'S WHERE YOU'LL LIKELY FIND THE BEST-VALUE PRODUCTS.

Though this might not be true 100% of the time, I've found it to be accurate far more often than not. This is another one of those tricks that supermarkets often sneakily employ: the products that earn them the most money (i.e. make you spend more!) will usually be right in your eyeline or at a level where they're easy to lazily grab. And where are the best-value products that I mention in the first tip? Right on the bottom shelf – almost on the floor! Needless to say, there are some great savings to be made down there (and sometimes on higher shelves too), so make sure you're always glancing down there at the prices too.

9. ALWAYS SHOP WITH A SHOPPING LIST.

Hands up if you've got into the habit of going to the supermarket to do a weekly shop without a shopping list? You end up not only very likely forgetting to buy ingredients you need for a specific meal, but also buying ingredients you don't need, because you're not even 100% sure what you're going to be making. These things are especially at risk of going to waste! Without the recipes you intend to make in front of you there and then, how are you supposed to ensure you have everything you need and nothing else? That's why, if you don't already, you should absolutely be in the habit of writing everything down for the recipes you need, having earmarked which ones you're going to be making across the week in advance. It also helps to reduce the likelihood of needing the next tip…

10. RESIST ANY IMPULSE BUYS YOU DON'T NEED.

Though we always talk about supermarkets in terms of grocery shopping, it can be easy to forget that they're actually packed with lots of other household items – some of which we need and a lot of which we really don't! There's everything from clothing to gardening sundries and expensive cosmetics, and that's before mentioning the eclectic 'middle aisles' in budget supermarkets.

It's not just going into the supermarket for a bag of carrots and coming out with an inflatable lilo that I'm referring to here. Supermarkets will often have brightly coloured promotions on the ends of supermarket aisles (nearer the front and middle of the shop) showcasing anything from new products to promotions on big brands. Again, if it wasn't on your list, do you really need it? The answer to that is up to you!

CROSS-CONTAMINATION

Naturally, there's one thing that has no exceptions whether you're cooking or baking gluten-free food on a budget or not: the need for managing cross-contamination. Fortunately, apart from investing in a good set of airtight containers to ensure safe food storage and potentially separate, brightly coloured utensils, the rest is more down to knowledge and encouraging best practice rather than equipment.

I split this best practice into four parts – sourcing, storing, preparing/cooking, and serving – as the consideration of each one is integral to the successful management of cross-contamination. So here's how to make it as easy as following steps 1, 2, 3... and 4!

1. WHEN SOURCING GLUTEN-FREE INGREDIENTS OR PRODUCTS, ENSURE THEY DON'T HAVE ANY GLUTEN-CONTAINING INGREDIENTS OR RELEVANT ALLERGEN WARNINGS.

Always remember to triple-check the ingredients list on any products used to ensure that they don't have any gluten-containing ingredients or relevant allergy warnings. Here's a list of common sources of gluten that you'll need to avoid:

- wheat
- barley
- rye
- oats
- spelt

Of course, even if a product doesn't have any gluten-containing ingredients, it can still be cross-contaminated through manufacturing methods. For example, even naturally gluten-free products like beansprouts or hazelnuts can sometimes have 'may contain' warnings that make them unsuitable for those with Coeliac disease. I've even seen 'may contain gluten' warnings on salt and pepper, so it's best to check everything!

Don't forget that a gluten-free product or ingredient doesn't always need a big 'gluten-free' label on it to be considered safe to eat – it just needs to have no gluten-containing ingredients and no 'may contain' warnings for gluten-containing ingredients. This is the case here in the UK, but check your country's Coeliac society website for specific guidance elsewhere in the world.

I've indicated each ingredient in this book as 'gluten-free' where commonly necessary. But it's still best to check the ingredients and allergy info on the packaging of every product you're using in particular.

2. WHEN STORING GLUTEN-FREE INGREDIENTS OR PRODUCTS, ENSURE YOU STORE THEM SEPARATELY FROM GLUTEN-CONTAINING FOODS.

Why? Because if a gluten-free product or ingredient comes into contact with gluten at any point, it's no longer gluten-free. So how can you minimize that risk? Here are a few common best practices:

- Firstly, once gluten-free products are removed from their packaging, they must immediately be stored separately from gluten-containing products. This can easily be achieved by using airtight containers. It's also wise to label the containers so it's clear to everyone in the household what's inside.

- Ideally, you'd keep gluten-free ingredients and products in a completely separate 'gluten-free cupboard' for ease and simplicity, if your kitchen allows.

- Don't forget about the fridge, too: a high-up shelf that's purely dedicated to gluten-free foods would be ideal. And don't neglect to remember the need for separate spreads like butter; after all, if you butter gluten-laden bread, then put the knife back into the butter, the butter is no longer gluten-free. For that reason, it's always a good idea to have separate spreads and condiments that are clearly labelled as being 'gluten-free only'.

3. WHEN PREPARING/ COOKING GLUTEN-FREE FOOD, ENSURE NEITHER THE FOOD NOR EQUIPMENT USED COMES/HAS COME INTO CONTACT WITH GLUTEN AT ANY POINT.

A large part of this involves any equipment used to prepare gluten-free food being freshly and thoroughly cleaned, especially if it has been used to prepare gluten-containing food in the past. From that point onwards, the same notion applies to any pots, pans or utensils involved in cooking it. You can happily use regular washing-up liquid and dishwashers to do this. Oh, and don't forget to consider the cleanliness of your work surfaces too – if gluten-containing bread has ever been sliced there or wheat flour has ever been thrown around, then please be extra thorough in your cleaning efforts!

Of course, I hope this goes without saying, but gluten-free food must be cooked entirely separately from gluten-containing food. Again, if even a speck of gluten comes into contact with that food at any point, it's no longer gluten-free!

Here are a few practical examples where the above translates into real-life use. This isn't an exhaustive list, but is enough to give you an idea of some common scenarios:

- **Do** clean utensils, pots, pans and chopping boards before using them to prepare gluten-free food. Ideally, you'd own utensils, pans, sieves (strainers) and boards that are solely dedicated to cooking gluten-free food.
- **Do** cover gluten-free food tightly with foil and cook it on separate trays, on a separate shelf, if ever cooking gluten-containing food in the same fan oven. This will prevent the likeliness of gluten being circulated with all the hot air.
- **Do** consider having separate small appliances that are dedicated for cooking gluten-free food, such as toasters and air fryers. Neither is particularly well suited to a thorough enough clean to prevent cross-contamination.
- **Don't** cook gluten-free food in the same pans on the hob, or on the same trays in the oven, as gluten-containing food. It should always be cooked entirely separately.

- **Don't** reuse oil that has been previously used to cook gluten-containing food when deep-frying.
- **Don't** place gluten-free bread in a toaster that has been used for gluten-containing bread.
- **Don't** cut gluten-free bread on a board that has been used for gluten-containing bread, unless thoroughly cleaned. Old boards with lots of deep cuts where gluten might be difficult to remove are best avoided.

4. WHEN SERVING GLUTEN-FREE FOOD, ALWAYS KEEP IT AS FAR AWAY FROM GLUTEN-CONTAINING FOOD AS POSSIBLE.

It would be a real shame to do all of the above successfully, then ruin it by serving the food with a spoon that you just used to serve from a plate full of gluten, or by serving everything on the same plate. Fortunately, managing cross-contamination while serving can be super simple:

- Use separate utensils to serve gluten-free food. Ideally they'd be brightly coloured to distinguish them from other utensils so guests don't use them interchangeably between other gluten-containing dishes. You might want to let them know this too!
- If you can, serve gluten-free food on different coloured plates to those used to serve gluten-containing food. That way, it's not only clear to everyone else which plates are gluten-free, but also you won't then forget which is which – accidents do happen!
- If any condiments or dips are being used, ensure the gluten-free diner has their own and that they're used purely for gluten-free spreading/dipping.

The moral of the story is that you can never be too careful! Never hesitate to visit the website of your country's Coeliac society for up-to-date info.

Though it's crucial that YOU understand all of the above cross-contamination knowledge, if you share a house with others or often visit other people's houses to eat, it's essential that they read these pages and know it too. We need underline everyone to understand in order to be happy, well and safe!

ESSENTIAL EQUIPMENT

As this is a recipe book that champions affordable, budget-friendly cooking, it would be a bit strange if I then demanded that you owned every different cooking pot, utensil, appliance and kitchen gadget under the sun, wouldn't it?

So here you'll find only the cooking equipment I've used in this book, which I have kept to an absolute minimum for obvious reasons. But not only is this all the gear you'll need for this book, it's also essentially a list of what I could happily cope with if I only had all of these things and nothing else. So in other words... essential equipment! This list assumes that you already have one sharp cooking knife, wooden spoons/spatulas, large baking trays, saucepans, frying pans, digital scales and an electric hand mixer.

ESSENTIAL COOKWARE + FOOD STORAGE

Not surprisingly, apart from the absolute essentials I've just mentioned, you won't need much in terms of extra equipment to be able churn out awe-inspiring budget-friendly winners as often as you please. So here are a few extra things that are super important that you'll definitely get your money's worth out of by using this book.

5.3 litre (5½ quart) large lidded pot or round lidded casserole dish (Dutch oven)

For the Big Batch Slow Cooking chapter, you'll need a generous-sized pot, as each of the recipes is made to serve around 6–8 people (or fewer with leftovers). The size is super important as these types of pot usually come in a smaller 3.3 litre (3½ quart) size or a larger size like this: trust me, in the smaller pot, you won't have a hope of fitting everything in that chapter in it! Mine is cast iron and is not only super versatile, as it can be used on both gas and induction hobs as well as in the oven, but I picked it up at the supermarket for a great price when compared to the big-brand cast-iron pots. You can also now buy lighter non-stick versions too, at excellent prices.

Large non-stick wok

The reason I specifically suggest a large one here is to ensure that you can make a generous amount of food in one cooking session, if needed, which is absolutely in the spirit of this book. See pillar 8 in my definition of budget-friendly cooking and baking on page 11 for why this is always a good idea!

Rectangular airtight containers (around 2.2 litres/2½ quarts each)

A key part of the Big Batch Slow Cooking chapter involves purposefully making too much food in order to create your own freezable ready meals each time you make dinner. But this concept isn't much good if you don't have a healthy amount of airtight containers in which to store them! I recommend around 2.2 litres (2½ quarts), rectangular specifically. Firstly because that's what I always use, but also because, in my experience, it's a great size and shape to ensure quick defrosting and reheating. Plus, they're a good size for the average freezer so you can stack them and use the space in your drawers efficiently.

ESSENTIAL BAKING TINS (PANS)

Though I'm often offered some super-fancy cookware these days (lucky me!) you might be surprised to learn that I still often use the same bakeware I've had for 10+ years. Despite just being super-affordable tins (pans) I bought in the supermarket, they're still going strong today and I find it very hard to stray away from them simply because they've never done me wrong!

Please remember, though: just because these are all of the different tins I use throughout this book, you're not expected to rush out and buy all of these immediately (as that would sort of defeat the whole concept). Though baking will often call for a variety of tins to accommodate all the different shapes and sizes of your creations, I've stuck to the most commonly used ones to ensure you have a decent chance at owning them already, and also so that you don't have to rush out and buy any expensive ones or obscure shapes and sizes.

Just please remember that even the cheapest baking tins will more than suffice and can last for years and years – there's absolutely no need to break the bank here! Moreover, it's the measurements of each tin that are far more important than spending a lot on them!

23 x 33cm (9 x 13in) rectangular baking tin

This is the tin I've used for all my traybakes for years and years and you'll need it for the lemon drizzle traybake (page 214). I also used two of these to make my big, rectangular Yorkshire pudding wraps (page 103).

900g (2lb) loaf tin

Again, this is an incredibly integral part of any small collection of essential bakeware, and I've lost count of the number of different loaf cakes I have made using mine. For this book, you'll need it for my chocolate banana bread (page 216), fruit tea loaf (page 222) and courgette and lime loaf cake (page 234).

12-hole cupcake tin

As this book shows, the amount of value you can get out of a humble cupcake tin often speaks for itself! You'll need one for my jam tarts (page 213), rainbow cupcakes (page 218), blueberry breakfast muffins (page 34), pizza muffins (page 59) and even my jaffa cakes (page 210).

6-hole silicone muffin tray

For my small batch blueberry breakfast muffins and pizza muffins, this'll come in especially handy if you're going to be baking them in the air fryer. And that's mainly because you won't have any hope of fitting a 12-hole cupcake tin into an air fryer no matter how determined you might feel!

23cm (9in) square baking tin

I call this my 'brownie tin' because that's what I most commonly make in it, but for this book it's perfect for everything from my depression cake (page 229) or golden syrup pudding cake (page 226) and even in the stuffing used for my Yorkshire pudding wraps (page 103).

22 x 16cm (8½ x 6¼in) medium rectangular ovenproof roasting dish

This is simply a medium-sized rectangular ovenproof dish that I often use for puddings to serve a small crowd. Mine is ceramic and I use it to make Eve's pudding (page 237).

20cm (8in) round baking tin

This tin is most commonly used for making round sponge cakes, but in this book you'll need one for one of my favourite desserts: peach almondine (page 232).

23cm (9in) loose-bottomed fluted tart tin

If you decide to make my lemon posset (page 242) into a full-on lemon tart to serve a crowd, you'll need one of these to support the pastry. I've used this many a time across my past books to make quiches and tarts, so hopefully this is one of the tins that you have already. However, it's not mandatory!

10cm (4in) round ramekins and microwave-safe pudding moulds

These super-affordable little pots can happily be used interchangeably as long as they're 10cm (4in) in diameter and, of course, microwave safe if that's where you're using them! I use these in my lemon posset (page 242), berry swirl no-bake cheesecake (page 238) and in my microwave spotted dick (page 244).

30 x 23cm (12 x 9in) Swiss roll tin

There's very little that's fancy about a Swiss (jelly) roll tin as it's essentially a specifically sized baking tray with slightly higher sides to hold the mixture. So in that sense, as long as you have a baking tray that's around the same size, you're good to go! I use this for my chocolate + caramel Arctic roll (page 247).

Round (or fluted) cookie cutter

Throughout this book I've used 5, 7 and 8cm (2, 2¾ and 3in) cutters, all from the same set of extremely humble plastic cutters that have served me well for years. Look for a set with all different sizes and you'll never need to buy them again! I use these for my jam tarts (page 213), lemonade scones (page 208) and party rings (page 224).

NOT MANDATORY BUT SUPER HANDY

In the spirit of being 'budget-friendly', it would be quite out of character for me to then send you out to buy an air fryer or slow cooker, wouldn't it? That's why, although there are chapters in this book dedicated to air frying and slow cooking, I've also provided alternative methods for those recipes (for the oven and/or hob) in case you don't own these small appliances already. So that makes both of these not mandatory for this book, although do check out pillar 7 (page 11) to read about why these low-running-cost appliances can be great savers.

9.5 litre (9½ quart) air fryer

Having released *Gluten Free Air Fryer* in the very recent past, an entire recipe book dedicated to cooking in an air fryer, this one might not surprise you. But as an appliance with a low running cost (when compared to an oven) and a famed ability to reduce cooking timings and therefore your time spent in the kitchen, it's also absolutely perfect for budget-friendly cooking. However, it didn't feel right making it an absolute essential for this book as they don't just magically appear in your kitchen for free! That's why, where possible, this book will include air fryer methods where possible, but will always endeavour to include alternative oven temperatures and timings too. So if you have an air fryer already, then feel free to use it, but you most certainly won't need to rush out and buy one especially for this book.

I specifically state this size air fryer, as the larger your air fryer, the more you can cook at once; this ensures you don't have to cook in batches and can enjoy lower running costs as a result.

6.5 litre (7 quart) slow cooker

The same applies for slow cookers as for air fryers, the only difference being that a slow cooker tends to have a considerably cheaper purchase cost than an air fryer. But as I just said, I didn't want to leave anyone in the situation where parts of this book would be useless to them if they didn't already own a slow cooker, so slow cooker methods are added alongside hob or oven temperatures/timings throughout this book. Again, if you have one, then feel free to use it! Please note the larger size of this slow cooker and head to page 171 to find out why I specifically state this.

Stick blender

This was one of the first kitchen gadgets I ever bought, not just because it's easy to use and clean, but because they've always been so incredibly affordable. I first bought mine to blitz up my veg and stock into soup, but in more recent years I've found it's fantastic for blitzing up ingredients into pesto or for making my own curry pastes. There's absolutely no need to break the bank for one of these – as long as it has two speeds, then that's all you'll ever need! Pay attention to the power specifications when buying, stated in watts. Mine is 200W, which is perfect for blending up cooked veg and nuts, but for anything tougher you'll need to opt for one with a little more power. Though you'll need one of these for recipes like my leek, potato and feta soup (page 178) and Mark's curry mee (page 164), I haven't used it extensively throughout this book.

Waffle maker

Of course, a waffle maker is mandatory if you want to make waffles (like my stuffed waffles on page 38). However, that's just one recipe in this book! So again, don't feel like you absolutely need to buy one ASAP – cheaper silicone waffle moulds can also work exceptionally well here too.

Digital food thermometer

Fortunately, you can pick one of these up online at an extremely affordable price these days and they come in handy whenever you want to check if your food is done or not, especially when cooking any kind of meat. With a digital food thermometer, you can check the exact internal temperature of whatever you're cooking and compare it to internal cooking temperatures over on page 255. The only exception to this rule is generally when cooking meat like chicken thighs or beef stewing steak, which both benefit from being overdone, or they can remain a little chewy. I suggest this handy device here as this book encourages the creation, storage and reheating of leftovers for cost-saving purposes; of course, ensuring you reheat said leftovers properly and thoroughly is important! And that's where a digital food thermometer can further remove all the guesswork, quickly demonstrating its usefulness and worth.

ESSENTIAL INGREDIENTS

ESSENTIAL COOKING INGREDIENTS

While I often use this part of my books to showcase all the essential dedicated gluten-free cooking ingredients you'll need throughout this book, as I've minimized their use wherever possible I've instead opted to showcase some of the naturally gluten-free 'super ingredients' you'll find regularly used. Don't get me wrong, you'll still need gluten-free soy sauce and gluten-free pasta occasionally, but this book assumes you already know what they are and where to find them – you can always check descriptions of these ingredients out in my previous books.

I call these cooking ingredients 'super', firstly because they're incredibly cost effective, secondly because their repeated use ensures you don't need to buy tons of other products for this book (like buying six different kinds of cheese – see pillar 6 on page 10), and lastly because all of them are key to transforming raw ingredients into your future favourite meals.

Vegetable oil in a spray bottle

With this book following on from my last book, *Gluten Free Air Fryer*, you'll notice that I've carried over a few nuggets of wisdom that were integral to those recipes. And vegetable oil in a spray bottle is one of them! While in that book this was mainly used to ensure an even spread of oil for maximum crispiness (which does still apply to this book in some cases), the main reason I've carried on using it here – whether I'm air frying or not – is because it's the most economical way to cook with oil. And cooking oil isn't cheap!

However, quick disclaimer: *please avoid buying vegetable oil in a spray bottle from supermarkets* – always fill your own spray bottle. Oil sold in ready-to-spray bottles costs literally five times the price than cooking oil in a normal bottle; worst of all, they purposefully manufacture the bottle so you can't even refill it without breaking it. Instead, just buy literally any 200ml (7fl oz) spray bottle, pour some oil into it and away you go. Oh, and please don't use low-calorie sprays instead of oil either, not just because they don't work as well as oil, but mainly because they're up to nine times more expensive than oil despite being essentially 50% actual oil, with the rest being water and thickeners.

Jar of jalapeños in brine

This is one of the most affordable ways to conveniently introduce spiciness to your food. Better still, jarred jalapeños add a bell-pepper-like flavour to your food that you won't get from dried chilli flakes or chilli paste. Even the brine from the jar comes in handy – gluten-free vinegars can be expensive and you've essentially got jalapeño-infused vinegar right there in the jar! Supermarket own-brand jarred jalapeños are reasonably priced, but look for larger jars down the international aisle, which will net you a larger total quantity for less money. Of course, ensure you avoid any in small jars by named brands – all you're doing is paying for the label and its in-your-face position in the supermarket!

Honey

This is a true hero ingredient when it comes to cooking from scratch on a budget, with the jarred supermarket value version being exactly the same price as caster (superfine) sugar, gram for gram. However, unlike sugar, which adds sweetness without any other distinct taste, honey can add tons of extra flavour when caramelized, which means it's a great substitute for times where I'd normally use light brown sugar, palm sugar or maple syrup when cooking, all of which are costlier by comparison (though their use isn't always avoidable when baking!). Jarred honey has a habit of crystallizing when exposed to oxygen (i.e. once opened) so if you find this is the case, simply place the jar in a bowl of hot tap water and give it a stir to bring it back to life. Also, if you find more of the honey gets stuck to your spoon than goes into your pan, give the spoon a little spray with cooking oil first – it'll slide right off! And remember – avoid the fancy, expensive stuff!

Mature Cheddar

It might seem a bit random that I've chosen to showcase cheese here, but as it's such a commonly used ingredient in this book I didn't have much choice! Its regular use isn't because I've suddenly taken a strong liking to it; supermarkets will always stock a 'budget' version of this cheese and it's one of the cheapest you'll find. However, unlike regular Cheddar, mature Cheddar adds so much extra flavour, so much so in fact that I use it instead of the far costlier Parmesan in my dishes. So expect to see this used very often whenever cheese is needed!

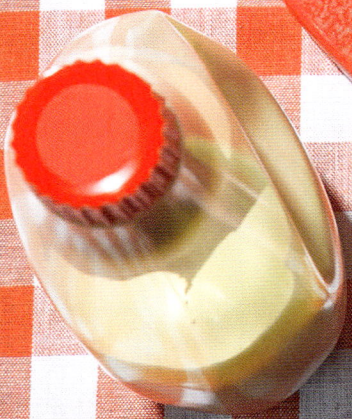

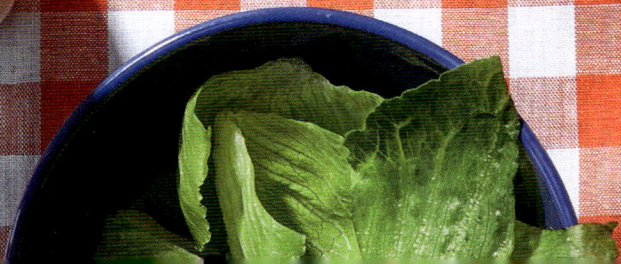

Frozen vegetables

Believe it or not, some pre-prepared frozen vegetables are cheaper than their fresh equivalent. However, do bear in mind that frozen vegetables aren't *always* cheaper so you'll need to compare the weight of fresh to frozen to be sure, though I've already done the hard work for you by including the cheaper, frozen versions in the recipes in this book.

Ginger paste

Though this isn't a 'budget ingredient' specifically, the fact you can often buy enormous jars of it makes it incredibly cost effective and convenient to use. Not only that, but the flavour it imparts in a dish is so significant that it's a 'super ingredient' in creating flavourful, budget-friendly food. Look in the world food or international aisles in supermarkets for the best-value, larger jars.

Spices + seasoning

Throughout this book, I've endeavoured to use the same small cell of spices, spice blends, dried herbs and seasoning over and over again. That means that not only can you buy them in larger quantities to start with (which will always be cheaper) but you'll be far less likely to end up with spices that you seldom use and that will expire. Here are my top five:

1. MILD CURRY POWDER

Curry powder is a mix of different spices that you can easily find and buy individually in supermarkets – the supermarket curry powder I use is a mix of cumin, coriander, turmeric, cassia, cardamom, fenugreek, nutmeg, black pepper and chilli powder. If you live in a country that doesn't have curry powder blends readily available, garam masala will do the trick in like-for-like quantities – especially as it's a blend of spices.

You might be surprised to hear that buying curry powder commonly costs less, gram for gram, than any of the individual spices used in its blend. Head to the international aisle for the cheapest price, where you'll find larger bags of curry powder that can easily be decanted into jars for future use – just be aware that they can be quite spicy if they aren't marked as being mild!

2. SMOKED PAPRIKA

This flavourful spice not only imparts a distinct, smoky bell-pepper flavour, but also a vibrant orange hue to your dishes. As always, buy a larger quantity if you can for a reduced price and be aware of the different variations paprika comes in: paprika, smoked paprika and hot paprika. Hot paprika has cayenne pepper added (and also, like plain paprika, doesn't have a smoky flavour) so bear that in mind if you don't like your food to be too spicy. I'd always recommend going for smoked paprika.

3. DRIED MIXED HERBS

The supermarket own brand blend I use is a mix of thyme, marjoram, parsley, oregano, sage and basil. While I enjoy cooking using specific herbs in my recipes, sometimes you can't beat this 'all-in-one' herb blend, which is perfect for everything from pizza to pasta, meatballs, risotto, chilli con carne, and more. I'd highly recommend buying larger amounts where possible, as not only is it incredibly versatile, it's not as potent as spices can be, meaning you'll use more and go through it faster.

4. CHINESE FIVE SPICE

Hands down, this is Mark's favourite, most-used spice and one that his mum always included in the stir fries, marinades and curries he enjoyed growing up. The one we use is a supermarket own-brand blend that contains star anise, cinnamon, fennel, black pepper and clove. It pairs perfectly with things like gluten-free soy sauce and many savoury dishes with a South East Asian influence or inspiration, which is how you'll see it used in the recipes in this book.

5. SALT + BLACK PEPPER

As salt and pepper are so common on tables across the world, it can be easy to forget just how important black pepper is as a cooking ingredient. As I've tried to keep the range of spices and seasoning to a minimum, you might notice that I use black pepper where I might otherwise have opted for cayenne or white pepper. That's because black pepper adds more than enough flavour and tongue-tingling heat to mean I don't end up asking people to buy spices they may not end up using all that often.

ESSENTIAL GLUTEN-FREE BAKING INGREDIENTS

There really isn't much getting around it when it comes to gluten-free baking: you need specialized, dedicated (and sometimes costlier!) gluten-free baking ingredients. However, that doesn't mean that you can't use them at all! By using these ingredients in the Bargain Bakes chapter alongside the cost savviness natively built into the recipes that live there, you'll find that delicious gluten-free bakes and desserts can be shockingly affordable to whip up.

Gluten-free plain (all-purpose) and self-raising flour

Most supermarkets used to stock their own brand of gluten-free flour blends, but this is a little less common to see than it used to be. However, when you see own-brand gluten-free flour blends down free-from aisles, make sure you use them! Though made from a blend of different naturally gluten-free flours and starches in varying quantities, you'll find that the ingredients in own-brand supermarket gluten-free flour blends are extremely similar to name-brand blends. For example, here are the ingredients lists for two different products:

Own-brand supermarket gluten-free self-raising flour blend: Rice Flour, Tapioca Starch, Potato Starch, Maize Flour, Raising Agents (Calcium Phosphate, Sodium Carbonates), Thickener (Xanthan Gum)

Name-brand gluten-free self-raising flour blend: Rice, Potato, Tapioca, Maize, Buckwheat, Raising Agents (Mono-Calcium Phosphate, Sodium Bicarbonate), Thickener (Xanthan Gum)

Though extremely similar in ingredients, supermarket gluten-free flour blends are often heavily discounted compared to name brands, with the price difference being as drastic as being able to buy two bags of supermarket own-brand gluten-free flour for the price of one name-brand bag.

Xanthan gum

If you've used my recipes before, you'll likely have come across this strange-sounding ingredient. Luckily it's just the name that's unusual as you'll easily source this in supermarket gluten-free or free-from aisles, where it's usually far cheaper than online. Luckily, we only ever need a small amount, so a small tub will last across many, many gluten-free bakes. It's essentially used as a binding agent that prevents gluten-free sponge cakes, biscuits and cookies from being too crumbly, so is absolutely essential in gluten-free baking!

Gluten-free baking powder

As you might know already, baking powder isn't always gluten-free because it's often bulked out with wheat flour. Luckily, you'll find that some of the 'big brand' baking powders in supermarkets are often gluten-free so they're easily sourced. However, though this book endeavours to dodge the use of 'big brand' products, there's an important caveat here: because these 'big brand' baking powders aren't dedicated gluten-free products per se (via their branding or placement in the supermarket) they won't have the dreaded 'gluten-free tax' added on to them, despite being gluten-free. That means that they're always likely to be cheaper than buying the 'free from' branded gluten-free baking powder, and we can take full advantage of that!

Gluten-free oats

Gluten-free oats can be a tricky topic, with some people with Coeliac disease experiencing cross-reactivity to them. That's why I've always endeavoured to minimize their use in my recipes so as not to exclude too many people too often. However, with gluten-free oats being a product where we have to pay extra for the pleasure of them not being cross-contaminated during manufacturing processes, that gave me an additional reason to minimize their use. Yet there's no denying that you'll most definitely need them for my blueberry breakfast muffins (page 34) and my oat and raisin/choc chip cookies (page 221), hence their inclusion here.

FAQ

These are some of the most common questions I've been asked concerning the budget-friendly recipes I've posted on social media before. Though I've already explained my own personal definition of a 'budget-friendly' recipe at the start of this book, that doesn't mean you might not have a few questions about how the recipes in this book fit into that or why I've made certain choices in certain ways. So hopefully this part answers anything extra you were wondering!

WHY ARE THESE RECIPES 'BUDGET-FRIENDLY'?

Because they use the pillars you'll find in my definition of budget-friendly cooking and baking over on page 8! To me, a recipe with cost saving in mind should take that mission as seriously as possible, but absolutely not at the expense of the taste, texture or visuals of the final dish. When you're gluten free, streamlining your spending is vital in order to offset the 'gluten-free tax' that's piled on top of our everyday essentials.

AREN'T THESE JUST NATURALLY GLUTEN-FREE RECIPES? OR JUST 'NORMAL' RECIPES SUBSTITUTED WITH GLUTEN-FREE INGREDIENTS?

I've always included naturally gluten-free recipes in my books because some of the best meals you could ever have never had gluten in them to start with. But this book and all of my others are always inspired first by foods we can't otherwise eat. See pillar 2 in my definition of budget-friendly cooking and baking on page 8 about why a mix of naturally gluten-free recipes and those which use specialized gluten-free products is key to effective budget cooking and baking.

WOULDN'T THIS RECIPE BE CHEAPER IF YOU DIDN'T USE 'X' INGREDIENT?

It goes without saying that the less you use, the cheaper the finished result will be. However, removing ingredients at random can affect the final dish in many undesirable ways. For example, if you simply removed meat from every dish in this book, not only would that remove a source of protein but you'd also find that the dish then didn't yield enough to serve as many people. You also might not fancy suddenly becoming vegetarian for the sake of cost! The same notion would apply to removing lentils, beans, pulses or veg from a dish too. Or what about if you removed certain spices? Well, you'd probably find the end result particularly bland!

The moral of the story here is that you can trust that I've substituted or rejigged all the costly ingredients for you! So what you're left with are all the affordable ingredients that need to be there, and nothing else. Plus, don't forget that you're expected to be using the savvy shopping tips on page 12 to ensure the ingredients that you do use are sourced as economically as possible.

WHY DO YOU STATE THE USE OF ONION OR LEEK IN MANY OF YOUR RECIPES? WHICH ONE SHOULD I USE?

You'll see that throughout the book, whenever I call for onion, I also suggest leek as an alternative. The answer to this question is simple: use onion if you can tolerate it, because it's cheaper! Mark and I both struggle to tolerate onion but find leek (mostly the green parts of it) to have no ill effects. So I've included leek as an alternative ingredient for those who suffer with the same problem we do!

WHY FROZEN VEG? WHAT IF I DON'T WANT TO USE FROZEN VEG?

As with most questions about why I used certain ingredients across recipes in this book, the answer will usually be this: because it's cheaper! Yep, that's right, some bags of frozen veg are actually cheaper than buying the fresh version and, better still, they come pre-chopped which saves you on prep. If you don't want to use frozen veg, you should know that you're missing out on a potential cost saving – but you should also know that that's totally fine! Simply use an equivalent amount of the fresh version.

I DON'T LIKE X, Y OR Z INGREDIENTS, WHAT CAN I USE INSTEAD?

You can use absolutely whatever else you'd prefer! If it's veg, use whatever you'd prefer that would reasonably cook in a similar amount of time or suits the cooking method. For example, if the recipe instructs roasting cauliflower in the oven but you'd prefer something different, you could also use an equivalent amount of broccoli, aubergine (eggplant), carrots, parsnips, sweet potato or butternut squash and the same spicing or any flavouring originally stated for the cauliflower. With veg, just ensure it's fork tender at the end, as all vegetables cook at different speeds, especially depending on how thin or thick you've sliced them.

If you're not a fan of lentils, pulses or beans, you should know that they're super ingredients because of their excellent nutritional values and exceptional value for money! But what if you can't tolerate them whatsoever? In that situation, you could replace them with more meat (if the recipe also includes meat), bearing in mind that this will increase the total cost of the dish. Alternatively, upping the quantities of veg would be fine too, though remember that this could mean less fibre and protein in the final dish.

Though I've balanced these recipes, that doesn't mean you can't change them and make them your own, especially if it's to suit your own dietary requirements.

WHY DON'T YOU STATE THE COST PER PORTION OF EACH MEAL?

I don't state an estimated price of how much each recipe would cost per portion simply because it wouldn't be accurate. The price of ingredients changes so quickly and so often that adding these figures would probably be less helpful than not including them at all.

I BOUGHT ALL THE INGREDIENTS FOR ONE OF THESE RECIPES + IT WASN'T PARTICULARLY CHEAP. WHY?

Any successful budget cooking or baking relies upon the steps that came before cooking. For example, in order to eat a delicious budget meal, you'd have needed a reliable budget-friendly recipe beforehand. And before you attempted said recipe, you'd have needed to source all the ingredients at the best possible prices using the savvy shopping tips on page 12. Of course, without savvy shopping, you could take the best budget recipe in the entire world, source all the ingredients from local farm shops, fancy supermarkets and the result would be far from a budget-friendly meal!

THIS RECIPE DOESN'T HAVE ADVICE ON HOW TO ADAPT IT FOR MY DIETARY REQUIREMENT. WHY?

The entire point of the key at the side of each recipe is to either indicate that the recipe is suitable for a variety of different dietary requirements, or if it's not, to provide information on how to adapt it. However, if a recipe requires so many alterations that it would essentially be an entirely different recipe, or it includes an ingredient that's so integral to the recipe that it can't be easily substituted, I won't provide advice for that particular dietary requirement.

However, this doesn't mean that it's impossible! My followers have had great success in making versions of my recipes to suit their dietary requirements, using ingenious ways I never thought were possible, and quite often they share the results in my Facebook group. So if you are finding yourself stuck and wanting to make a particular recipe, but there isn't any advice for adapting it to your dietary requirement, you could always join my Facebook group and see if anyone has had success in adapting it before. Alternatively, you can also ask for any tips or advice on adapting it too!

FREEZING + DEFROSTING GUIDE

As you'll see in pillar 8 of my definition of budget cooking and baking on page 11, purposefully planning the use of your leftovers can be a huge time and cost saver, and I absolutely encourage you to read that first so you have an understanding of why you should even bother with this bit! And that's because your freezer (which is using power all the time, I might add!) can play a huge part in reducing how often you cook, while saving you money at the same time.

However, if you're like me, your freezer might at one point have been full of random bits of unlabelled leftovers that leave you with little actionable clue of how to get it onto plates ASAP... and in some cases you likely have even less of a clue as to what some things in your freezer even are! So sadly, in the freezer is where they stay, for who knows how long?

That's why, to put an end to that, I've endeavoured to give freezing and defrosting guidance for as many recipes as possible; that way, not only do you know how to store and freeze them, but you also know how to reheat them and get them onto plates quickly. It's very likely you've been directed here from a recipe thanks to the freezer key, so here is where you'll find all the answers.

SOUPS, STEWS + CURRIES

To freeze, once cooled, portion out leftovers into medium airtight containers and freeze for up to 3 months.

To defrost, place the container in the microwave for 3–4 minutes at full power (900W) with the lid on. Transfer the frozen block to a large, lidded pot and pour over a splash (around 5 tablespoons) of boiling water. Place over a high heat and bring the water back to boiling. Then reduce the heat to medium, pop the lid on and simmer for 25–30 minutes, using a wooden spoon to break the block into smaller chunks within the last 10–15 minutes. Continue to simmer with the lid removed for around 5 further minutes to thicken, if needed.

If using a particularly huge airtight container, you'll likely need to microwave it for an extra 1–2 minutes and cook it for an extra 10–15 minutes after the lid has been placed on.

RISOTTO + RICE DISHES

Follow the advice for soups, stews and curries, simmering for the final 5 minutes (lid removed) to ensure each grain of rice is defined and the dish isn't too wet or stodgy. Stir as little as possible until the end, otherwise you'll break all the rice and turn it to mush!

PASTA DISHES

Follow the advice for soups, stews and curries but stir as little as possible until the end – otherwise you'll break all the pasta into small bits! If reheating a pasta bake, I recommend you also pop the reheated dish into the oven at 180°C fan/200°C (400°F) for 15 minutes or air fryer at 200°C (400°F) for 8–10 minutes to crisp up the top once more.

SPONGE CAKES

To freeze, once cooled, ideally slice and store in airtight containers and freeze for up to 3 months.

To defrost, remove from the container and allow to defrost at room temperature on a wire rack for 2 (smaller slices) to 4 (larger or whole cakes) hours.

CUPCAKES

To freeze, once cooled and iced (frosted), freeze on a baking sheet for 1–2 hours. Once the buttercream is solid, transfer to airtight containers and freeze for up to 3 months.

Defrost at room temperature on a wire rack for 2–3 hours.

BISCUITS + COOKIES

To freeze, once cooled, store in airtight containers and freeze for up to 3 months.

To defrost un-iced biscuits and cookies, remove from the airtight container and either reheat in the air fryer from frozen at 160°C (320°F) for 5 minutes or in the oven at 180°C (350°F) for 8–10 minutes. To defrost iced biscuits, allow to defrost at room temperature on a wire rack for around 2 hours.

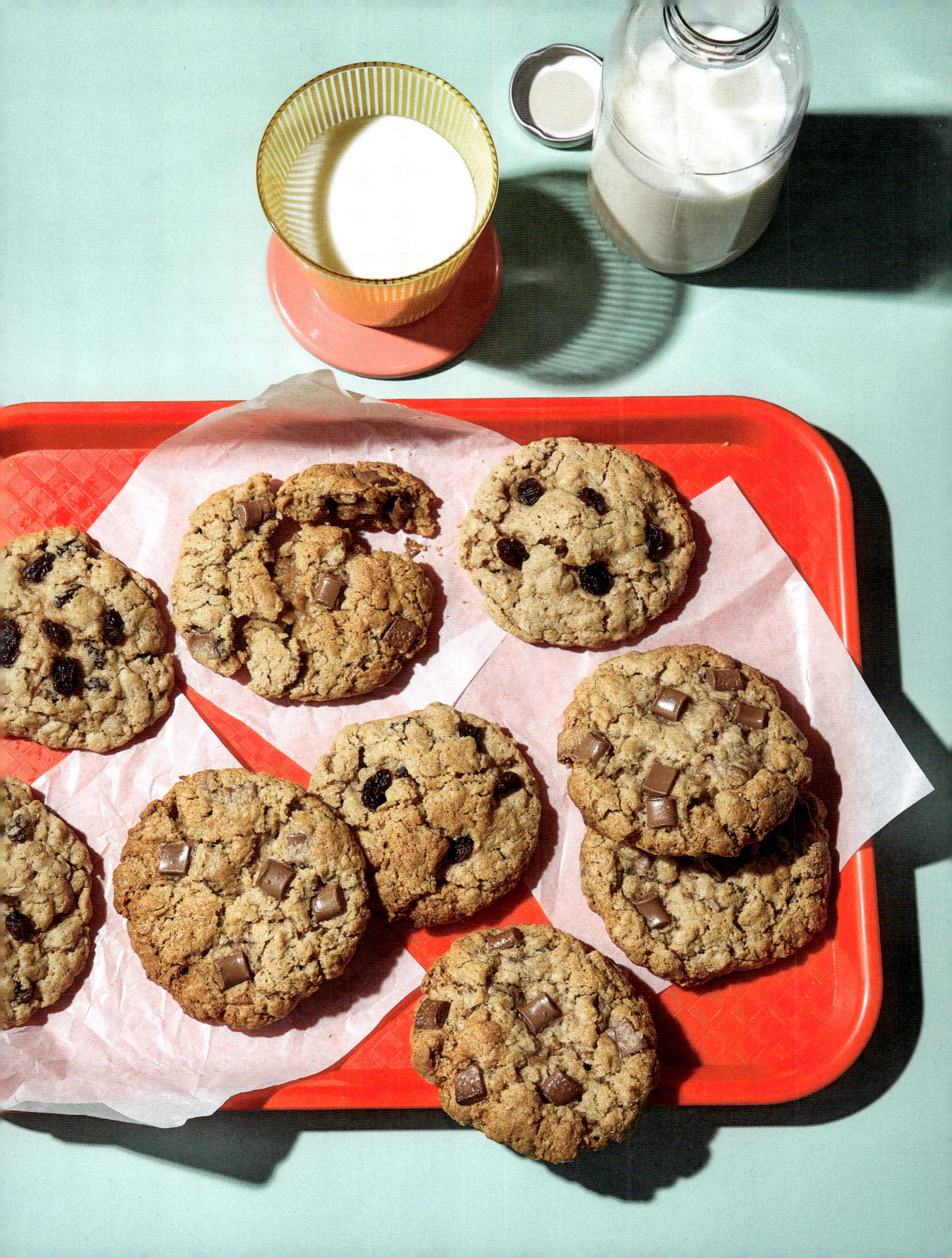

KEY

Just as a handy reminder for those still in disbelief: yes, everything in this entire book is gluten-free!

But it's also incredibly important to me that as many people can enjoy my recipes as possible. That's why I've labelled all of my recipes to clearly indicate whether they're dairy-free, lactose-free, low lactose, vegetarian, vegan or low FODMAP (as well as whether they're freezable or not too).

Even if a recipe isn't naturally suitable for all dietary requirements, watch out for the helpful notes by the key. These will indicate any simple swaps you can implement in order to adapt that recipe to your dietary requirements, if possible.

Please note that making swaps due to dietary requirements can obviously affect the final cost of each dish, depending on which and how many changes you need to make! Fortunately, no matter which products you swap in to make a recipe suitable to your dietary requirements, all of the savvy shopping tips will more than help to ensure you source these swaps for the best prices.

Here's a breakdown of the labels I'll be using so you know what they look like and exactly what I mean when I use them:

DF DAIRY-FREE

This indicates that a recipe contains zero dairy products. Ensure that no ingredients used have a 'may contain' warning for traces of dairy and double-check that everything used is 100% dairy-free.

LF LACTOSE-FREE

Lactose-free? Isn't that the same as dairy-free? No, it definitely isn't! For example, lactose-free milk is *real* cow's milk with the lactase enzyme added, so while it's definitely not dairy-free, it is suitable for those with a lactose intolerance. The 'lactose-free' label indicates that a recipe is naturally lactose-free or uses lactose-free products. Please ensure all ingredients and any convenience products used are lactose-free.

LL LOW LACTOSE

Ingredients like butter and harder cheeses (such as Cheddar and Parmesan) are incredibly low in lactose. That means that people with a lactose intolerance should have no problems tolerating them. So for those ingredients, you won't necessarily need a special 'lactose-free' equivalent. Of course, recipes that use these ingredients aren't technically 'lactose-free', so they'll be labelled as low lactose for clarity. Please ensure all ingredients and any convenience products used are lactose-free or very low in lactose.

V VEGGIE

This indicates that a recipe is both meat-free and fish-free. I've provided simple vegetarian swaps where necessary and possible. Please make sure all products and ingredients used are veggie-friendly.

VE VEGAN

This indicates that a recipe contains no ingredients that are derived from animals. Please make sure all products and ingredients used are vegan-friendly.

F LOW FODMAP

This indicates that one serving of the finished recipe is low FODMAP. The low FODMAP diet was specifically created by Monash University in order to help relieve the symptoms of IBS in sufferers.

A couple of quick side notes:

Whenever I mention spring onions (scallions) in this book, I mean the green parts <u>only</u> for FODMAP reasons. Also, garlic-infused oil is low FODMAP, as long as it's clear and doesn't have visible bits of garlic floating in it. Ensure any products used (such as spices, seasonings or sausages, for example) are free of onion and garlic powder – these tend to be common ingredients in spice blends. You'll easily find low FODMAP convenience products – such as stock cubes and curry powder – online.

Though this book features the use of onion and garlic, you'll always find an alternative to onions (leeks, green parts only) and garlic is often optional; if not, the FODMAP key will suggest using a specific amount of garlic-infused oil instead.

A cost-conscious ingredient used within a lot of recipes in this book is frozen sliced mixed (bell) pepper. However, due to each colour of pepper having a different safe FODMAP serving size (75g/2⅔oz for green, 43g/1½oz for red, 38g/1⅓oz for orange, 35g/1¼oz for yellow) and them all being mixed together in the packet, this product isn't easily controllable for the elimination phase of the diet. As such, in the FODMAP key for the recipes that use this product, I've given the alternative of using all green peppers (not frozen) or a specific weight instead; just remember to thinly slice them first! A given weight of ingredients like this ensures that once you divide the finished dish between the amount of people it serves, the amount of green pepper per person will be 75g (2⅔oz) or less; a safe low FODMAP serving size. However, if you use more peppers than specified or enjoy more than the given portion size per person, this might then exceed the safe FODMAP serving size limit; so it's always a good idea to weigh the ingredient out and stick to the serving size suggestions per person.

For the recipes that don't have a FODMAP key, that doesn't mean it's impossible to make them low FODMAP! It's more likely that there are simply too many changes needed for me to list. If you're feeling determined, you can always check the safe FODMAP serving sizes of each ingredient in a recipe using the Monash FODMAP app.

Brief disclaimer: You should always start the low FODMAP diet in consultation with your dietician. Please ensure all ingredients and any convenience products used are low FODMAP. All FODMAP serving sizes were correct at the time of writing. As Monash University regularly tests the FODMAP levels of different foods, these quantities might change over time as new research emerges. For example, in my previous books the low FODMAP serving size given for avocado was 30g (1oz), but new research by Monash University means this has now been updated to 60g (2¼oz). Be sure to check their website every now and then for the latest info.

❄ FREEZABLE

This indicates that the finished dish is freezable and will include all relevant freezing and defrosting/reheating advice next to the freezer key, found at the side of each recipe. However, as many of the recipes in this book ended up with near identical freezing/defrosting advice (and they were getting a bit lengthy!) you might find that this key often instead refers you to the freezing + defrosting guide over on page 28. There you'll find freezing/defrosting advice that applies to many of the finished dishes in this book, such as stews, soups and curries, pasta dishes and even leftover cakes, cupcakes and biscuits too.

Providing specific information on not only how to preserve leftovers in the freezer (and how long you can store them for) is obviously very much in the nature of this book in order to prevent food and money going to waste. However, unlike in my previous books, I've now also endeavoured to share specific steps on how to defrost and reheat dishes so you can get them back onto plates ASAP; because the goal of preventing waste hasn't been achieved until that part actually happens!

The Big Batch Slow Cooking chapter also purposefully encourages the creation of leftovers in order to take advantage of the benefits of bulk buying as well as cutting down on how much time and electricity you spend cooking. And without the freezer, that chapter wouldn't be possible! So please ensure you've cleared out a little space in your freezer ready for use with this book.

LUNCH +
ON-THE-GO

When it comes to lunch, whether you're enjoying it at home, at work or out and about, a gluten-free lunch usually means two things. First of all, if it's a sandwich, that means forking out for the cost of gluten-free bread, which as we all know can incur a huge premium over 'normal' bread. And, secondly, if you're hoping to grab a convenient gluten-free lunch out in the wild, finding a safe, suitable and affordable option can be a challenge... if not an impossibility!

And that's why this chapter aims to tackle both problems simultaneously. Not only will you find so many easy, simple, flavourful, quick-to-throw-together options that aren't simply a filling slapped between two costly slices of bread, but almost all of them make amazing lunchbox legends too as they're delicious hot or cold. And, trust me, if you make your mobile lunch using the recipes in this chapter, it's more than likely that what you've brought with you will be far more appealing than any gluten-free option you'll find when you're out and about, and that's before even considering cost comparison.

Of course, it's common knowledge that a packed lunch is a cost-effective way to dodge the premium added to dining out or buying on-the-go convenience products, so this chapter will continue to make use of highly budget-friendly ingredients to drive the cost down even more. So without further ado: let them eat lunch!

SMALL BATCH BLUEBERRY BREAKFAST MUFFINS

Makes 6

Prep 10 mins

Oven 16 mins or
Air Fryer 14 mins

V

DF Use dairy-free milk.

LF Use lactose-free milk.

F Use lactose-free milk and maple syrup instead of honey.

VE See dairy-free advice and use light brown sugar instead of honey.

❄ Once cooled, freeze for up to 2–3 months in airtight containers. Allow to defrost on a wire rack at room temperature for 2–3 hours. To reheat, air fry at 200°C (400°F) for 5–6 minutes.

TIPS

The lemon juice isn't for flavour, it's to react with the bicarb to ensure the muffins are full of lots of airy bubbles that make the texture of the muffins super light. So make sure you include it!

Don't push the blueberries right to the bottom of the muffins – if the bottom of the muffin is just a layer of blueberries, then it will all stick to the cases!

So often when I have to catch the train at the crack of dawn, I rely on having something pre-made that I can eat on the go; more often than not, it's gluten-free cereal and/or nut bars, oaty biscuits or whatever I bought from the 'free-from' aisle (sometimes at eye-watering prices!). However, the more early starts I had, the more I'd end up buying, and the costs quickly added up. So to alleviate my reliance on more expensive convenience products, I started making these oaty muffins with bursting blueberries in advance: I keep them in the freezer or in an airtight container ready for the morning!

- 100g (¾ cup) gluten-free self-raising flour
- 25g (¼ cup) gluten-free oats, plus an extra 3 tsp for sprinkling on top
- ½ tsp bicarbonate of soda (baking soda)
- 110ml (½ cup minus 2 tsp) milk
- 60ml (¼ cup) vegetable oil
- 40ml (2½ tbsp) honey
- 1½ tsp vanilla extract
- Grated zest of 1 lemon and 1 tbsp lemon juice
- 85g (3oz) blueberries

To cook in an oven, preheat the oven to 180°C fan/200°C (400°F).

Combine the flour, oats and bicarb in a large bowl. In a large jug (pitcher), combine the milk, oil, honey, vanilla, lemon zest and juice. Add the wet ingredients to the dry and whisk in until smooth. Line 6 holes of a muffin tray with cupcake cases (ensure the tray will fit in your air fryer if planning on cooking in the air fryer).

Fill each case to around three-quarters full, ensuring the mixture is evenly split between all 6 cases. Top each with 4–5 blueberries and very gently push them in, then sprinkle each with ½ teaspoon of oats. Bake in the oven for 15–16 minutes or until golden on top. Transfer to a wire rack to cool completely.

To cook in an air fryer, heat the air fryer to 170°C (340°F). Fill the cases as directed opposite, then air fry for 12–14 minutes or until golden on top. Transfer to a wire rack to cool completely.

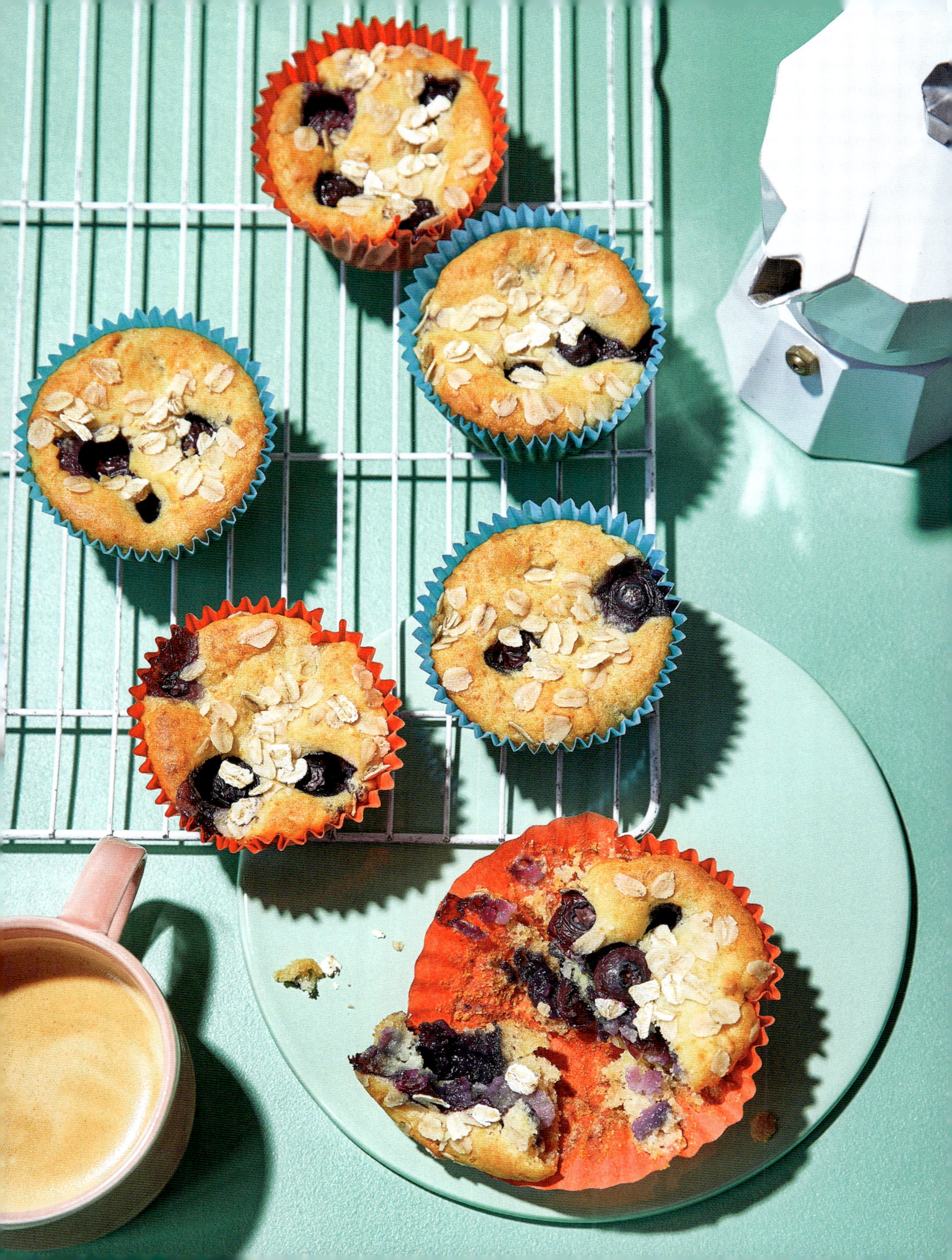

BUTTERMILK PANCAKES 3 WAYS

Serves 4 (makes 16)

Prep 15 mins

Hob 15 mins

In contrast to the pancake recipes I've shared in the past, these even fluffier and lighter pancakes use buttermilk. Not only does it give a unique, buttery flavour but it also reacts with the bicarb (baking soda) to ensure you get lots of bubbles in your batter to keep things light as a cloud. Of course, if you'd rather use milk you're more than welcome to (and you can get an extremely similar effect), but you absolutely must add the lemon juice and allow the milk to rest until thickened. Without the lemon juice, your milk won't thicken and the batter will be way too runny.

(V)

(DF) Use dairy-free milk mixed with lemon juice instead of buttermilk, and dairy-free chocolate chips, if using.

(LF) Use lactose-free milk mixed with lemon juice instead of buttermilk and lactose-free chocolate chips, if using.

(F) See lactose-free advice, and use no more than 35g (1¼oz) ripe banana or 140g (5oz) blueberries per person. Serve with maple syrup instead of honey.

(❄) Once cooled, store in an airtight container and freeze for up to 3 months. Air fry from frozen for 5–6 minutes at 200°C (400°F).

- 300g (2¼ cups) gluten-free self-raising flour
- 3 tbsp caster (superfine) sugar
- 1 tsp bicarbonate of soda (baking soda)
- 4 large eggs
- 460ml (2 cups minus 1¼ tbsp) buttermilk, **or** 400ml (1⅔ cups) milk, mixed with 6 tbsp lemon juice and rested for 10–15 minutes until thickened
- Vegetable oil spray
- Maple syrup or honey, to serve

For blueberry pancakes
- 300g (10½oz) blueberries

For banana pancakes (pictured)
- 4–5 ripe bananas, thinly sliced

For choc chip pancakes
- 160g (5½oz) milk chocolate chips

TIP

To create slices of caramelized banana for an added topping (as seen in the photo opposite) simply roll 2cm (¾in) slices of ripe banana in caster (superfine) sugar until lightly coated. Fry over a medium heat for 3–5 minutes in a pan generously sprayed with vegetable oil. Flip the slices and fry for a further 1 minute until caramelized and golden on both sides.

In a large bowl, combine the flour, sugar and bicarb. In a large jug (pitcher), combine the eggs with the buttermilk or milk and lemon mixture. Create a well in the flour bowl, then pour in the egg mixture while whisking thoroughly. After 30 seconds of whisking, the consistency should be smooth, like thick cream, not runny like water. Allow the batter to rest for 5–10 minutes.

Place a large frying pan over a medium heat and generously spray the base with vegetable oil. Once hot, pour in enough batter to form as many 10cm (4in) rounds as will fit without touching.

Immediately scatter 1 tablespoon of blueberries, 5–6 slices of banana or 1 teaspoon of chocolate chips onto each pancake. Fry for about 3 minutes until golden brown on the underside and the edges are starting to look less wet, then flip and fry for a further 1½ minutes. Remove the cooked pancakes to a plate and stack up, then repeat until all the batter has been used.

Serve stacked, with maple syrup or honey (as a more affordable alternative), drizzled over.

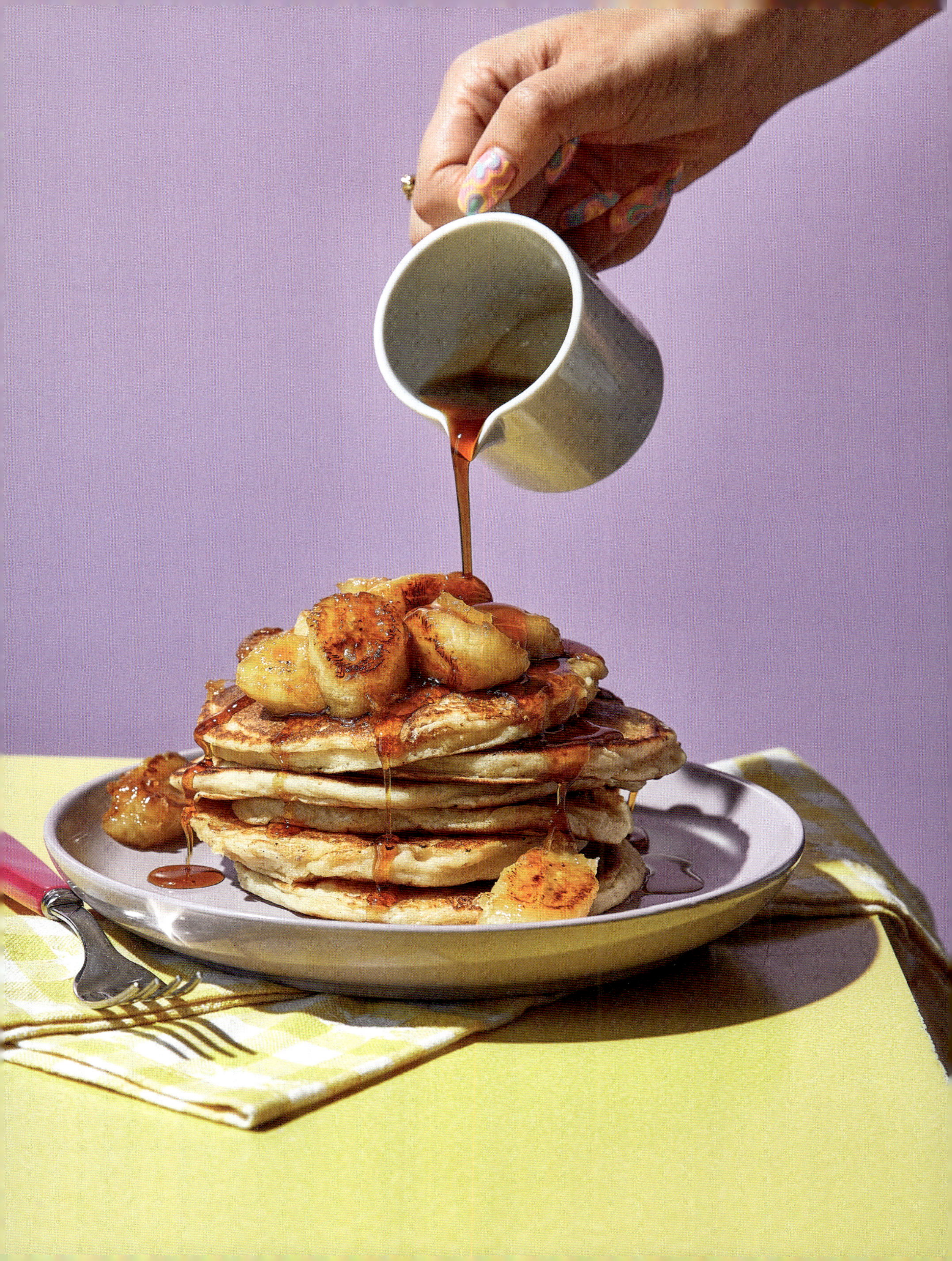

STUFFED WAFFLES 3 WAYS

If there's one lunch option I wish I had seen on my travels, it'd have to be savoury, stuffed gluten-free waffles. That's why I'm sharing my three fave versions, each stuffed with one of my favourite fillings. Now, while I'm not instructing you to rush out and buy a waffle maker especially to make this, I will advise you that they're usually very affordable and the kind of thing you might find down the middle aisle in budget supermarkets. They vary a little in terms of how hot they get and how fast they cook, so use the timings below as a guide – essentially, when it's golden and crisp on both sides, it's done!

Makes 3–4
Prep 5 mins
Waffle Maker 10 mins

V Make the cheese and chive waffles.

DF Use dairy-free milk.

LL Use lactose-free milk.

F See low lactose advice. For pizza waffles, use FODMAP-friendly pepperoni. For tuna crunch, serve no more than 60g (2¼oz) of avocado per person and use all green (bell) peppers instead of mixed colours.

❄ Once cooled, store in an airtight container and freeze for up to 3 months. Air fry from frozen for 8–10 minutes at 200°C (400°F).

TIP

If the waffles stick to your waffle maker, try spraying the top and bottom with a little vegetable oil before you pour in the batter. My waffle maker is non-stick so I don't really need to, but with a cast-iron one this step is essential.

- 150g (1 cup plus 2 tbsp) gluten-free self-raising flour
- 1 tsp dried mixed herbs, if making pizza waffles
- ½ tsp gluten-free baking powder
- 1 tsp salt
- 280ml (1¼ cups) milk
- 1 large egg

For pizza waffles

- 4 tbsp passata (sieved tomatoes)
- 5 slices of pepperoni, finely chopped
- Small handful of thinly sliced or grated mozzarella
- 4–6 small basil leaves
- Large handful of rocket (arugula), to serve

For tuna crunch

- 1 x 145g (5oz) can of tuna in spring water, drained
- 50g (1¾oz) mixed frozen sliced (bell) peppers, defrosted and finely chopped
- Small handful of thinly sliced or grated mozzarella
- Small handful of roughly chopped spring onion (scallion) greens
- ½ medium avocado, thinly sliced, to serve

For cheese and chive (pictured)

- Small handful of finely chopped chives
- ½ handful of thinly sliced or grated mozzarella
- ½ handful of grated mature Cheddar
- 2 large eggs, each fried in a few sprays of vegetable oil, to serve

Turn the waffle maker on so it starts heating up.

In a large bowl, combine the flour, dried herbs (if making pizza waffles), baking powder and salt. Add the milk, crack in the egg and whisk until smooth. Allow to rest for 5 minutes or so while the waffle maker heats up.

Once the waffle maker has heated, pour in just enough of the batter to cover the base (into as many separate waffle recesses your machine has). Then close the lid, keep it closed for around 2 minutes, then open and add the fillings.

For pizza waffles, spoon on the passata, then scatter on the pepperoni and mozzarella. Pour on another measure of the batter so that it covers the filling, then place the basil leaves on top of the batter. Close and cook for a further 3 minutes, until golden all over. Remove and keep warm while you make the rest. Serve with rocket.

For tuna crunch, spread out the tuna, scatter on the peppers, mozzarella and spring onion. Pour on another measure of the batter so that it covers the filling, then close and cook for a further 3 minutes until golden all over. Remove and keep warm while you make the rest. Serve with avocado.

For cheese and chive, scatter on the chives, mozzarella and Cheddar. Pour on another measure of the batter so that it covers the filling, then close and cook for a further 3 minutes until golden all over. Remove and keep warm while you make the rest. Serve with a fried egg.

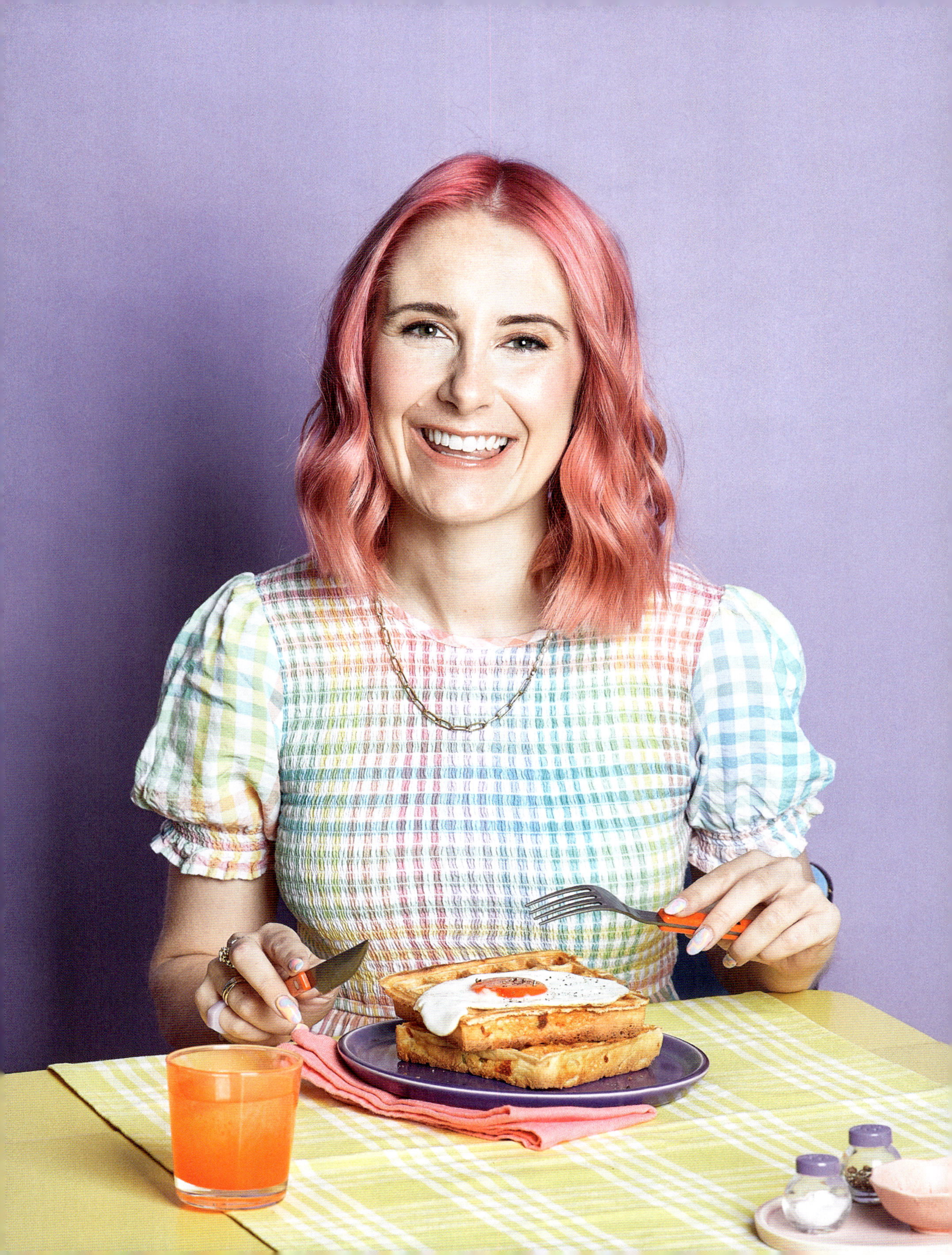

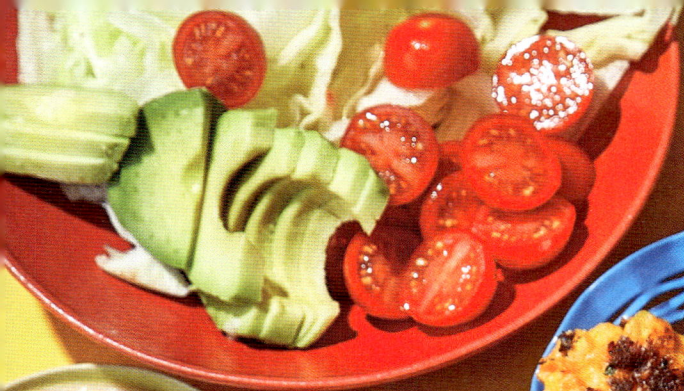

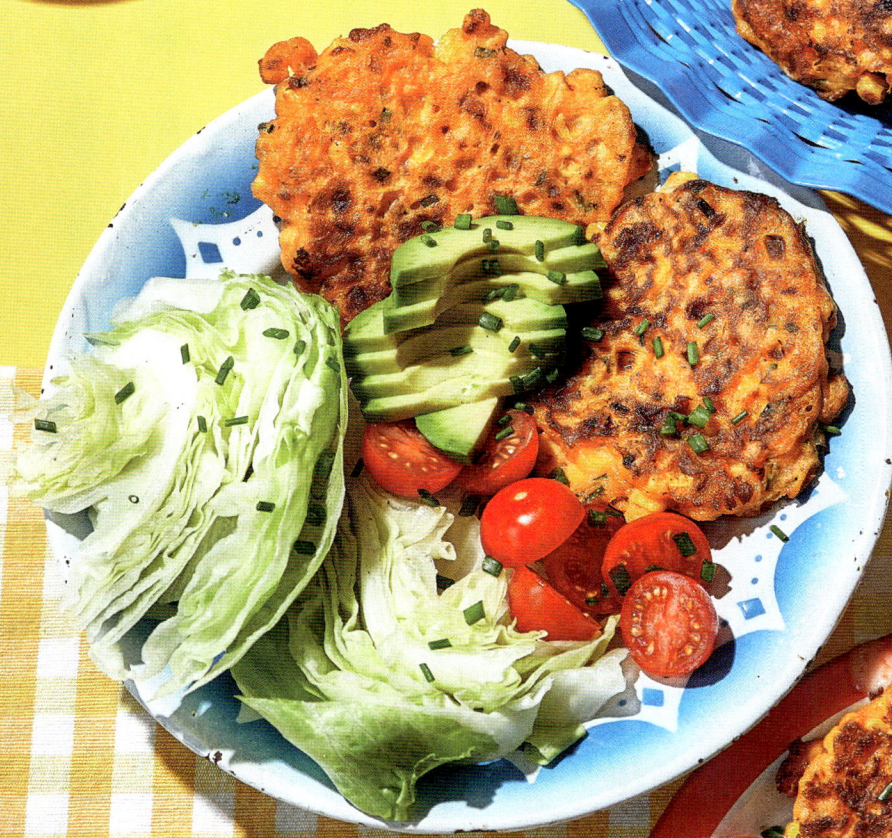

CHILLI CHEESE CORN FRITTERS

With a mild kick of chilli, charred cheese and sweetcorn that tastes like it just came off the BBQ, these fritters are more than fit for topping, dipping, chopping up in a salad or simply just enjoying as they are! Whether you eat them piping hot, fresh from the pan or air fryer, or completely cold (fresh from the lunchbox!) at your desk, you'll be 100% confident that nobody else's lunch tastes quite this awesome.

Serves 4 (makes 10–12)

Prep 5 mins

Hob 25 mins or
Air Fryer 20 mins

V

DF Use dairy-free milk and dairy-free cheese.

LI Use lactose-free milk.

VE See dairy-free advice and combine 2 tbsp flaxseed mixed with 6 tbsp water (allow to rest for 10 minutes); use the resulting mixture in place of the eggs. Use vegan-friendly mayo.

❄ Once cooled, store in an airtight container and freeze for up to 3 months. Air fry from frozen for 7–8 minutes at 200°C (400°F) until crisp on the outside.

- 150g (1 cup plus 2 tbsp) gluten-free self-raising flour
- 2 large eggs
- 100ml (generous ⅓ cup) milk
- 500g (1lb 2oz) drained canned or frozen sweetcorn
- Small handful of chives, very finely chopped, plus an extra small handful to serve
- 1 tbsp tomato purée (paste)
- 2 tsp chilli paste or 2 tsp dried chilli flakes
- 1 tsp salt
- ½ tsp ground black pepper
- 100g (3½oz) mature Cheddar, grated
- Vegetable oil spray

To serve (optional)
- 1–2 medium avocados, thinly sliced
- 12 cherry tomatoes, halved
- 1 iceberg lettuce, quartered into wedges
- 4 tbsp sweet chilli sauce (ensure gluten-free)
- 4 tbsp mayonnaise
- 1 tbsp water

Add the flour to a large bowl. Use a fork to beat the eggs and milk together in a jug (pitcher). Pour half the wet mixture into the flour and mix with a wooden spoon until smooth, then add the rest of the wet mixture and mix again.

Stir through the sweetcorn, chives, tomato purée, chilli paste or flakes, salt, pepper and grated cheese.

To cook on the hob, place a large frying pan over a medium heat and generously spray with oil. Once heated, spoon one heaped wooden spoonful of the mixture per fritter into the pan (I managed to cook 4 in my 30cm/12in pan) and flatten down into slightly less than 1cm (½in) thick, round patties using the back of the spoon. Spray the tops generously with oil.

Fry for 4–5 minutes until the underside is golden brown (lift it up a little and peek underneath to check), then slide a spatula underneath, ensuring the entire fritter is supported, and flip. Press down firmly with the back of the spatula and fry for a further 3–4 minutes or until the underside is golden brown too. Respray the pan with oil and repeat with any remaining mixture.

To cook in an air fryer, spoon heaped wooden spoonfuls of the mixture onto 12cm (4¾in) squares of non-stick baking parchment and flatten down into slightly less than 1cm (½in) thick, round patties using the back of the spoon.

Heat the air fryer to 200°C (400°F). Place as many of the fritters in the air fryer as will fit without any touching and spray generously with oil. Air fry for 5 minutes, then carefully flip and peel off the baking parchment before spraying generously with oil once more. Air fry for a further 4–5 minutes until golden brown on top. Respray the air fryer with oil and repeat with any remaining mixture.

To serve, if you like, top the fritters with avocado and tomato, and serve with a wedge of lettuce on the side. Combine the sweet chilli sauce, mayo and water in a small dish, then drizzle over everything and sprinkle over the chives.

POTATO 'TATTIE' SCONES

Whether you call them tattie scones, potato scones or potato farls, there's one thing that never changes: they're an absolute joy to eat at any time of the day! These classic pan-fried or griddled thin and crispy potato thins are perfect for topping, and with the bulk of the ingredients being ever-affordable potatoes, you simply can't go wrong.

Makes 12
Prep 10 mins
Hob 40 mins
Hob + Air Fryer 35 mins

LL **V**

DF Use a (hard) dairy-free alternative to butter.

VE See dairy-free advice and serve with pan-fried frozen mushrooms instead of poached eggs.

F Serve no more than 60g (2¼oz) of avocado per person. Use a FODMAP-friendly chilli jam.

❄ Once cooled, freeze for up to 2–3 months in airtight containers. Reheat in the air fryer from frozen at 200°C (400°F) for 3–4 minutes.

TIP

Although optional, this recipe assumes you're familiar with poaching eggs. If you choose to serve my tattie scones with poached eggs and you've never poached them before, I'd highly recommend watching a short video online before you launch into it.

I always crack each individual egg into a small bowl, then gently pour it into the simmering water from the bowl; it's easier, safer and helps to stop the white spreading too much. I usually poach 2–3 eggs at the same time depending on how big my pan is (they need a quite a lot of space). When the egg white closest to the yolk looks cooked, use a slotted spoon to delicately lift it onto a plate of kitchen paper to drain, then serve.

For the tattie scones

- 500g (1lb 2oz) potatoes, peeled and cut into roast-potato-sized chunks
- 30g (1oz) butter, plus an extra 4 tsp for frying, or vegetable oil spray, for air frying
- 110g (¾ cup plus 1½ tbsp) gluten-free plain (all-purpose) flour, plus extra for dusting

To serve (optional)

- 2 medium avocados, halved and thinly sliced on the diagonal
- 6 large eggs, each poached in a medium pan of boiling water (with 1 tbsp white wine vinegar added to the water) for 3–4 minutes, then removed with a slotted spoon
- 6 tbsp chilli jam

Boil the chopped potatoes in a pan of well salted water for 10–12 minutes, then drain well, return to the pan and allow to dry off a little.

Mash the butter into the potatoes then stir through the flour gradually until a dough is formed. Split the dough into 3 portions. On a lightly floured surface, roll out one portion into a large circle around 5mm (¼in) thick. Carefully place a small side plate (about 21cm/8¼in diameter) on top of the dough and cut around it using a sharp knife, then cut the circle into quarters.

To cook on the hob, place a large frying pan over a medium heat and add 1 teaspoon of butter. Once melted (don't let it burn!), use a silicone brush to spread it over the base of the pan. Carefully lower as many scones as will fit into the pan and fry on each side for around 3–5 minutes until lightly golden on both sides. Repeat with the rest of the dough, using an extra teaspoon of butter to fry each batch in.

To cook in an air fryer, heat the air fryer to 180°C (350°F). Generously spray the base of the air fryer basket or crisping tray with oil. If you have an air fryer with 2 drawers, use both. Carefully place as many scones as will fit in the air fryer basket without touching and generously spray with oil. Air fry for 8 minutes, turning them over halfway. They should be cooked through and lightly golden on both sides. Repeat until you've cooked all of the scones, respraying the basket or crisping tray, and the scones, with oil.

Enjoy straight away while still warm or enjoy cold, optionally with sliced avocado, poached eggs and a dollop of chilli jam.

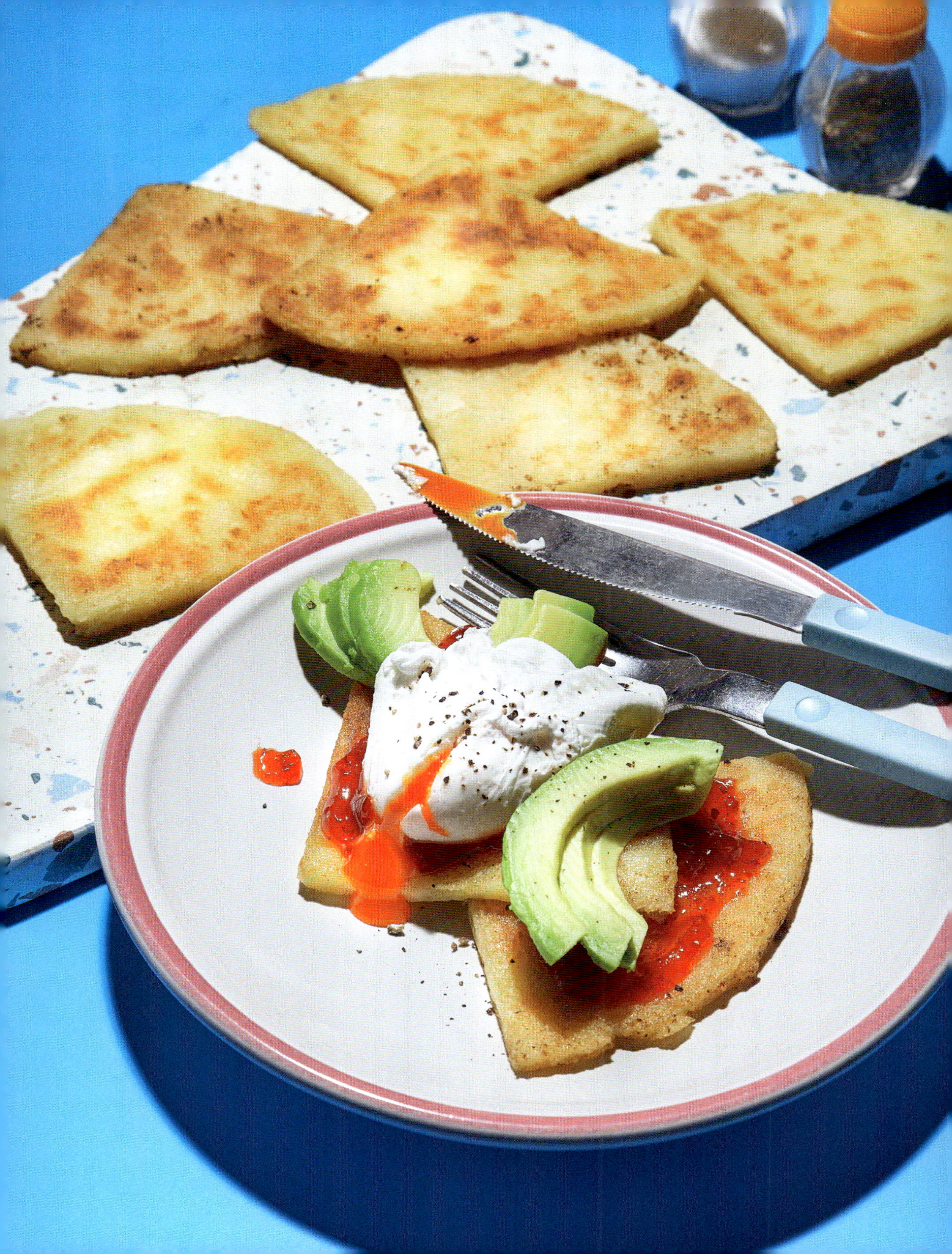

SMOKY BACON NAAN

Though this might seem like a completely random idea, it was inspired by an amazing Indian restaurant in London that serves classic English breakfast options with their own unique spin on them. The only problem is that none of the things I'd like to order are gluten-free! And if I could eat anything, this would be the first thing I'd order. But until they offer a gluten-free naan (I'm not holding my breath!) I will happily enjoy this instead. Expect crispy bacon wrapped in a soft, fluffy naan with a little cream cheese and chilli jam to boot.

Makes 4

Prep 15 mins

Air Fryer 10 mins or
Hob 10 mins

V Omit the bacon and replace with gluten-free veggie sausages (cooked according to packet instructions and halved lengthways).

DF Use a thick dairy-free yoghurt instead of Greek, and dairy-free milk and cream cheese.

LF Use lactose-free Greek yoghurt, milk and cream cheese.

F See lactose-free advice and use a FODMAP-friendly chilli jam.

❄ Once cooked and cooled, freeze for up to 3 months. Air fry from frozen at 200°C (400°F) for 6–7 minutes until crisp.

For the naan bread
- 225g (1¾ cups) gluten-free self-raising flour, plus extra for dusting
- 90g (½ cup minus 1 tbsp) Greek yoghurt
- 60ml (¼ cup) milk
- 1 large egg
- 1 tsp salt
- 2 tsp nigella seeds (optional)
- Vegetable oil spray

For the filling
- 4 tbsp cream cheese
- 4 tbsp tomato chilli jam
- 8 rashers of smoked back bacon, air fried for 7–8 minutes until crisp
- Small handful of coriander (cilantro) leaves, roughly chopped (optional)

Add the naan ingredients, except the oil (giving the yoghurt a good stir before adding) to a large bowl. Mix thoroughly, using a spatula, to ensure there are no hidden clumps of yoghurt-coated flour. As it starts to come together, use your hands to bring it together into a slightly sticky ball.

Knead briefly in the bowl until smooth and combined but still a little sticky and loose.

Transfer the dough to a medium sheet of lightly floured non-stick baking parchment. Divide the dough into 4 equal portions and roll each into a ball. Place 3 of the dough portions back in the bowl.

Using floured hands, gradually push the dough down into a naan shape until it's about 2–3mm (⅛in) thick, ensuring it's not thicker or thinner in certain areas; keep lightly flouring your hands whenever it starts to stick to them.

Repeat until you have 4 flattened naan, each on its own sheet of parchment. Use a pair of sharp scissors to trim the parchment around the naan, ensuring you leave no more than 1cm (½in) excess parchment.

To cook in an air fryer, heat the air fryer to 200°C (400°F). Lift one naan on baking parchment into the air fryer (or as many as will comfortably fit at once) and generously spray with oil. Air fry for 5 minutes, flipping halfway (discard the parchment after flipping) and lightly spray with oil once again; after flipping it should puff up and bubble. Repeat for any remaining naan that wouldn't fit into the air fryer.

To cook on the hob, place a frying pan over a medium-high heat. The pan may get hotter the longer you have it on, so bear in mind that you may need to reduce the heat slightly for your final naans. Slap the flattened dough into the hot, dry frying pan with the parchment facing up. After around 30 seconds or so, remove the parchment and spray generously with oil. Once the base has browned in places, flip over using a spatula and fry for a further 30 seconds, spraying generously with oil once more. Repeat until you've used up all your dough.

To serve, spread cream cheese on the left side of each naan, and on the right side spread the tomato chilli jam. Add the crispy bacon, followed by a few coriander leaves, if using, then fold shut.

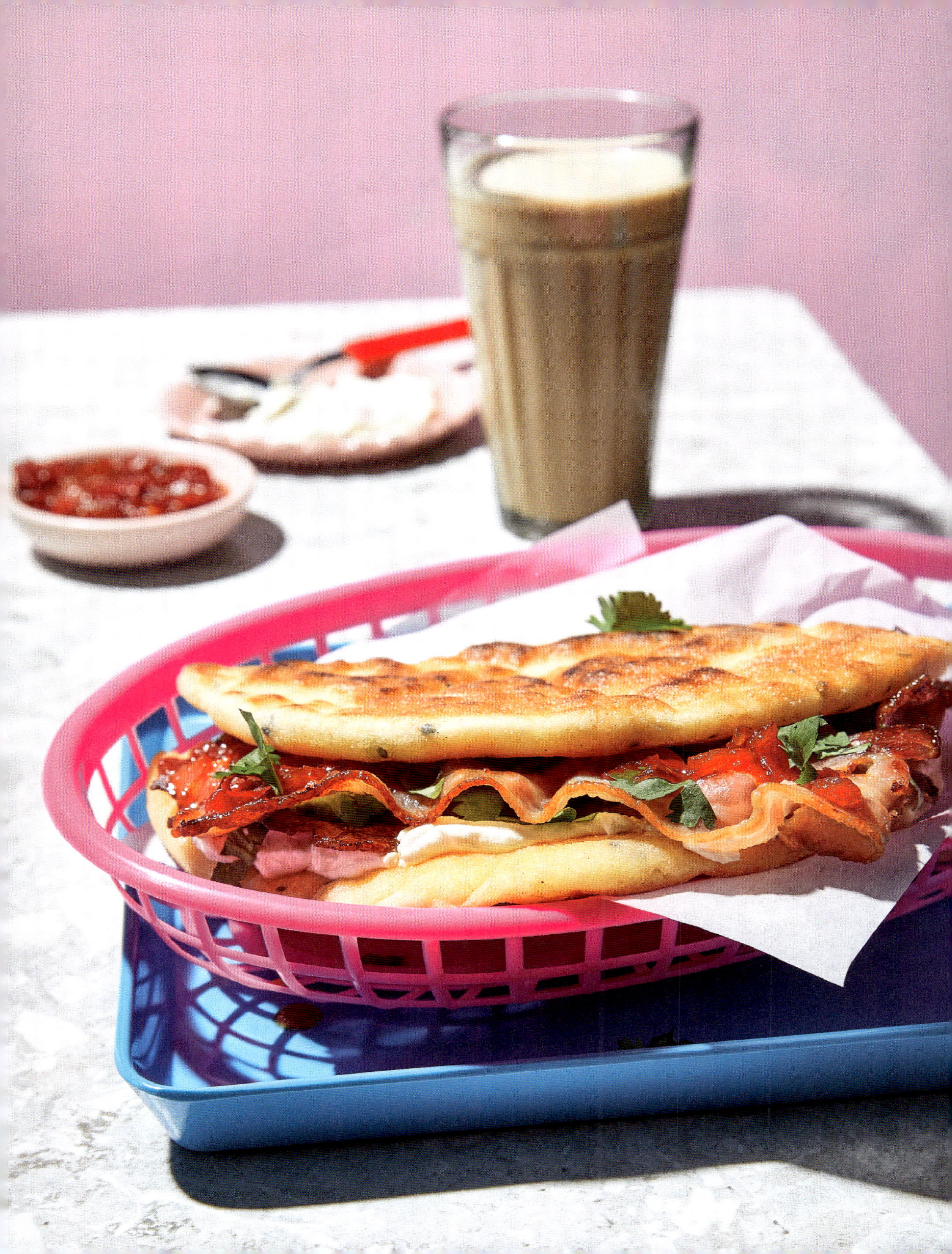

CHEDDAR + MUSHROOM LENTIL SLICE

Serves 4

Prep 10 mins

Hob + Oven 40 mins or
Hob + Air Fryer 35 mins

This satisfyingly cheesy baked lentil dish lives here in the lunch chapter, as not only is it absolutely delicious hot or cold, but after it's cooled a little, you can cut it into easy-to-serve slices like a crustless quiche. And, in reality, you should very much treat it that way! Enjoy it with a side salad or maybe a little coleslaw at home or from a tupperware box if you're out and about – it's totally up to you!

LL **V**

DF Use dairy-free cheese.

VE See dairy-free advice.

❄ Once cooled, slice and store in airtight containers in the freezer for up to 2–3 months. Allow to defrost completely in the fridge, then reheat in the air fryer for 4–5 minutes at 200°C (400°F).

TIPS

If cooking on the hob, remember: the larger your pot, the thinner the finished bake will be. A 20–25cm (8–10in) pot is the sweet spot for nice, thick slices!

If cooking in the air fryer, using the largest roasting or baking tin that will fit in your air fryer is key; ideally a 20cm (8in) round or rectangular tin. If you don't have a tin this big, you can always split the mixture to make two smaller portions.

- Vegetable oil spray
- 100g (3½oz) frozen chopped onion **or** ½ medium leek, finely chopped
- 500g (1lb 2oz) frozen sliced mushrooms
- 1 tsp salt
- ½ tsp ground black pepper
- 1 tsp Dijon mustard
- 1 tsp dried mixed herbs
- 3 tbsp cornflour (cornstarch) or potato starch
- 2 x 400g (14oz) cans of lentils, drained
- 125g (4½oz) mature Cheddar, grated
- 50g (1¾oz) mozzarella, grated or thinly sliced

Spray the base of a large ovenproof (if cooking in the oven) pot with oil and place over a medium heat. Once hot, add the onion or leek and fry until the onion is browned or the leek has softened. Add the mushrooms and fry until liquid is released, then continue to fry until the liquid has completely evaporated.

Add the salt, pepper, mustard, mixed herbs, cornflour or potato starch and lentils, then stir briefly until everything is mixed well. Stir in the grated Cheddar and simmer until you're left with a nicely thickened, sticky mixture.

To cook in an oven, preheat the oven to 200°C fan/220°C (425°F). Use the back of a spoon to pat everything flat into an even layer, then scatter on the mozzarella. Bake in the oven for 24–28 minutes or until the cheese on top is golden brown. Allow to cool for 10–15 minutes – it'll firm up and be easier to slice once cooled.

To cook in an air fryer, heat the air fryer to 200°C (400°F). Transfer the mixture to your largest available roasting or baking tin that'll fit into your air fryer. Use the back of a spoon to pat everything flat into an even layer, then scatter on the mozzarella. Air fry for 18–22 minutes or until the cheese on top is golden brown, then allow to cool for 10–15 minutes.

Slice and serve alongside a side salad and salad cream.

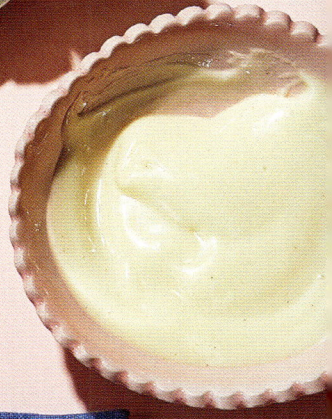

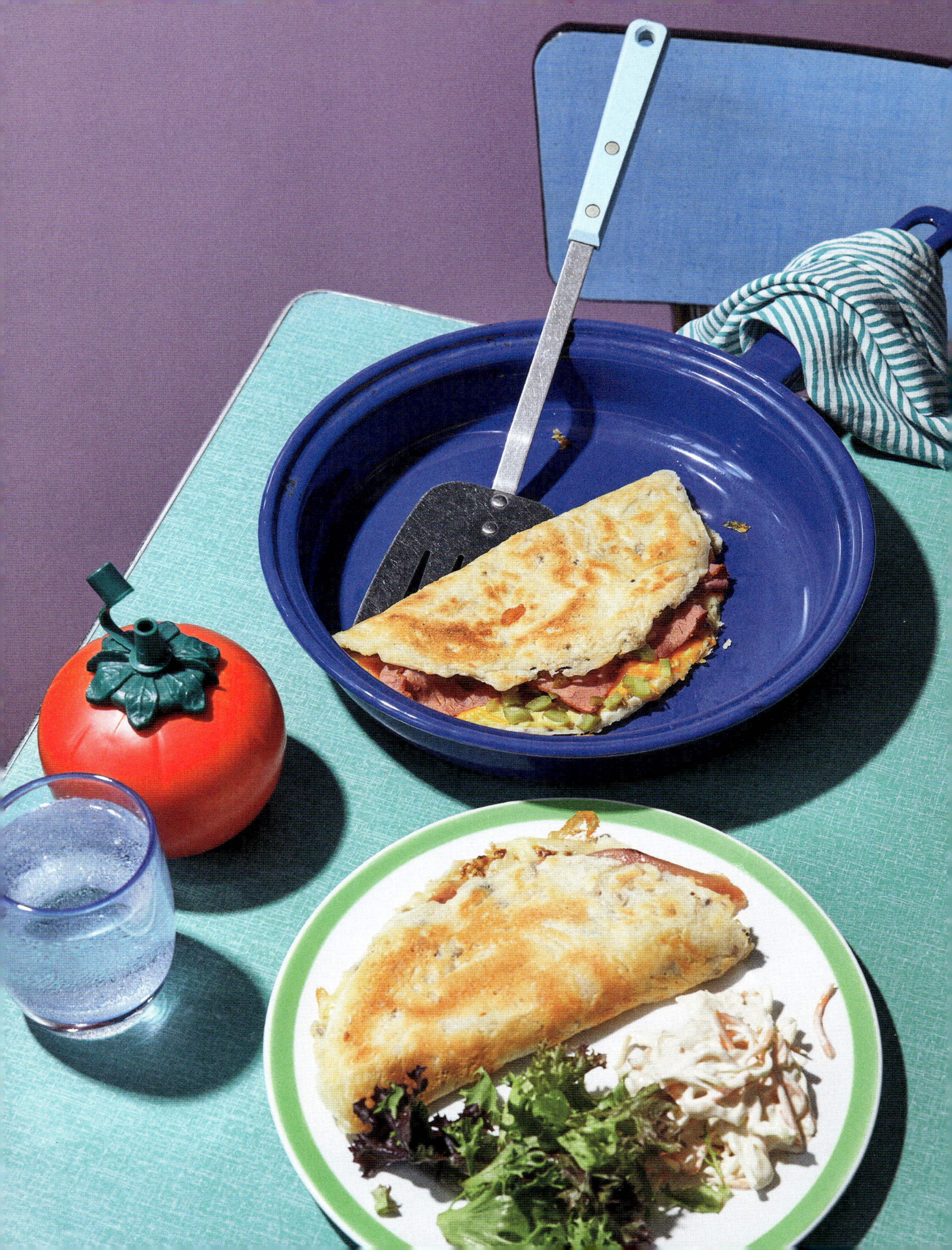

EMERGENCY PAN SANDWICH 3 WAYS

Makes 2
Prep 2 mins
Hob 10 mins

DF Use a thick dairy-free yoghurt instead of Greek yoghurt, and dairy-free cheese.

LL Use lactose-free Greek yoghurt.

F See low lactose advice.

V Make the mozzarella and tomato pan sandwich.

VE Combine dairy-free and veggie advice.

❄ Once cooled, store in an airtight container and freeze for up to 3 months. Air fry from frozen for 8–10 minutes at 200°C (400°F) until piping hot in the middle.

Just like my emergency stuffed crust pizza (see page 75), this recipe will always be there for you when absolutely nothing else is! My light and fluffy frying pan flatbread is cooked, fried and folded right there in the pan, meaning there's minimal washing up and, naturally, it can be made in a flash. It's essentially like a toastie but in a puffy, cloud-like flatbread; best of all, you won't need to use any slices of costly gluten-free bread to make this. It's delicious hot or cold, so once cooled, you can simply pop it into an airtight container and take it wherever you go. I like to have mine with coleslaw and a side salad.

- Vegetable oil spray
- 40g (4¾ tbsp) gluten-free self-raising flour
- 30g (2 tbsp) Greek yoghurt or natural yoghurt
- 35ml (2 tbsp plus 1 tsp) water
- Pinch of salt
- 1 tsp mixed seeds, such as sunflower, pumpkin, sesame and golden flaxseeds (optional)

For ham and cheese
- 30g (1oz) mature Cheddar, grated
- 2 slices of ham
- ¼ tsp wholegrain mustard

For mozzarella and tomato
- 1 small tomato, cut into 5mm (¼in) slices
- 30g (1oz) mozzarella, grated

For the New Yorker (pictured)
- 2 slices of pastrami
- 30g (1oz) red Leicester cheese, grated
- ¼ tsp Dijon mustard
- 1 slice of gherkin, finely diced

Place a 23cm (9in) frying pan over a medium heat. Generously spray with oil.

Add the flour, yoghurt, water, salt and mixed seeds, if using, to a large bowl and mix until a smooth, thick, spreadable batter is achieved.

Place half the dough mixture in the pan and use the back of a wooden spoon to spread it into an even circle, about 5mm (¼in) thick, that covers most of the base of the pan. Fry for a few minutes, then check the underside – if it's golden, add the filling of your choice to one side of the flatbread and fold shut like a book. Fry until the cheese has all melted, then flip and fry until golden brown on both sides. Remove from the pan and repeat with the remaining dough, spraying the pan with oil once more.

HOMEMADE SOFT FLOUR WRAPS

Makes 9
Prep 15 mins + 10 mins resting
Hob 20 mins

If you've been searching for an easy gluten-free tortilla wrap recipe, – since the prices of gluten-free supermarket versions are simply too outrageous – then look no further. Once you've got your psyllium husk (source it online and ideally make sure it says 'blonde' somewhere on the listing), this recipe is simple. You'll only need a small amount of it for this recipe, and the brand I buy online is exceptionally reasonable and comes in 300g (10½oz) packets, meaning you can make this recipe 14 times for over 100 wraps! If you're in need of a little inspiration for easy on-the-go lunch options to pair with these, then I've shared three of my favourites below.

DF LF F V VE

❄ Once cooled, freeze for up to 2–3 months. Reheat in the air fryer from frozen at 200°C (400°F) for 2–3 minutes or for a couple of minutes in a pan on the hob.

Note: The dietary keys do not take into account the three filling suggestions, so use your own judgement here depending on your own dietary requirements!

TIP

Each filling suggestion is enough to fill one wrap, though bear in mind that you won't need the entire quantity of karaage popcorn chicken to fill one wrap – save the rest for future wraps or lunches.

See the tip on page 190 for advice on weighing out the dough portions using digital weighing scales to ensure consistency of size. Remember to use the portion measurements given here though.

- 210g (1½ cups) gluten-free plain (all-purpose) flour, plus extra for dusting
- ½ tsp salt
- 20g (¾oz) blonde psyllium husk
- 300ml (1¼ cups) warm water
- 25ml (1½ tbsp) vegetable oil

For a fridge-raid folded wrap

- Small handful of cooked chicken, ham or roasted veggies
- Small handful of lettuce or rocket (arugula)
- ¼ medium avocado
- 15g (½oz) mature Cheddar, grated
- 2 tsp sweet chilli sauce (ensure gluten-free) or mayonnaise

For a beat-up egg sarnie wrap

- 2 eggs
- 15g (½oz) mature Cheddar, grated
- Pinch each of salt and pepper

- Drizzle of vegetable oil
- 1 slice of ham

For a fried chicken wrap (pictured)

- 2 tsp mayonnaise
- Small handful of chopped lettuce
- 5 cherry tomatoes, sliced
- 1 quantity of karaage popcorn chicken (see page 64), or any leftover cooked chicken
- Drizzle of sweet chilli sauce (ensure gluten-free)

In a large bowl, combine the flour, salt and psyllium. Pour in the warm water and oil and mix together thoroughly. Use either a spatula or (ideally) an electric hand mixer and mix for 2 minutes, or an extra minute longer if mixing by hand with a spatula. The mixture will seem quite loose at first, but the more you mix, the more it comes together and thickens up. Once the mixture is more of a sticky, thicker dough, cover and allow to rest for 10 minutes to help the dough hydrate.

The dough should now be soft and very slightly sticky, but nowhere near as sticky as before. Sprinkle the dough with a small amount of flour and knead briefly in the bowl, using floured hands, to further bring it together.

Portion the dough out into 45–50g (1½–1¾oz) portions for smaller wraps, or 75–80g (2½–2¾oz) for larger wraps. You can adjust the weight depending on what size works for you and how much you intend to fill them.

continued overleaf

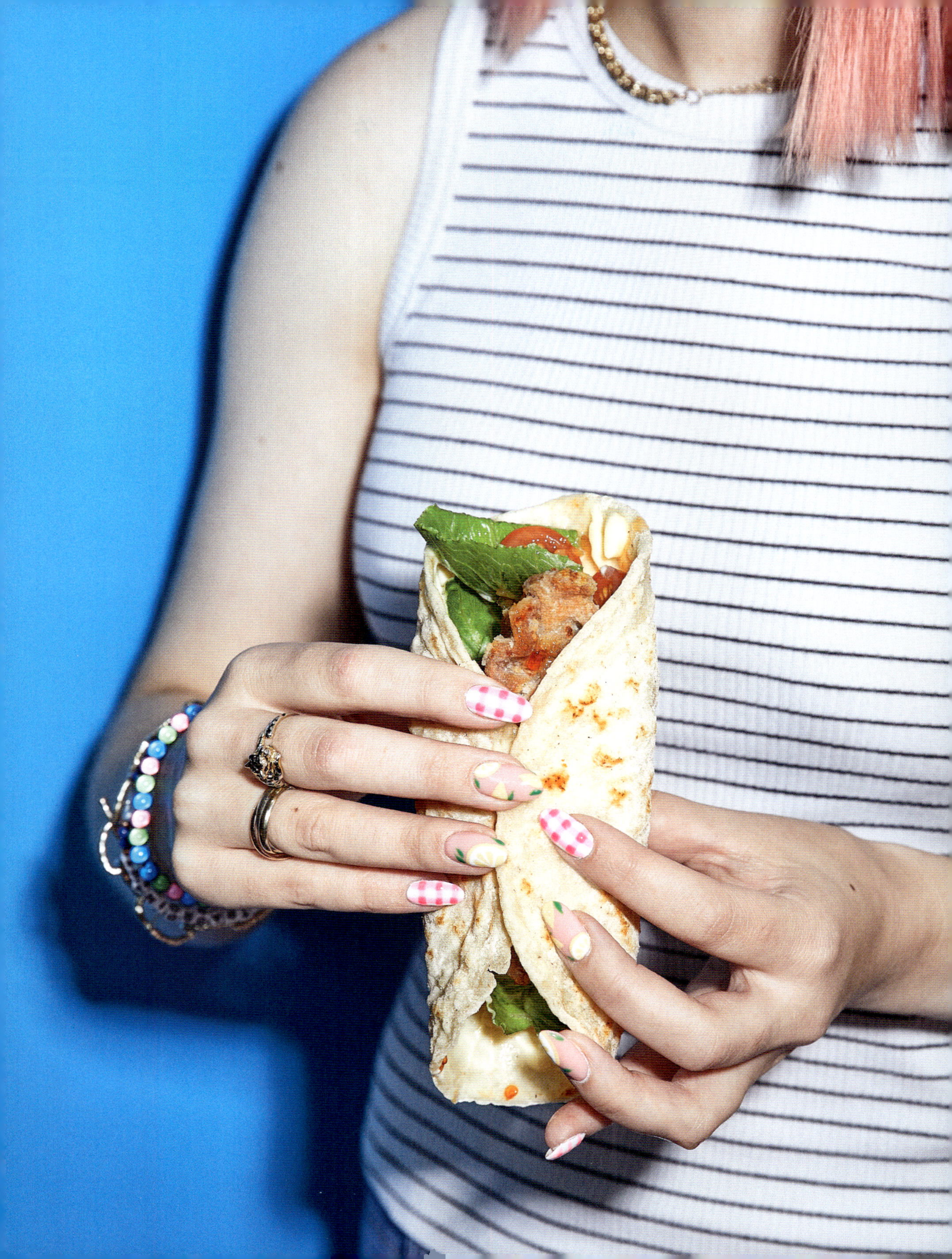

Place a portion of the dough between two 20cm (8in) square pieces of non-stick baking parchment and roll it into a circular shape, around 1mm thick, or as thin as possible. You can also use a tortilla press for this part if you have one. If using a tortilla press and the dough is still a little too thick, you can manually roll it further using a rolling pin while it's still between the 2 sheets of parchment

Place a large frying pan over a medium-high heat. Once hot, peel one sheet of parchment from the top of the flattened/rolled out wraps. Transfer to your pan, using the remaining parchment to lower it in, tortilla side down. After 10–15 seconds, carefully peel off the parchment – use a spatula to ease it off if it helps.

The wrap should start to get little bubbles on the surface if the pan is hot enough. Cook until the underside starts to lightly colour, for 1–2 minutes, then flip and cook on the other side for a minute or so more.

Remove from the pan and wrap in a clean tea towel (dish cloth) while you repeat with the rest of the dough, reusing the same baking parchment to do so. (Covering the wraps in the tea towel helps them become more flexible and soft).

I've provided three different ways of using the wraps for lunch to the right (see the filling tip on the previous page) but do just use them however you would usually use them: for lunches or dinners from fajitas to wraps in lunchboxes and everything around and in between!

For a fridge-raid folded wrap (if you made large wraps)

Use a sharp knife to cut up the middle of the wrap, just to the centre, then place different fillings into each quarter of the wrap. Fold each section over the top of the previous and then either enjoy straight away cold or ideally heat on both sides in a pan until the wrap is golden, the fillings are hot and any cheese has melted.

For a beat-up egg sarnie wrap

Beat the eggs in a jug (pitcher) and stir in the grated cheese and the salt and pepper. Place a frying pan (a similar size to your wrap) over a medium heat with the drizzle of oil and, once hot, add the beaten egg to the pan, allowing it to spread out all around the pan. Cook for a couple of minutes until the egg has basically set, then place your wrap on top of it and gently press down. Cook for a further 30 seconds or so before inverting it all onto a plate. Place back in the pan but with the wrap on the bottom this time, place the ham on top (or any other fillings of choice) and carefully fold shut like a book. Allow to cook on both sides for a few minutes until the wrap is starting to colour, then lift out of the pan, cut into two and enjoy straight away.

For a fried chicken wrap (pictured)

Place a wrap on a plate and spread the mayonnaise over it in a thin layer. Down the centre of the wrap, add a layer of chopped lettuce, chopped cherry tomatoes and the chicken, then drizzle with some sweet chilli sauce. Roll the wrap up, folding in the sides, and enjoy.

NOT ANOTHER BORING SALAD 3 WAYS

If you relate to the title of this recipe, then I can certainly say that this one was written for you. Hands up if you've been in a position where an uninspired salad dish is the only thing that's gluten-free on the menu; or even worse, hands up if you've ever been served an extremely bland side salad that's essentially just leaves in a bowl. I am now typing this one handed because my other is currently raised in the air. Fortunately, these three salad variations are here to restore your faith. Each one is jam-packed with protein, maximum flavour and a variety of textures to keep you guessing. This is the first salad recipe I've ever published in a book, so I was sure to make it an awesome one! It makes use of the air fryer to prepare any ingredients that need cooking, though feel free to do these simple things on the hob (frying bacon/chicken or croutons and boiling the eggs) if you don't have one.

Serves 3
Prep 10 mins
Air Fryer 10–20 mins

DF Make the chicken, bacon and avocado or the tuna and jammy eggs variations.

LL If making the crispy chickpea and whipped feta variation, use lactose-free Greek yoghurt.

F Make the chicken, bacon and avocado (use maple syrup instead of honey) or tuna and jammy eggs variations and serve no more than 60g (2¼oz) avocado per person.

V Make the crispy chickpea and feta salad variation.

- Vegetable oil spray
- Salt and ground black pepper

For the salad
- ½ iceberg lettuce, shredded
- 30g (1oz) rocket (arugula), watercress, or lamb's lettuce
- 30g (1oz) spinach leaves
- 1 medium carrot, grated (optional)
- ½ cucumber, cut into 5mm (¼in) cubes (optional)
- 6–8 cherry tomatoes, halved

For the croutons
- 2 slices of frozen gluten-free bread
- 4 small pinches of dried mixed herbs

For chicken, bacon and avocado with a honey mustard dressing
- 2 small chicken breasts, cut into long strips 1.5cm (⅔in) wide
- 2 rashers of smoked back bacon
- 60g (¼ cup) honey
- 1½ tsp wholegrain mustard
- 1½ tsp white wine vinegar
- 1 medium avocado, diced

For tuna and jammy eggs with a lemon pepper dressing
- 3 large eggs
- 100g (scant ½ cup) mayonnaise
- 1 tsp Dijon mustard
- Grated zest of 1 lemon and juice of ½

- 2 x 145g (5oz) cans of tuna in spring water, drained
- 1 medium avocado, diced (optional)

For crispy chickpea and whipped feta dressing (pictured overleaf)
- 1 x 400g (14oz) can of chickpeas, drained
- 1 tsp dried mixed herbs, plus ½ tsp for the whipped feta
- 200g (7oz) feta-style salad cheese
- 150g (⅔ cup) Greek yoghurt
- Grated zest of ½ lemon
- 1 tbsp honey
- 100g (3½oz) jarred roasted red (bell) peppers, finely chopped

Toss all the prepared salad ingredients in a bowl and set aside.

Now prep the croutons. Heat the air fryer to 200°C (400°F). Lay both slices of bread out on a plate and spray generously with oil. Sprinkle a pinch of salt, pepper and mixed herbs over each. Flip over and repeat. Air fry for 8–9 minutes until crisp, hardened and golden on the outside (if your bread isn't frozen, halve the cooking time). Transfer to a board and chop into 1cm (½in) cubes. Set aside.

For a chicken, bacon and avocado salad

Heat the air fryer to 200°C (400°F). Generously spray the base of the air fryer basket or crisping tray with oil. If you have an air fryer with 2 drawers, you'll likely need to employ both, so grease both if necessary.

continued overleaf

Add the chicken to a bowl, season with ½ teaspoon each of salt and pepper, and spray well with oil. Mix briefly, then add the chicken and bacon to the air fryer, making sure everything is touching as little as possible. Air fry for 7–8 minutes or until the chicken is a little golden at the edges and the bacon is super-crisp, then remove. Finely chop the bacon.

Meanwhile, for the dressing, mix together the honey, wholegrain mustard, white wine vinegar and a pinch of salt in a small dish.

To serve, add the chicken to a (clean) large bowl alongside the avocado, followed by the prepared salad and croutons. Drizzle the dressing over everything, cover with a plate and shake from side to side until everything is well coated. Plate up and scatter over the crispy bacon.

For a tuna and jammy eggs salad

Heat or preheat the air fryer to 150°C (300°F). Place the eggs into the air fryer and air fry for 8–9 minutes, then remove and leave until cool enough to handle, before peeling.

Meanwhile, mix together the mayonnaise, mustard, half the lemon zest, the lemon juice, a pinch of salt and ½ teaspoon of pepper in a small dish.

To serve, add the drained tuna to a large bowl alongside the avocado, followed by the prepared salad and croutons. Drizzle the dressing over everything, cover with a plate and shake from side to side until everything is well coated. Plate up, scatter over the remaining lemon zest, halve the eggs and place 2 halves on the side of each plate.

For a crispy chickpea and whipped feta salad

Add the chickpeas (ensure they're as dry as possible) to a large bowl, followed by the mixed herbs and ½ teaspoon each of salt and pepper. Spray well with vegetable oil, then shake the bowl from side to side until they're all well coated.

Heat or preheat the air fryer to 200°C (400°F). Add the coated chickpeas to the air fryer and cook for 10–11 minutes or until browned in places and a little crunchy on the outside.

Meanwhile, add the block of feta-style cheese, yoghurt, lemon zest, honey, ½ teaspoon of dried mixed herbs, ¼ teaspoon of salt and ½ teaspoon of pepper to the empty bowl (no need to clean it). Use a stick blender to blend until smooth – plunge the blender into the block of feta first in short pulses to help break it up first.

To serve, plate up the prepared salad and scatter over the chopped roasted red pepper and the croutons. Drizzle the whipped feta over each portion and divide the crispy chickpeas between each plate.

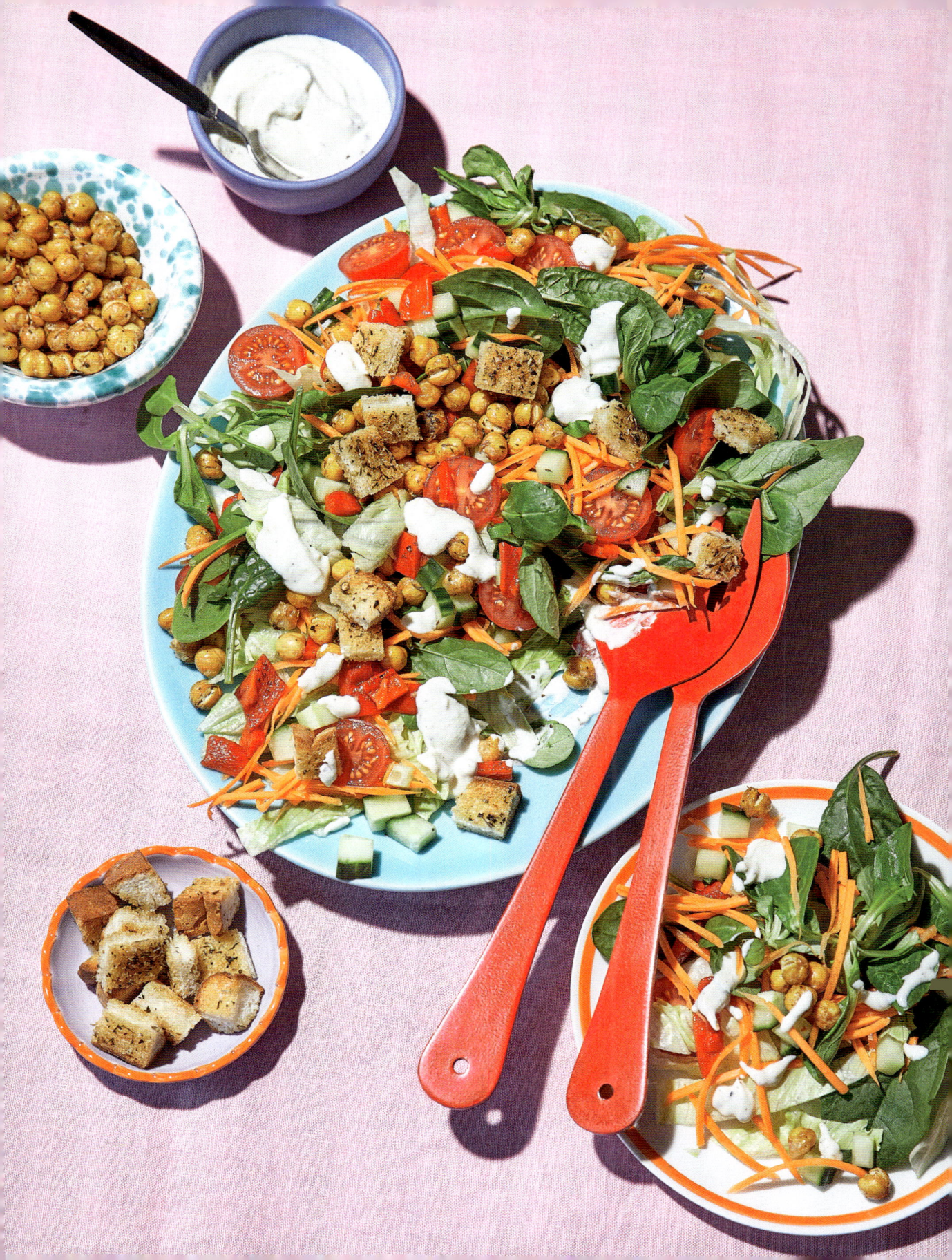

HAWAIIAN-STYLE HULI HULI CHICKEN POKE BOWL

Serves 3–4

Prep 10 mins + 15 mins marinating

Hob + Air Fryer/Grill (Broiler) 20 mins

I am a huge poke bowl fan (pronounced 'poh-kay' to rhyme with 'okay'), so I'm super excited to share my own tribute to this dish, which celebrates its Hawaiian roots with fruity, sticky, smoky and sweet chicken and pineapple.

DF **LF**

F Use light brown sugar instead of honey, 1 tbsp garlic-infused oil instead of garlic paste and no more than 60g (2¼oz) avocado per person.

V Use 400–500g (14–17oz) firm tofu, cut into 1cm (½in) strips, instead of chicken.

VE See veggie advice, and use light brown sugar instead of honey, and vegan-friendly mayo.

❄ Once the chicken has cooled, store in airtight containers in the freezer for up to 2–3 months. Allow to defrost completely in the fridge, then reheat in the air fryer for 5–7 minutes at 200°C (400°F). Check the internal temperature with a digital food thermometer against those given on page 255.

TIP

As sushi rice is quite costly, I use a little cheat to make any old rice sticky: just add a little starch!

- 500–600g (1lb 2oz–1lb 5oz) skinless, boneless chicken thighs or breast, cut into 1cm (½in) strips
- 2 tbsp tomato purée (paste)
- 4 tbsp gluten-free soy sauce
- 3 tbsp rice wine vinegar
- 4 tbsp honey
- ½ tsp dried chilli flakes
- 3 tsp cornflour (cornstarch) or potato starch
- 1 tsp ginger paste
- 1 tsp garlic paste (optional)

- 1 x 227g (8oz) can of pineapple rings in juice, including the juice
- Vegetable oil spray, for air frying

For the cheat's sushi rice

- 400ml (1⅔ cups) boiling water
- 3 tbsp caster (superfine) sugar
- 2 tbsp rice wine vinegar
- ½ tsp salt
- 200g (1 cup plus 2 tbsp) long-grain rice
- 1½ tbsp cornflour (cornstarch) or potato starch

To serve

- 100g (scant ½ cup) mayonnaise
- 1 tsp sweet chilli sauce (ensure gluten-free)
- 2 medium avocados, halved, thinly sliced then fanned out a little
- 150g (5½oz) edamame beans **or** ½ lettuce, shredded
- 1 carrot or cucumber, pared into long, thin strands using a julienne peeler

Add the chicken, tomato purée, soy sauce, vinegar, honey, chilli flakes, cornflour or potato starch, ginger, garlic, if using, and three-quarters of the pineapple juice to a large bowl. Mix well, then add the pineapple rings. Cover and refrigerate for 15 minutes and up to 12 hours.

For the rice, add the water, sugar, vinegar and salt to a pot that has a lid and bring to the boil. Once boiling, add the rice, pop on the lid and reduce the heat to low. Cook for 20 minutes, then take off the heat and stir in the cornflour or potato starch. Keep warm with the lid on. Meanwhile, cook the chicken.

To cook the chicken in an air fryer, heat the air fryer to 200°C (400°F). Spray the base of the basket or crisping tray with oil. If you have an air fryer with 2 drawers, you should use both.

Air fry thighs for 10 minutes and breasts for 5 minutes, then brush both sides with the marinade and flip. Air fry thighs for another 5 minutes, or breasts for another 2 minutes, then add the pineapple. Air fry thighs for a final 5 minutes and breasts for a final 4 minutes, until the chicken is a little black in places.

To cook the chicken under the grill, set the grill (broiler) to high. Place the chicken and pineapple on the rack of a grill pan lined with foil. Grill breasts for 8 minutes and thighs for 12 minutes, turning halfway, until the chicken is black in places. Rest the chicken for 10 minutes. Slice the pineapple into chunks.

Mix the mayonnaise and sweet chilli sauce in a bowl. Divide the rice between bowls, then top with avocado, edamame beans or lettuce, carrot or cucumber, and some chicken and pineapple. Drizzle with sauce and serve.

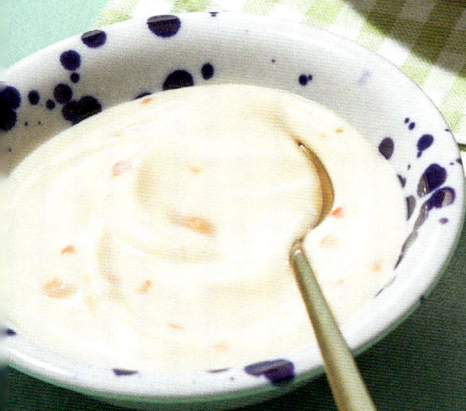

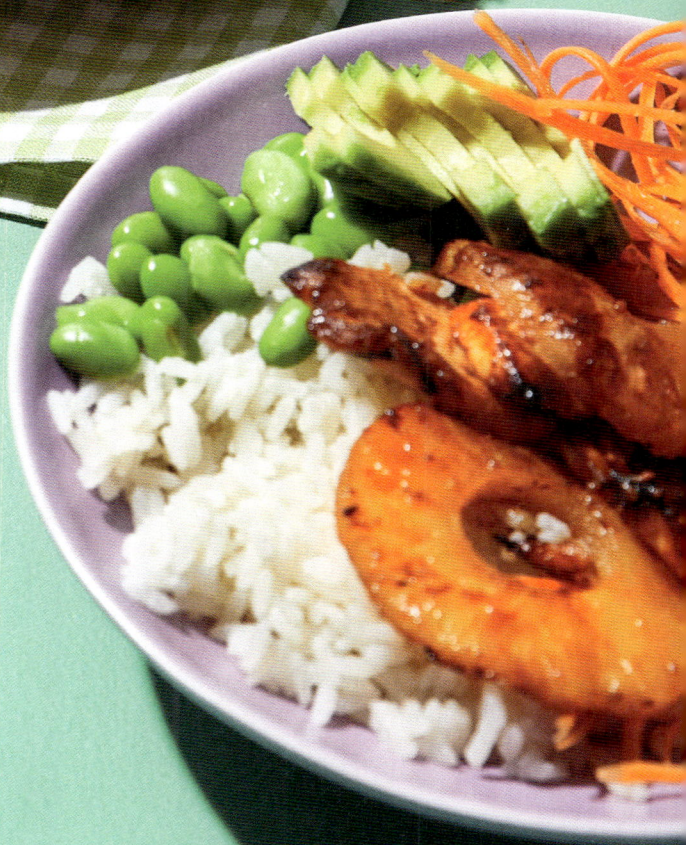

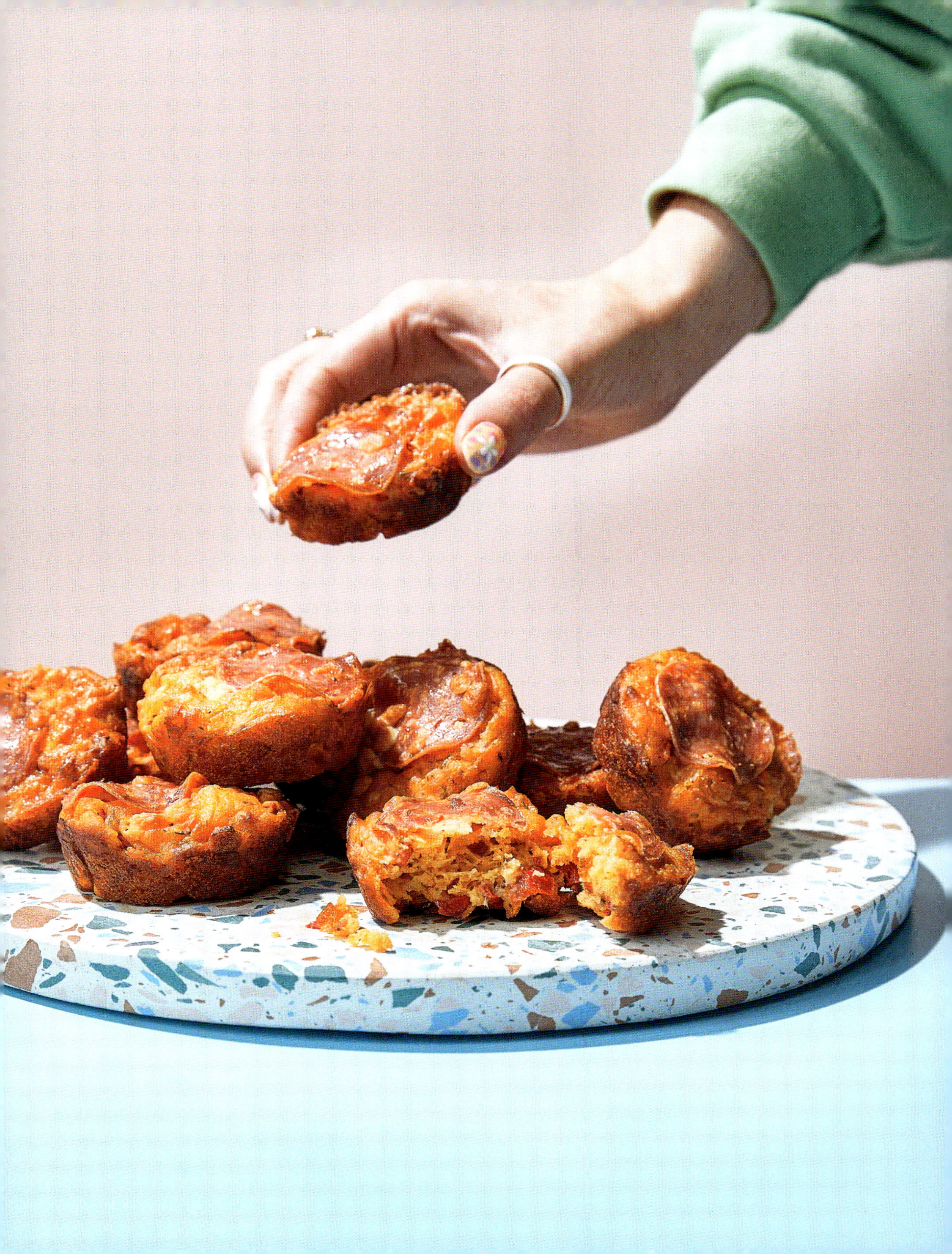

PIZZA MUFFINS

Out-and-about lunches don't get much easier than this to pack up, transport and eat! Delicious hot or cold, these savoury muffins are like biting into a pizza cloud, infused with herbs, roasted red peppers, tomato and topped with cheese and crispy pepperoni. Of course, like with any good pizza recipe, feel free to top these with whatever you like!

Makes 12

Prep 10 mins

Oven 18 mins or
Air Fryer 14 mins

DF Use dairy-free milk and cheese.

LL Use lactose-free milk.

F Use lactose-free milk and FODMAP-friendly pepperoni. One muffin is a safe low FODMAP serving size.

V Omit the pepperoni and top with more finely chopped red (bell) pepper.

VE Combine the dairy-free and veggie advice and replace the egg with gluten-free egg replacement powder.

❄ Once cooled, freeze for up to 2–3 months in airtight containers. Allow to defrost on a wire rack at room temperature for 2–3 hours. To reheat, air fry at 200°C (400°F) for 5–6 minutes or until the tops are crisp again.

- 130g (1 cup) gluten-free self-raising flour
- 1½ tsp gluten-free baking powder
- 2 tsp dried mixed herbs
- Pinch each of salt and freshly ground black pepper
- 1 medium egg
- 150ml (⅝ cup) milk
- 2 tbsp garlic-infused oil
- 1 tbsp tomato purée (paste)
- 50g (1¾oz) jarred roasted red (bell) pepper, very finely chopped
- 60g (2¼oz) mature Cheddar, grated
- Vegetable oil spray
- 12 slices of pepperoni (or your preferred pizza topping)

Add the flour, baking powder, mixed herbs, salt and pepper to a large bowl and briefly mix until combined.

Crack the egg into a jug (pitcher), then add the milk, garlic-infused oil and tomato purée and beat with a fork until smooth.

Pour the wet ingredients into the dry and whisk until it forms a smooth batter, then add the red pepper and cheese, reserving a small handful of the cheese for later. Mix in until evenly dispersed.

To cook in an oven, preheat the oven to 200°C fan/220°C (425°F). Generously spray the holes of a 12-hole muffin tray with oil, then spoon the mixture equally between each muffin hole. Sprinkle each with the reserved grated cheese, then top with a slice of pepperoni. Bake in the oven for 15–18 minutes or until the cheese on top is golden.

To cook in an air fryer, heat the air fryer to 180°C (350°F). Generously spray the holes of two 6-hole silicone muffin trays with oil – ensure they fit into your air fryer first! Spoon the mixture equally between each muffin hole. Sprinkle each with the reserved grated cheese and top with a slice of pepperoni. Ensure you press the pepperoni slices into the mixture a little, otherwise they can fly about in the air fryer! Place as many of the muffin trays into the air fryer as will fit and air fry for 12–14 minutes or until the cheese on top is golden.

Transfer to a wire rack to cool to room temperature or just warm. Enjoy warm or cold.

PASTA SALAD 3 WAYS

Serves 2
Prep 2 mins
Hob 15 mins

DF **LF** **F**

V Make the tomato and roasted red pepper pasta salad variation.

VE See veggie advice.

❄ Once cooled, store in airtight containers in the freezer for up to 2–3 months. Allow to defrost completely in the fridge, then reheat in the microwave for 3–5 minutes at full power until piping hot, gently stirring halfway.

First of all, this certainly isn't a fancy salad by any means – it's actually a recreation of the pasta salad pots I used to enjoy before being gluten free, which I would buy from the supermarket! But if any of you have ever tried to eat cold gluten-free pasta, you might have found it to be very hard and quite unpleasant! That's because gluten-free pasta is often made from corn and rice, which are two very hard, starchy grains; when they cool, they almost set. But with this recipe, you'll be able to take any old gluten-free pasta and ensure it's perfect for these three variations on a classic pasta salad. I've found that gluten-free pasta made from a blend of corn, rice and brown rice (check the ingredients on the back of the packet) works especially well.

- 1 tbsp vegetable oil
- 200g (7oz) gluten-free dried pasta

For tuna mayo (pictured)
- 150ml (⅝ cup) mayonnaise
- 1 x 145g (5oz) can of tuna in spring water, drained
- 4 tbsp drained canned sweetcorn
- 1 tbsp finely chopped chives
- ½ tsp Dijon mustard

- ½ tsp salt
- ½ tsp ground black pepper

For chicken and bacon
- 70g (2½oz) leftover cooked chicken, cut into 5mm (¼in) dice
- 2 rashers of smoked back bacon, air fried for 7–8 minutes until crisp, then finely chopped
- ½ tsp dried mixed herbs
- Pinch of salt
- ½ tsp ground black pepper

For tomato and roasted red pepper
- 100ml (generous ⅓ cup) passata (sieved tomatoes)
- 50g (1¾oz) jarred roasted red (bell) pepper, finely chopped
- ½ tsp tomato purée (paste)
- 1 tsp dried mixed herbs
- 1 tsp salt
- ½ tsp ground black pepper

TIPS

Using a large pan will help to avoid overcrowding the pasta, which almost always results in the pasta getting stuck together! The vegetable oil also helps to prevent the pasta from sticking together.

To avoid the pasta being super-hard when cold, it's imperative to overcook it. I would never normally advise this as it's more liable to break, but the rest of the method is written with this in mind!

A wooden spoon is much less likely to damage the overly softened pasta than a metal spoon, but you still need to mix it gently. Get your wooden spoon right to the bottom of the bowl and gently/slowly bring that to the top, then repeat a few times until all the pasta is coated.

Gluten-free orzo also works especially well in this recipe.

For **tuna** or **chicken pasta salad**, add all the ingredients for your chosen variation to a large bowl and mix well until everything is evenly dispersed. For **tomato and roasted red pepper pasta salad**, add all the ingredients to a small frying pan, mix well and simmer for 15 minutes, then transfer to a large bowl.

Grab your largest saucepan and fill it with water to about an inch below the top. Add the oil to the water. Bring to a rolling boil, then add the pasta and cook for 2 minutes longer than the packet states. It should look nicely swollen and a little paler than you'd normally look for (see **TIPS** opposite). Drain and allow to cool for no more than 1 minute.

Add the very slightly cooled pasta to the bowl with the other salad ingredients and use a wooden spoon (see **TIPS** opposite) to gently stir in the pasta until it's nicely coated – then stop!

Serve straight away or, if enjoying at a later time, allow to cool completely, then store in airtight containers in the fridge for up to 3–4 days. Allow to return to room temperature before enjoying for the best pasta texture.

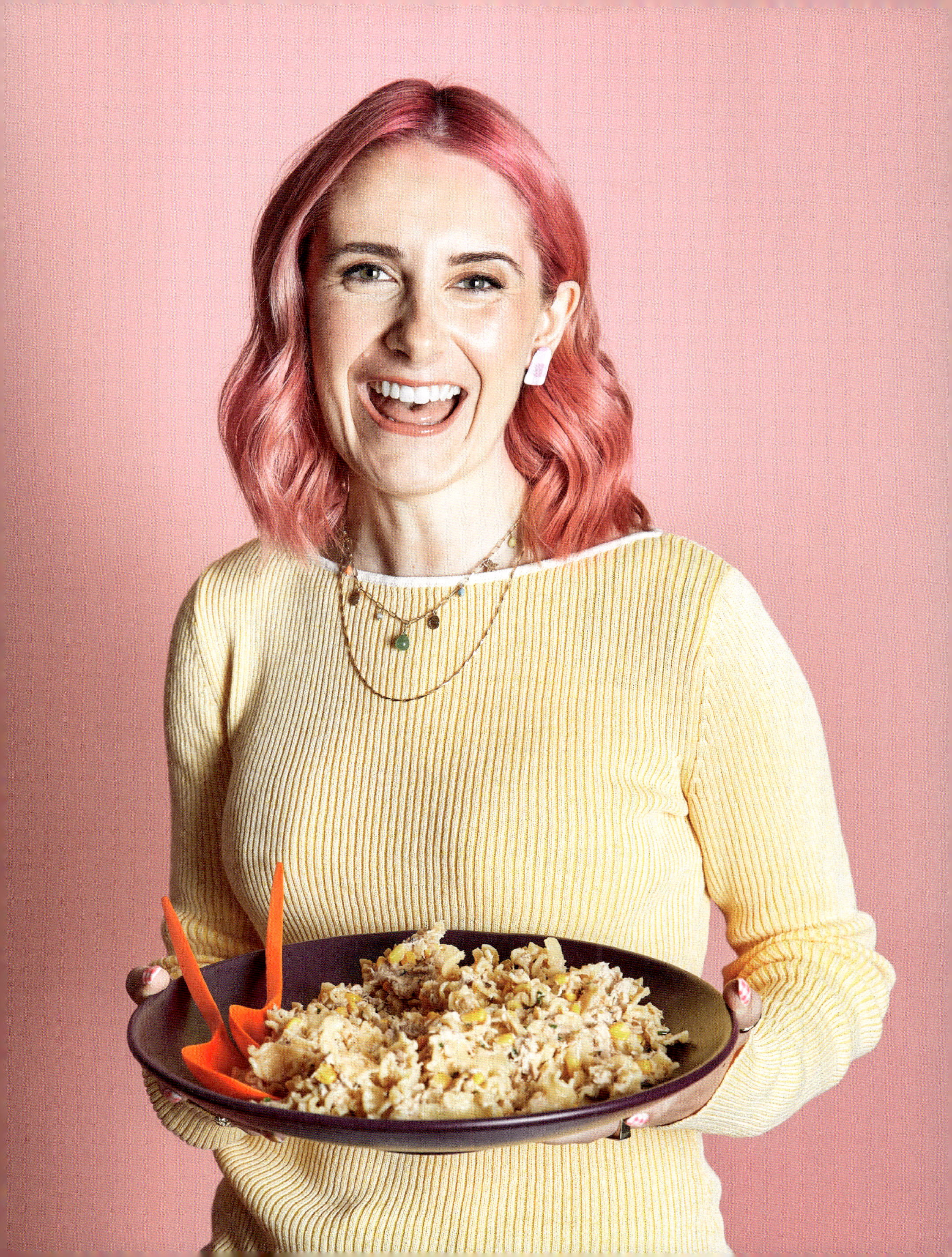

AIR FRYER FAVOURITES

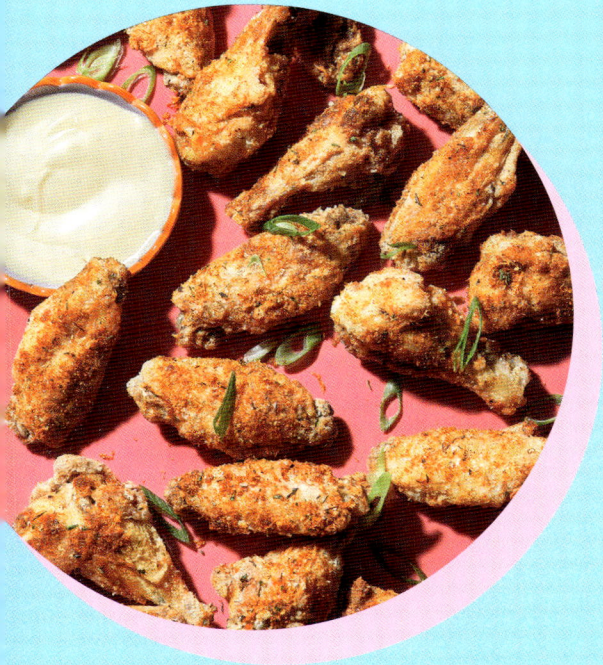

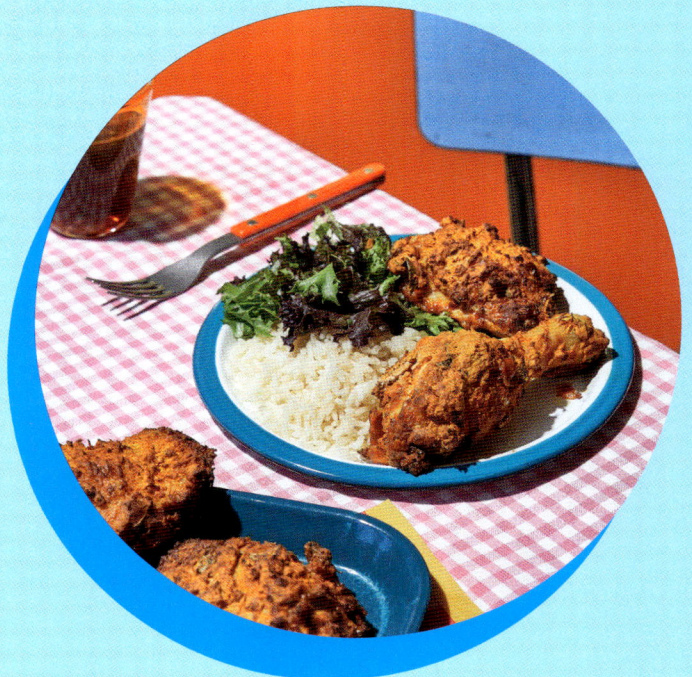

Since championing low-running-cost appliances is a key part of my definition of budget-friendly cooking and baking (see pillar 7 on page 11 for more info), it was an inevitability that the ever-popular air fryer deserved its own chapter in this book.

So here it is! Yet you might be surprised to find that this chapter certainly isn't the only place in this book that you'll find air fryer cooking temperatures and timings; I've actually included them for every recipe where it was possible and made sense! So definitely don't think that using your air fryer is restricted to this chapter alone.

And although this chapter is obviously here to showcase even more of my tantalizing air fryer favourites, it actually mainly exists to serve as a reminder that if you have an air fryer already, you should absolutely be using it for this book! But, as requiring everyone to rush out and buy an air fryer didn't feel very much in the spirit of the book, you'll also find alternative cooking methods suggested throughout this chapter. I really wanted this book to be as accessible and flexible as possible, which is why you've somehow now got an exciting and eclectic air fryer chapter where an air fryer is actually entirely optional!

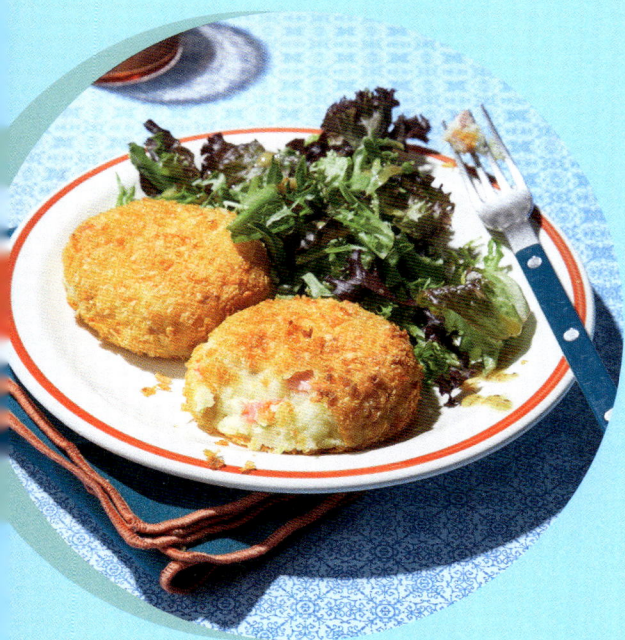

KARAAGE POPCORN CHICKEN

Serves 4
Prep 10 mins + 1 hour marinating
Air Fryer 15 mins
Hob 6 mins

This recipe went down so well on social media that I absolutely had to include it here. Essentially, this is my version of Japanese fried chicken, which not only yields tender, juicy chicken, but a super-crispy, crunchy coating. Unlike with most fried chicken where all the flavour is in the coating, in Japan they usually do it the other way around, by marinating the chicken with tons of flavour instead.

DF **LF**

F Omit the garlic paste or replace with 1 tbsp garlic-infused oil.

V Use 500g (lb 2oz) firm tofu, cut into 3cm (1¼in) chunks, instead of chicken.

VE See veggie advice.

❄ Once cooled, store in an airtight container and freeze for up to 3 months. Air fry from frozen for 8–10 minutes at 200°C (400°F). Check the internal temperature with a digital food thermometer against those given on page 255.

TIP

While you won't find potato starch in supermarkets, it's quite common to find in health food shops, Chinese supermarkets (ensure there's no 'may contain' warnings) and, of course, online too. I've tried this recipe using cornflour (cornstarch) and it wasn't anywhere near as crispy or crunchy – hence why potato starch is the way to go!

- 600g (1lb 5oz) boneless, skinless chicken thighs, cut into 5cm (2in) chunks
- 2 tsp ginger paste
- 2 tsp garlic paste (optional)
- 3 tbsp rice wine vinegar
- 3 tbsp gluten-free soy sauce
- 1 tsp ground black pepper
- 3 tsp lemon juice
- 120g (¾ cup) potato starch
- Vegetable oil spray

Add the chicken to a bowl, followed by the ginger paste, garlic paste, if using, vinegar, soy sauce, black pepper and lemon juice. Stir until everything is well coated, then cover and refrigerate for at least 1 hour and up to 12 hours. For best results, I usually do around 8 hours if I have the time.

When ready to cook, place the potato starch in a medium bowl, and have a plate ready. Take each piece of chicken and roll it around in the starch until well coated, then place on the plate.

To cook in an air fryer, heat the air fryer to 200°C (400°F) and generously spray the base of the air fryer basket or crisping tray with oil.

Place as many chicken pieces in the air fryer as will fit without touching (use both drawers if your machine has two) and spray well with oil. Air fry for 12–14 minutes, turning them halfway, until golden and crisp.

Once done, optionally allow the chicken to cool for 5–10 minutes, then air fry for another 2–3 minutes. This makes the coating even crisper! Remove from the air fryer and serve alongside your favourite dips.

To cook on the hob, add enough oil to a large frying pan so it is around 1cm (½in) deep. Place over a medium heat for 7–10 minutes or until it reaches 180°C (350°F). If you don't have a digital food thermometer to check the temperature, you can use the wooden spoon-handle test: place the handle in the oil and observe the oil around it – if bubbles form around the wood and rise up, then it's ready. Line a large plate with kitchen paper, ready for later.

Take the coated chicken and carefully lower it into the hot oil using a pair of small tongs – it should sizzle nicely. Cook (in batches if needed) for 8–10 minutes, turning halfway, or until the crispy coating starts to turn golden. Remove with a slotted spoon and place on the plate lined with kitchen paper.

Once done, optionally fry the chicken again for another 2 minutes. This makes the coating even crispier!

Allow to rest for 5–10 minutes, ideally on a wire rack, then serve alongside your favourite dips, or use in my homemade soft flour wraps over on page 50.

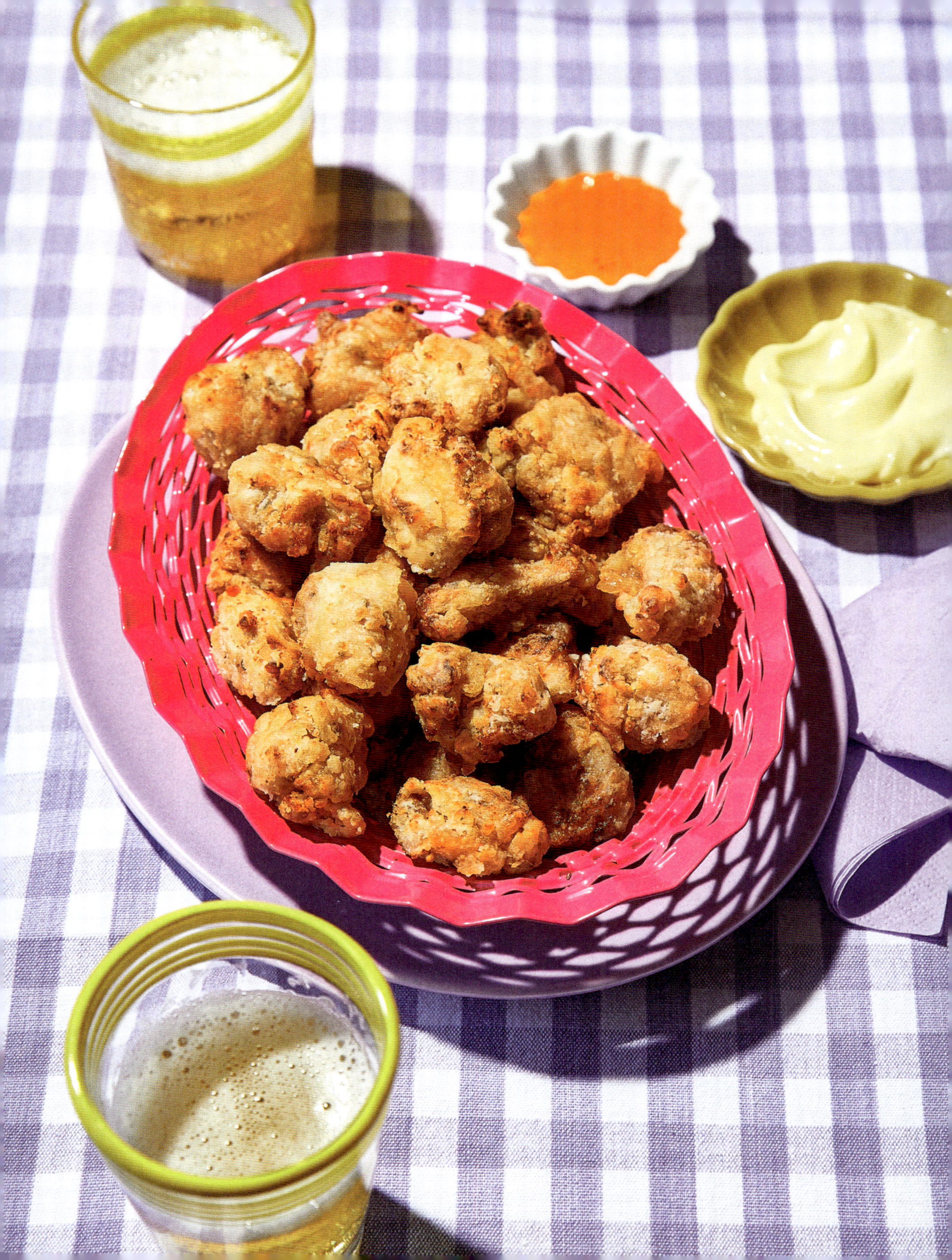

MARK'S MALAYSIAN-STYLE FRIED CHICKEN
(AYAM GORENG)

Serves 4

Prep 10 mins + 30 mins marinating

Air Fryer 22 mins or
Oven 50 mins

DF Use a thick dairy-free yoghurt.

LF Use lactose-free yoghurt.

F Omit the garlic paste and use lactose-free yoghurt.

✳ Once the chicken has cooled, store in airtight containers in the freezer for up to 2–3 months. Allow to defrost completely in the fridge, then reheat in the air fryer for 8–9 minutes at 200°C (400°F). Check the internal temperature with a digital food thermometer against those given on page 255.

On my first trip to Malaysia, I was overwhelmed by the sheer volume of crispy, spicy, golden fried chicken ready to order for all the locals alongside their Nasi Lemak. Sadly, this fried chicken infatuation didn't have a happy ending as I never found a gluten-free version! However, Mark instead made me his own version when we got home and, after one bite, it was the 'happily ever after' I needed! Serve with rice and a side salad.

- 4 skin-on, bone-in chicken thighs and 4 drumsticks
- Vegetable oil spray

For the marinade
- 1 tbsp ginger paste
- 1 tbsp garlic paste (optional)

- 2 tbsp mild curry powder
- 1 tbsp smoked paprika
- 1 tsp chilli powder
- 1 tbsp dried curry leaves
- 1 tsp salt
- ½ tsp ground black or white pepper
- 3 tbsp natural or Greek yoghurt

For the crispy coating
- 3 tbsp gluten-free self-raising flour
- 4 tbsp cornflour (cornstarch) or potato starch

Add the chicken pieces to a large bowl, followed by the marinade ingredients. Mix well until the chicken is coated and the spices are evenly dispersed. Cover and marinate in the fridge for 30 minutes or up to 12 hours.

Remove the chicken from the fridge and add the crispy coating ingredients to the bowl, then mix until the chicken is well coated.

To cook in an air fryer, heat the air fryer to 200°C (400°F). Generously spray the base of the air fryer basket or crisping tray with oil. If you have an air fryer with 2 drawers, you'll likely need to employ both, so grease both if necessary.

Place as many chicken pieces as will fit in the air fryer basket without touching and generously spray with oil, ensuring

any white floury patches disappear. Air fry the drumsticks for 15–16 minutes and thighs for 20–22 minutes, turning them over halfway and spraying any remaining floury patches with oil once turned. They should be golden brown and crisp.

To cook in an oven, preheat the oven to 180°C fan/200°C (400°F). Generously spray a large baking tray with oil.

Marinate and coat the chicken as directed above, spread out on the baking tray and generously spray with oil, ensuring any white floury patches disappear. Bake in the oven for 35–40 minutes for drumsticks and 45–50 minutes for thighs, turning them over halfway and spraying any remaining floury patches with oil, until golden brown and crisp.

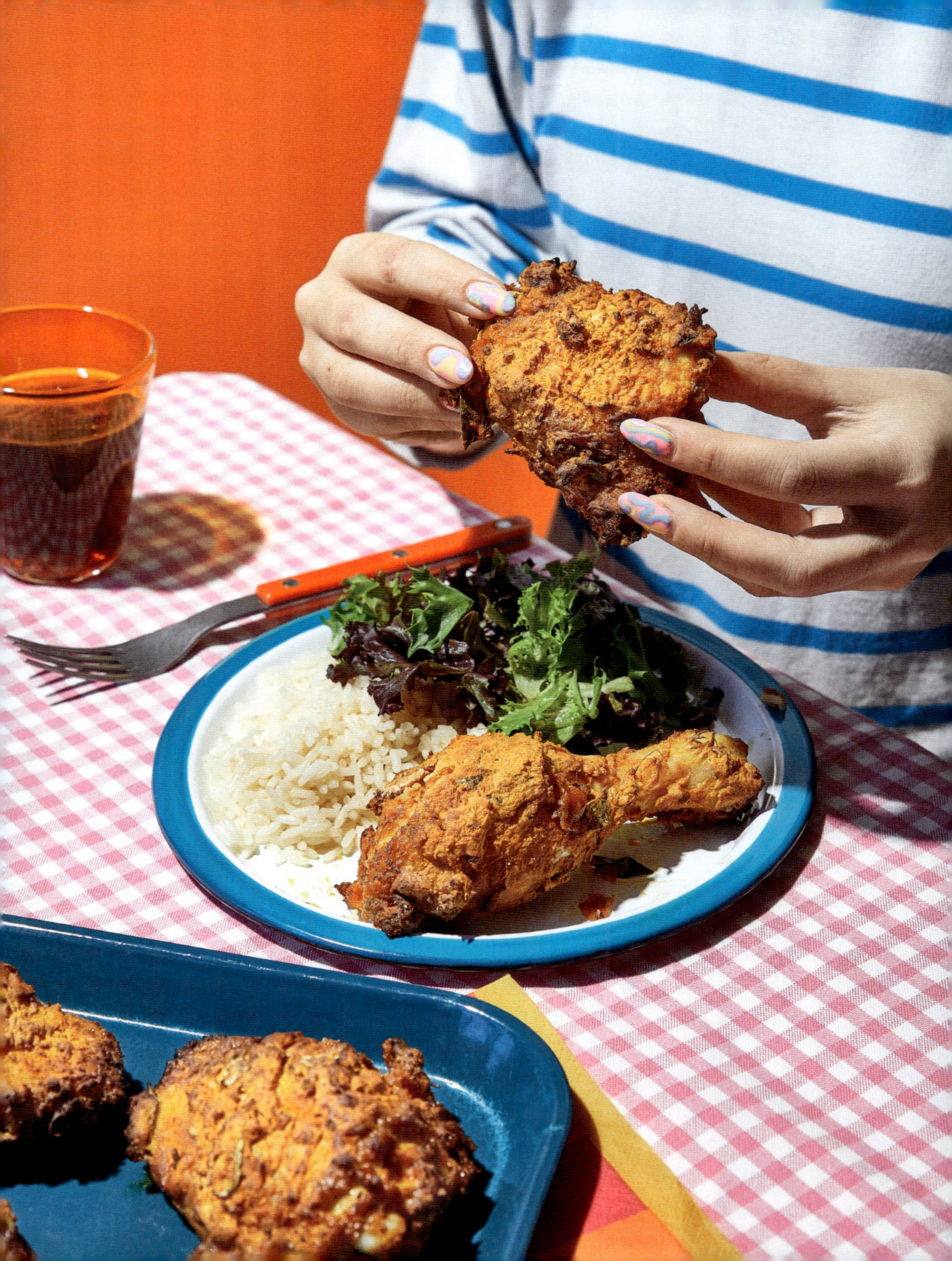

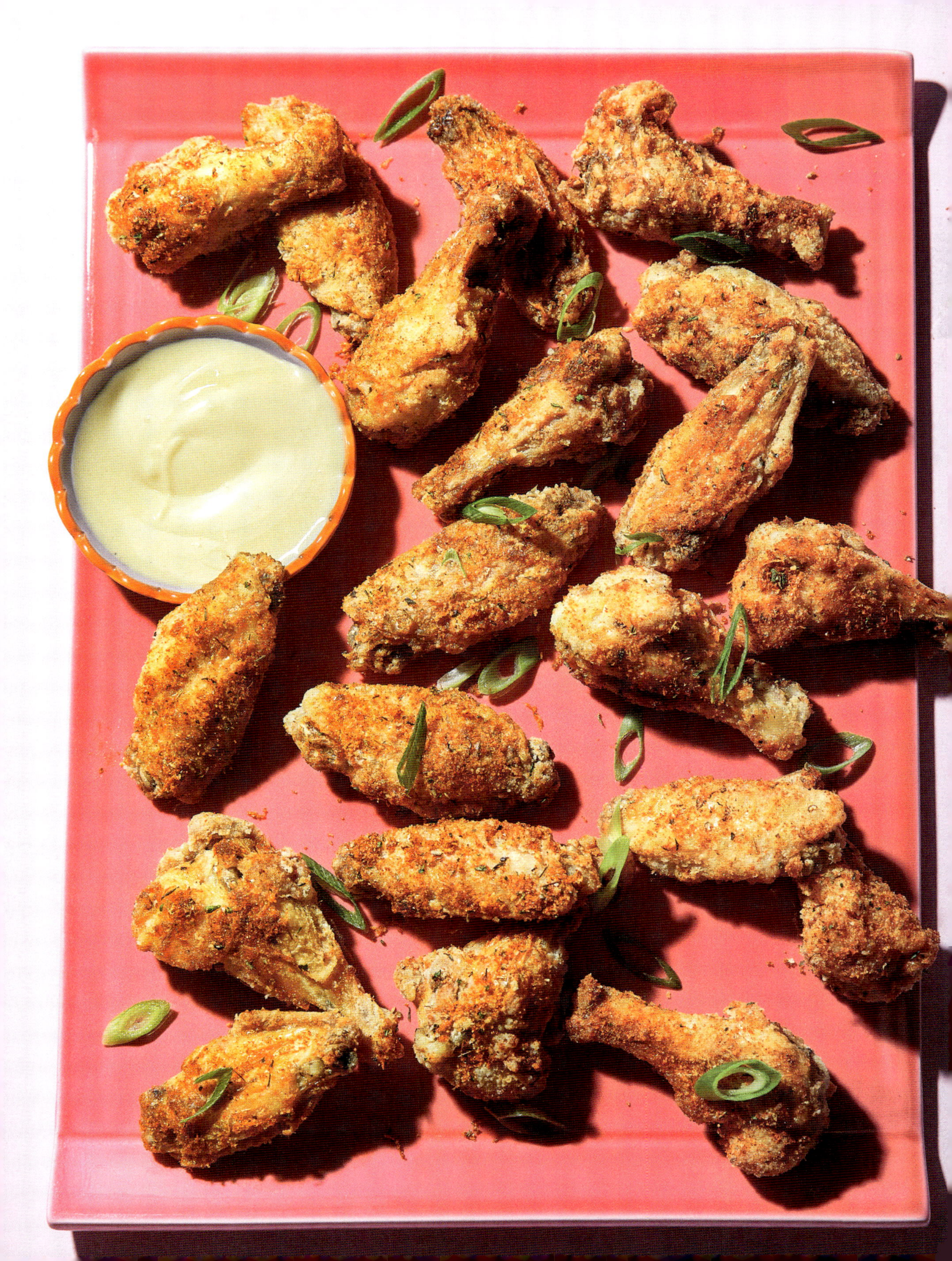

LOUISIANA-STYLE CAJUN CHICKEN WINGS

Serves 4

Prep 5 mins

Air Fryer 18 mins or
Oven 30 mins

DF **LF**

F Use maple syrup instead of honey.

❄ Once the chicken has cooled, store in airtight containers in the freezer for up to 2–3 months. Allow to defrost completely in the fridge, then reheat in the air fryer for 8–10 minutes at 180°C (350°F). Check the internal temperature with a digital food thermometer against those given on page 255.

Without a doubt, chicken wings are the cheapest cut of chicken in supermarkets, and fortunately for us, it couldn't be easier to transform them into a main course that everyone will be requesting you make again and again. This recipe is my 'secret weapon' when it comes to friends and family coming over to eat: with crispy, light batter on each wing and a sweet, mildly spicy and sweet dry rub that's seriously addictive, these are sure to disappear fast! Serve as a main alongside fries, wedges, mashed potato or sweet potato fries.

- 1kg (2lb 3oz) chicken wings, halved at the joint and tips removed
- 3 tbsp vegetable oil, plus a little oil spray
- 3 tbsp gluten-free plain (all-purpose) flour or cornflour (cornstarch)
- 1 tsp gluten-free baking powder (optional)
- ½ tsp salt

- ½ tsp ground black pepper
- Small handful of spring onion (scallion) greens, thinly sliced

For the spice mix
- 1 tsp smoked paprika
- ½ tsp mild curry powder or ground cumin
- 1 tsp dried mixed herbs
- ¼ tsp cayenne pepper

- 1½ tsp light brown sugar
- ¼ tsp salt
- Grated zest of 1 lemon

For the honey mustard dip
- 100g (generous ⅓ cup) mayonnaise
- 1½ tbsp honey
- 1½ tbsp Dijon mustard
- 1 tbsp lemon juice

TIP

Sometimes you can buy chicken wings that are already prepared (with the tips– the part without any meat – removed, and halved at the joint) which makes life so much easier. However, sometimes you can't! Luckily, it's easy to prepare them yourself at home with a large, sharp kitchen knife – I'd highly recommend watching a short video online first if you've never done it before so you know exactly where to cut.

If you don't have cayenne pepper, you can use an equivalent amount of black pepper, dried chilli flakes or chilli powder.

Add the chicken wings to a large bowl followed by the oil, flour, baking powder, if using, salt and pepper. Mix well until everything is evenly dispersed and the chicken is well coated.

Combine the ingredients for the spice mix in a small bowl, ensuring there are no clumps of spices or sugar, and set aside. In another small bowl, combine the ingredients for the honey mustard dip and set aside.

To cook in an air fryer, heat the air fryer to 200°C (400°F). Generously spray the base of the air fryer basket or crisping tray with oil. If you have an air fryer with 2 drawers, use both. Place as many of the prepared wings in the air fryer (basket or crisping tray in) that will comfortably fit without touching,

then air fry for 16–18 minutes until crisp and golden, flipping each wing over after 10 minutes. Repeat with the remaining wings.

To cook in an oven, preheat the oven to 200°C fan/220°C (425°F). Line a grill (broiler) pan with foil, place the wire rack on top, then add the chicken wings. Cook in the oven for 25–30 minutes, until crisp and golden, flipping them over halfway.

Transfer the cooked wings to a large serving plate and use a teaspoon to sprinkle half the spice mix on top, then lightly toss the wings about a bit until coated. Repeat with the rest of the spice mix, top with spring onion greens and serve with the honey mustard dip.

HAM + CHEESE CRISP BAKES

While the free-from supermarket versions of these aren't usually outrageously sky-high in price, they're far from the best value for your money; often you'll get two small ones that only serve one person even though the packet swears it serves two. So if you always feel a little short changed when you buy these, definitely give this recipe a go. They're usually largely potato based, so they actually work out as being incredibly cheap to make! Serve with a leafy dressed salad.

Serves 4 (makes 8)

Prep 10 mins + 15 mins chilling

Hob + Air Fryer 25 mins or
Hob + Oven 40 mins

- Vegetable oil spray
- 100g (3½oz) frozen onion **or** ½ medium leek, finely chopped
- 900g (2lb) Maris Piper potatoes, peeled and cut into 2cm (¾in) cubes
- 200g (7oz) mature Cheddar
- 1 tsp salt
- ½ tsp ground black pepper
- 120g (4oz) sliced ham, roughly chopped
- 5 tbsp gluten-free plain (all-purpose) flour
- 2 large eggs
- 2 tbsp milk
- 130g (4½oz) gluten-free cornflakes, crushed in a bowl using the end of a rolling pin

DF Use dairy-free cheese and dairy-free milk.

LL Use lactose-free milk.

F Use leek (green parts only) instead of onion, gluten-free breadcrumbs instead of cornflakes, and use lactose-free milk.

V Use a small handful of thinly sliced spring onions (scallions), instead of ham.

❄ Once cooled, store in an airtight container and freeze for up to 3 months. Air fry from frozen for 17–20 minutes at 180°C (350°F), turning halfway.

TIP

See the tip on page 76 for advice on weighing out portions of the potato mixture using digital weighing scales to ensure consistency of size. Remember to use the portion measurements given here though.

Spray the base of a large frying pan with oil and place over a medium heat. Once hot, add the onion or leek and fry until the onion is browned or the leek has softened. Remove from the heat and set aside.

Meanwhile, boil the potatoes in a large pan of boiling water for around 15 minutes, until completely cooked through. Drain and transfer to a large bowl.

Transfer the cooked onion or leek to the bowl with the potatoes and mash well with a potato masher until smooth. Add the cheese, salt and pepper and mash again to combine everything. Stir through the ham and transfer to the fridge to chill for 15–30 minutes (this will make the mixture much easier to form).

Divide the mixture into 8 equal portions (about 150g/5½oz each) and, on a board, flatten into thick patties.

Spread the flour over a dinner plate; crack the eggs into a small bowl, add the milk and beat; then spread the crushed cornflakes out onto a second dinner plate.

Take one patty and roll it around on the flour plate until lightly dusted on all sides. Next, coat well in the egg mixture, then roll around on the cornflake plate until tightly coated. Repeat until all the patties are coated.

To cook in an air fryer, heat the air fryer to 200°C (400°F) and generously spray with oil. Place as many crisp bakes as will comfortably fit in the air fryer without touching, spray generously with oil and air fry for 10–12 minutes or until the cornflakes are golden and crisp.

To cook in an oven, preheat the oven to 200°C fan/220°C (425°F). Generously spray a baking tray with oil, then place the crisp bakes on the tray and generously spray with oil once again. Bake in the oven for 20–25 minutes until golden.

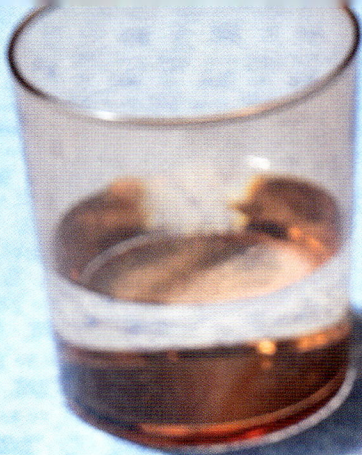

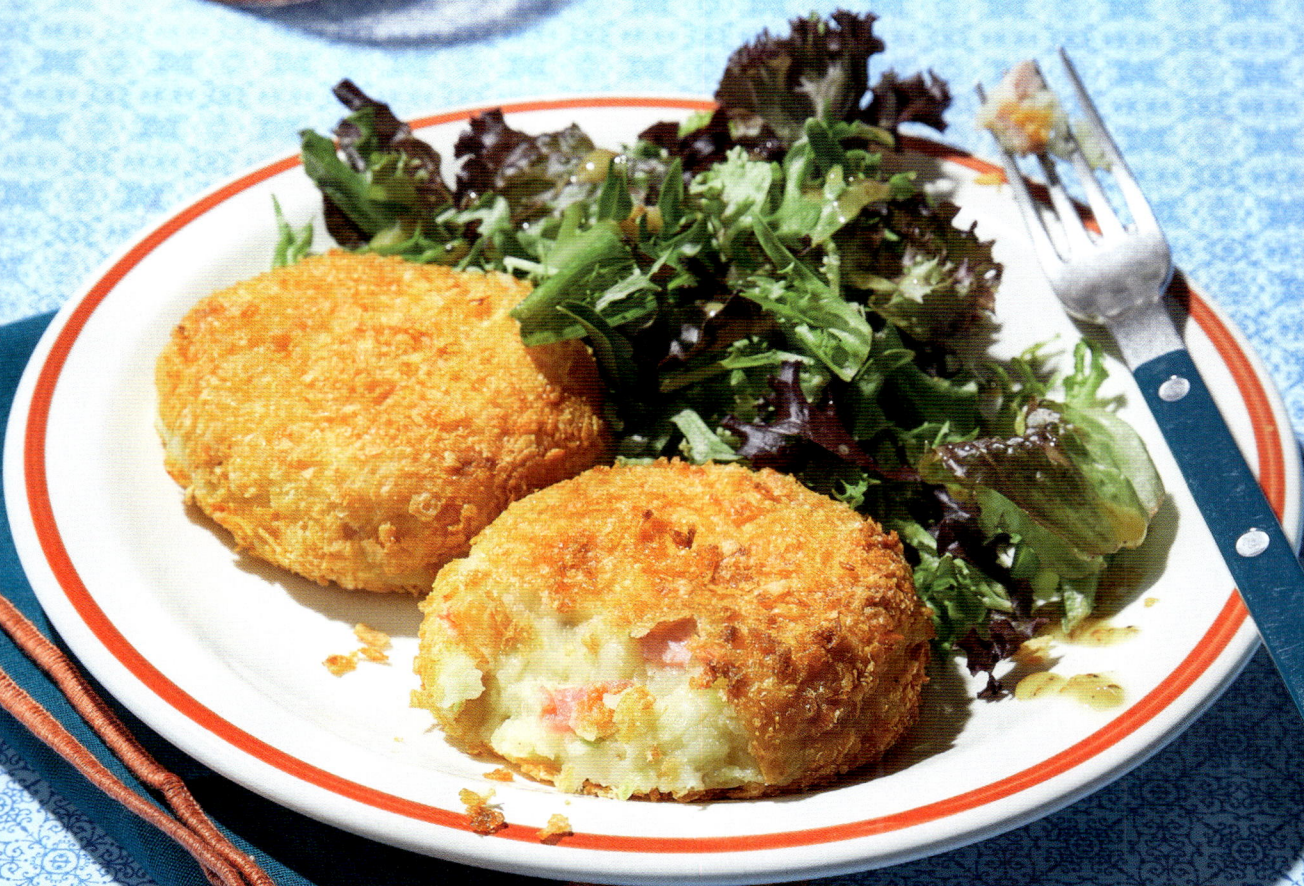

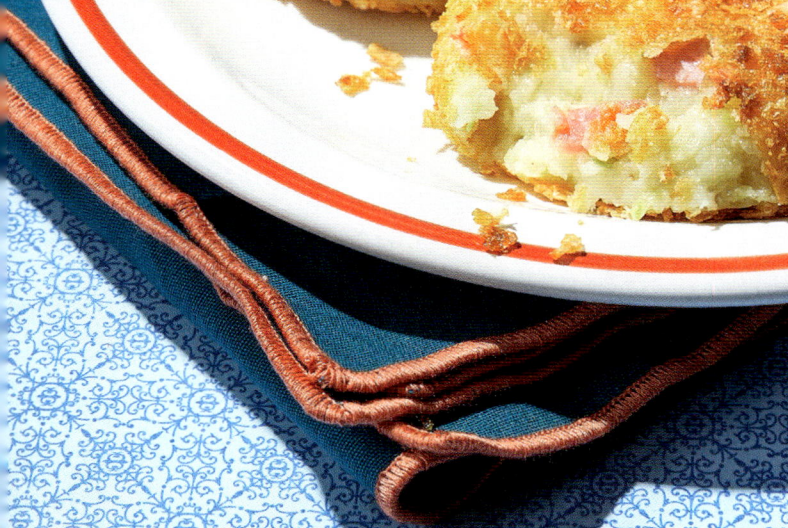

CHEESE + CHIVE CRISPY PANCAKES

If reading this title hits you with a bout of excitement mixed with nostalgia, then you've come to the right place. I've kept things super simple here, but feel free to experiment with your own fillings too. Serve with mashed potato, gluten-free gravy and peas.

Serves 4 (makes 8)

Prep 15 mins

Hob + Air Fryer 25 mins or
Hob + Oven 30 mins

V

DF Use dairy-free milk and cheese.

LL Use lactose-free milk.

F See low lactose advice and use gluten-free breadcrumbs instead of cornflakes.

❄ Once cooled, store in an airtight container and freeze for up to 3 months. Air fry from frozen for 8–10 minutes at 200°C (400°F).

- Vegetable oil spray
- 110g (generous ¾ cup) gluten-free plain (all-purpose) flour
- 2 large eggs
- 190ml (generous ¾ cup) milk

For the coating
- 4 tbsp gluten-free plain (all-purpose) flour
- 1 tsp salt
- ¼ tsp ground black pepper
- 2 large eggs
- 2 tbsp milk
- 100g (3½oz) gluten-free cornflakes, crushed until fine in a bowl using the end of a rolling pin

For the filling
- 1 x 125g (4½oz) ball of mozzarella, sliced
- 150g (5½oz) mature Cheddar, grated
- ½ bunch of chives, finely chopped

Spray a small frying pan with oil and place over a medium heat. While you wait for it to heat up, mix together the flour, eggs and milk in a large bowl, whisking well until smooth (it should be the consistency of thin cream). Transfer to a jug (pitcher).

Pour enough pancake batter into the pan to three-quarters cover the base, then tilt the pan to cover the rest of the base. Fry for 1–2 minutes before flipping and frying for a further 30 seconds. Transfer to a plate and repeat until all the batter is used (it should make 8 pancakes), spraying the pan with more oil between each one.

Combine the flour, salt and pepper for the coating on a large dinner plate. Beat the eggs and milk with a fork, then transfer to another large, deep plate. Place the cornflakes on a third large plate. Lastly, steal 1 tablespoon of the flour mixture and 2 tablespoons of the egg mixture from the prepared plates and combine together in a small dish (this will act as your 'glue').

Place some mozzarella, Cheddar and chives on the lower half of each pancake, leaving a 1cm (½in) gap around the bottom edge. Brush the flour and egg slurry around the bottom edges, then fold the pancakes over and press down firmly to seal.

Keep the folded pancakes as flat and as supported as possible while handling them. One by one, coat the sealed pancakes in the flour, then in the egg, and finally in the cornflakes, pressing around the edge to seal once more.

To cook in an air fryer, heat the air fryer to 200°C (400°F) and generously spray the basket or crisping tray with oil. Place as many coated pancakes in the air fryer as will fit without touching (use both drawers if your machine has two) and spray well with oil. Air fry for 7–9 minutes until golden, crisp and puffed up. If considerably puffed up, once removed from the air fryer, pierce a hole in the top and flatten with a spatula. Repeat for any remaining coated pancakes.

To cook in an oven, preheat the oven to 200°C fan/220°C (425°F). Generously spray a large baking sheet with oil, then place as many coated pancakes on it as will comfortably fit without touching. Spray well with oil once more and bake in the oven for 10–12 minutes until golden and crisp.

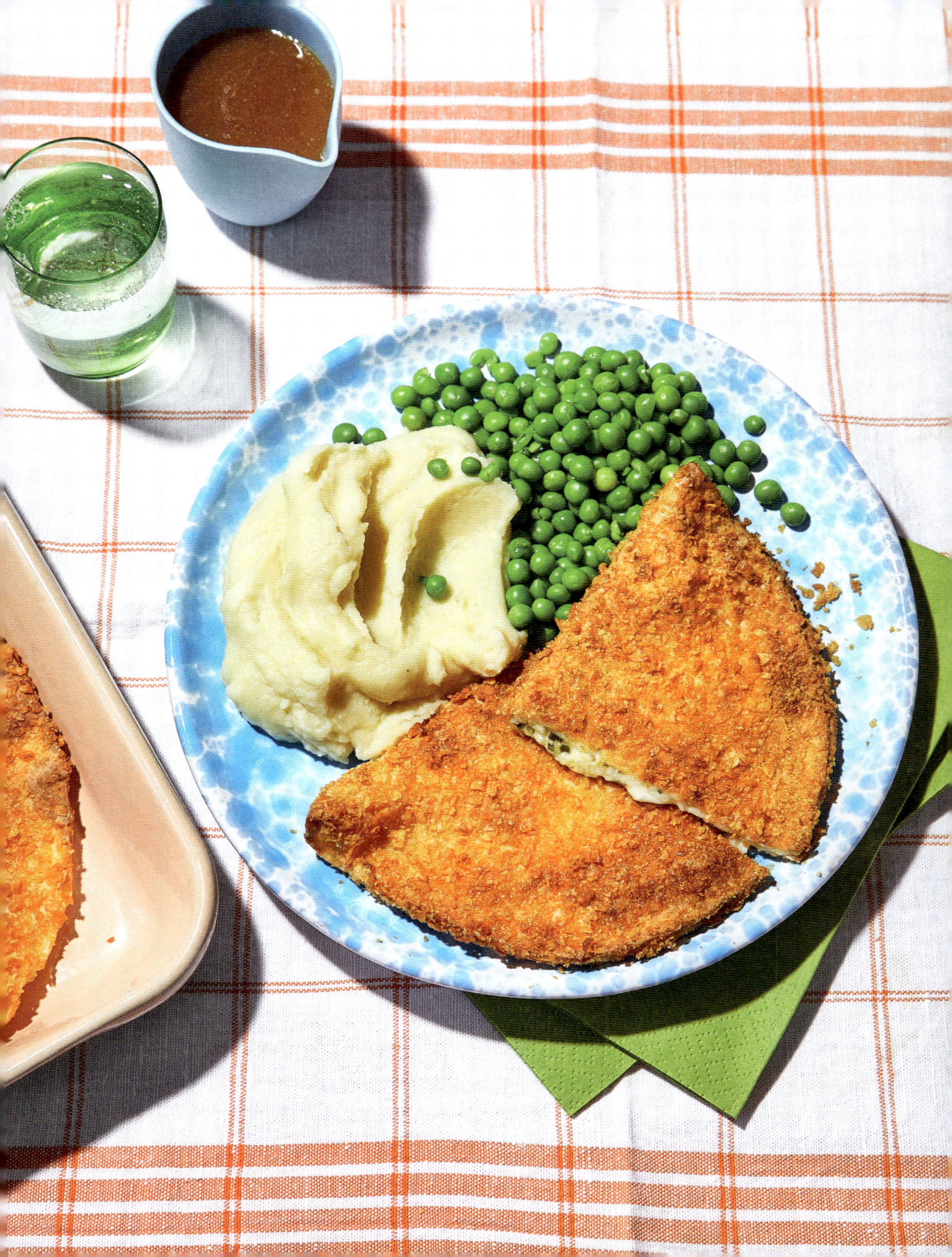

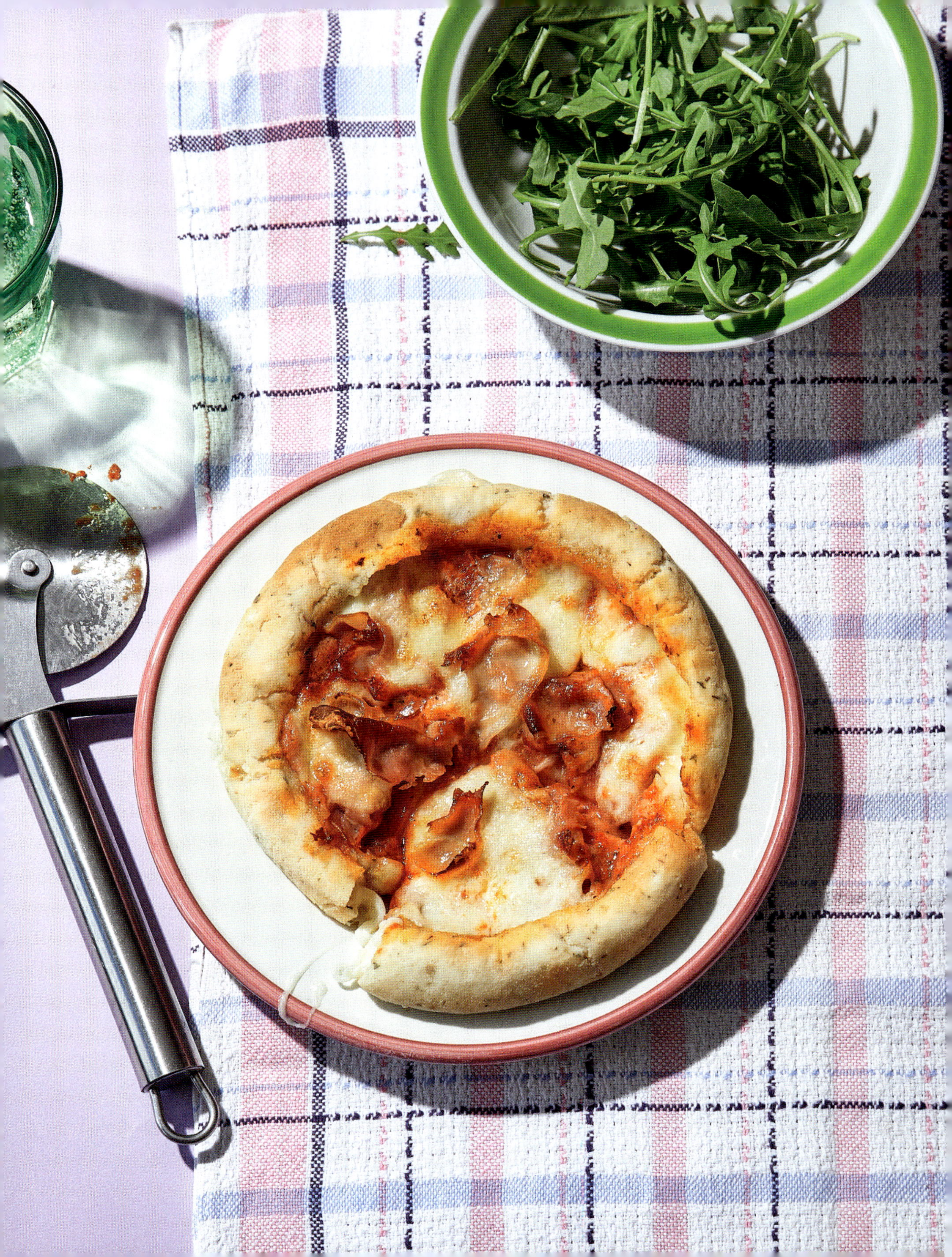

EMERGENCY STUFFED-CRUST PIZZA

Makes 1 small pizza

Prep 15 mins

Air Fryer 7 mins or
Oven 11 mins

Only a gluten-free person truly understands the necessity and meaning of an 'emergency pizza'. This is essentially a recipe for one exceptionally awesome stuffed crust pizza that can be made in next to no time with very few ingredients, in your air fryer. Crisis averted!

DF Use a thick dairy-free yoghurt and grated dairy-free cheese instead of mozzarella sticks and slices.

LL Use lactose-free Greek yoghurt.

F Use lactose-free Greek yoghurt and FODMAP-friendly toppings.

V Use veggie-friendly toppings.

VE See dairy-free advice and use vegan-friendly toppings.

❄ Once cooled, store in an airtight container and freeze for up to 3 months. Air fry from frozen for 4–5 minutes at 200°C (400°F).

TIP

The key to a crispy base is to first of all ensure the dough is rolled as thinly as possible. Secondly, don't overload each base with sauce and toppings, as this can make the base more 'bready' than crispy.

- 40g (4¾ tbsp) gluten-free self-raising flour, plus extra for dusting
- 20g (1½ tbsp) Greek yoghurt (or thick natural yoghurt)
- 2 tbsp water
- ¼ tsp dried mixed herbs
- Pinch of salt

- ½ x 210g (7½oz) ball of mozzarella, cut into sticks 0.5 x 3cm (¼ x 1¼in), plus an extra few slices to top
- Toppings of your choice, such as pepperoni, tuna, thinly sliced (bell) peppers, ham, pineapple etc.

For the pizza sauce
- 3 tbsp passata (sieved tomatoes)
- ¼ tsp garlic-infused oil
- Pinch of dried mixed herbs
- Small pinch each of salt and pepper

Add the flour, yoghurt, water, mixed herbs and salt to a large bowl. Mix thoroughly, ensuring there are no hidden clumps of yoghurt-coated flour. As it starts to come together, use your hands to bring it together into a slightly sticky ball. Knead the dough briefly in the bowl until smooth, combined and no longer sticky. Dough still too sticky? Add a little more flour. Dough looks too dry? Add a little more water.

Transfer the dough to a sheet of non-stick baking parchment that's comfortably larger than your air fryer basket or oven baking tray.

Lightly flour a rolling pin and roll out the dough into a circle or rectangle that is 2–3mm (⅛in) thick. Re-flour the rolling pin as necessary to stop it from sticking.

Place small sticks of mozzarella all around the edge of the pizza base and fold the edge of the dough over the mozzarella. Tuck the edge of the dough just under the mozzarella and gently press to seal. Trim the baking

parchment around the pizza base, leaving a little excess around the edges.

Combine all the pizza sauce ingredients in a small bowl. Spread onto the base, right up to the crust. Add the mozzarella slices, followed by any toppings of your choice – if air frying, ensure you press any lighter toppings like pepperoni in a little, otherwise they can fly about!

To cook in an air fryer, use the parchment to lift the pizza base into the air fryer basket. Heat the air fryer to 200°C (400°F) and air fry for 7 minutes or until the mozzarella is golden and the toppings are nicely seared. Remove using a spatula.

To cook in an oven, preheat the oven to 240°C fan/260°C (500°F) or as hot as your oven will go. Use the baking parchment to lift the pizza onto the baking tray, then add the mozzarella, followed by the toppings of choice. Bake in the oven for 10–11 minutes or until the mozzarella is golden and the toppings are nicely seared.

FIRECRACKER FISHCAKES

Serves 4 (makes 8)

Prep 10 mins

Hob + Air Fryer 25 mins or
Hob + Oven 50 mins

Without a doubt, fish is probably the most expensive protein we regularly eat, and until recently I thought there was just no way around it. I often use basa fillets instead of cod (as they're around half the price) but even the price of basa keeps creeping up and up. But I've recently discovered what's labelled as 'white fish fillets' (usually pollock) in the freezer aisle, which is currently half the price of basa. So celebrate that nugget of knowledge by making these super-simple fishcakes.

DF Use dairy-free milk.

LF Use lactose-free milk.

F Use maple syrup instead of honey and gluten-free breadcrumbs instead of cornflakes.

❄ Once cooled, store in an airtight container and freeze for up to 3 months. Air fry from frozen for 17–20 minutes at 180°C (350°F), turning halfway. Check the internal temperature with a digital food thermometer against those given on page 255.

TIPS

I use gluten-free cornflakes (usually a bit cheaper and more readily available) to coat my fishcakes, but you could also use gluten-free breadcrumbs instead.

Digital weighing scales can make portioning out exactly 115g (4oz) of the potato mixture incredibly easy, ensuring that each fishcake is exactly the same size and that they'll cook at the exact same speed. Simply put the bowl containing the filling on the scale and press the 'zero' button to set the weight to '0'. Once you remove the filling, the scale will now show you how much you've removed, so you can continue to portion it out until the scale reads -115g (-4oz). Simply press the 'zero' button again and portion out once more. You can use this method when portioning out the mixture for my crisp bakes (page 70) and other recipes throughout this book too.

- Vegetable oil spray
- 520g (1lb 2½oz) frozen white fish fillets
- 600g (1lb 5oz) Maris Piper potatoes (about 3 medium), peeled and cut into 2cm (¾in) cubes
- 3 tbsp fish sauce
- 20g (¾oz) jarred jalapeños, chopped
- 1 tbsp ginger paste
- 2 tbsp honey
- 2 tbsp gluten-free plain (all-purpose) flour
- ¼ tsp ground black pepper

For the coating

- 3 tbsp gluten-free plain (all-purpose) flour
- 1 large egg, beaten with 3 tbsp milk
- 130g (4½oz) gluten-free cornflakes, crushed in a bowl using the end of a rolling pin
- 1 tbsp dried mixed herbs
- ½ tsp dried chilli flakes

To cook in an air fryer, heat the air fryer to 200°C (400°F). Spray the base of the basket or crisping tray with a little oil. Add the frozen fish and air fry for 10 minutes, until cooked through, then allow to rest in the air fryer with the lid open or the drawer ajar.

Meanwhile, boil the potatoes in a large pan of boiling water for about 15 minutes, until completely cooked through. Drain, transfer to a large bowl and mash until smooth.

Add the fish sauce, jalapeños, ginger paste, honey, flour and black pepper to the potato and mix until smooth, then stir in the fish – it should flake as you do so, but don't over-mix, to ensure that the fish stays in bite-sized chunks.

Divide the mixture into 8 equal balls (115g/4oz each) and flatten into thick patties on a board.

Spread the flour for the coating on a plate. Combine the beaten egg and milk on a large, deep plate. Combine the crushed cornflakes, mixed herbs and chilli flakes on a third plate.

One by one, coat the patties in the flour, then in the egg, and finally in the cornflakes, pressing them on tightly.

Heat the air fryer to 200°C (400°F) and spray with oil. Place as many fishcakes as will comfortably fit in the air fryer without touching, spray with more oil and air fry for 10–12 minutes or until the cornflakes are golden and crisp.

To cook in an oven, preheat the oven to 180°C fan/200°C (400°F). Lightly spray a baking tray with oil, add the frozen fish and bake for 15–20 minutes, then allow to cool on the tray. Increase the oven temperature to 200°C fan/ 220°C (425°F) and generously spray a (clean) baking tray with oil.

Boil, drain and mash the potato, then combine with the other ingredients as directed opposite and follow the steps to portion out and coat the fishcakes.

Place the coated fishcakes on the baking tray and generously spray with oil once again. Bake for 25–30 minutes, or until golden and crisp.

AIR FRYER FAVOURITES

76

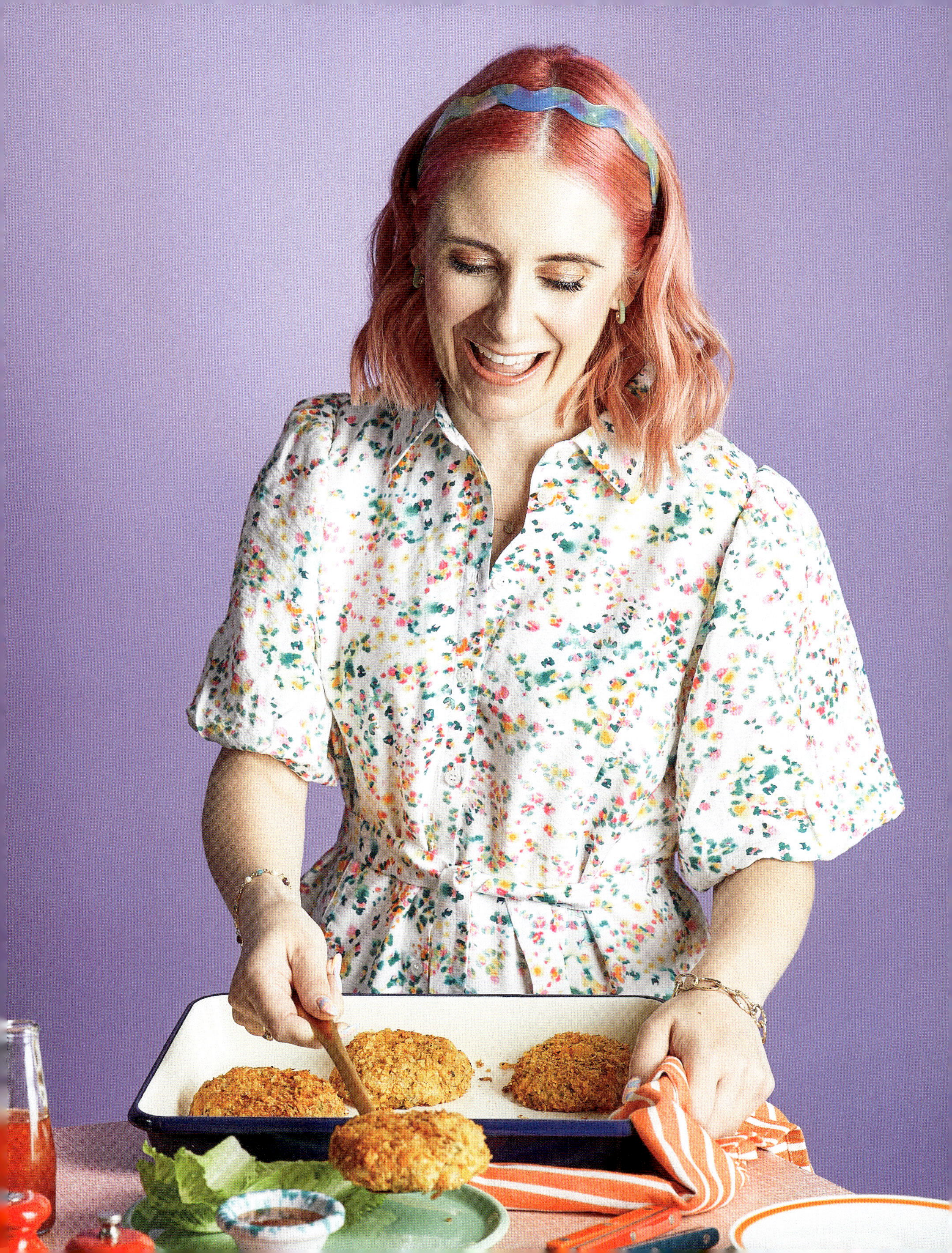

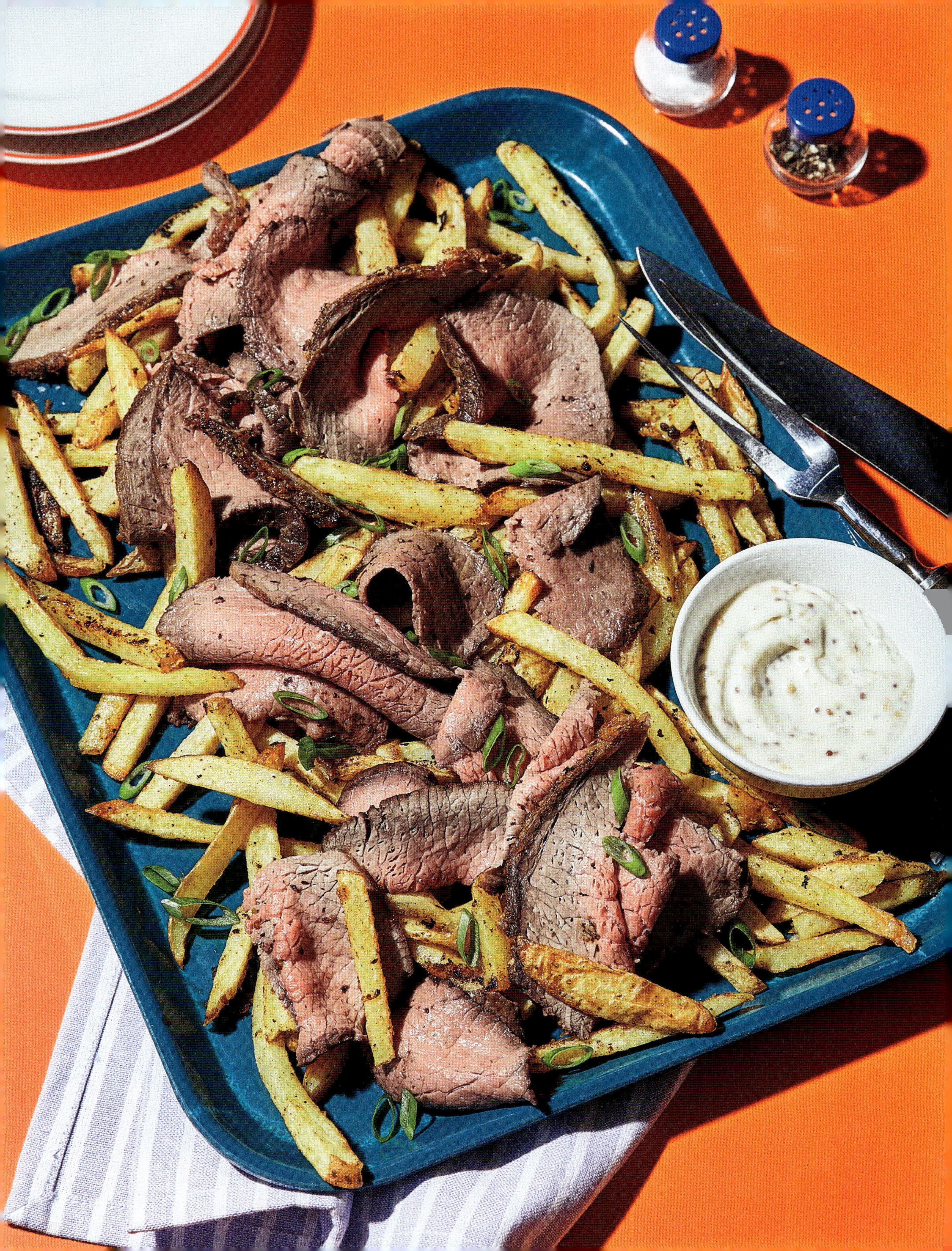

ROAST BEEF

While you're more than welcome to use this recipe and serve up your roast beef the traditional way, this is my new go-to. With tender shavings of roast beef, mildly spicy 'dirty' chips and a mustard dip, it's a nice change from a Sunday roast! Ensuring the beef is a little pink in the middle is a must for me (you can always cook yours for a little longer if you'd prefer) and is a great tactic to get the best texture out of one of the most affordable cuts of roasting beef.

Serves 4–5

Prep 5 mins

Air Fryer 1 hour 10 mins or **Hob + Oven** 55 mins

DF **LF** **F**

❄ Once cooled, store the beef and chips in separate airtight containers, then freeze for up to 2–3 months. Air fry the chips from frozen at 200°C (400°F) for around 10–15 minutes. Allow the steak slices/shavings to fully defrost in the fridge, then air fry at 180°C (350°F) for 3–4 minutes. Check the internal temperature with a digital food thermometer against those given on page 255.

TIPS

The timings for cooking the roast beef joint are given assuming it has been cooked straight from the fridge. If you've removed the beef joint from the fridge prior to cooking and allowed it to come up to room temperature, reduce the cooking time by around 5 minutes.

If cooking a smaller beef roasting joint, reduce the time by 3 minutes per 100g (3½oz) for the air fryer, or 6 minutes per 100g (3½oz) for the oven.

Remember, the key to cooking crispy chips in the air fryer is to ensure they're not piled up too much and well shaken/regularly turned in the air fryer basket. Oh, and the oil in the coating helps out a lot too, so don't scrimp there!

- 1kg (2lb 3oz) beef roasting joint (topside, top rump or silverside)
- Vegetable oil spray
- 1 tsp salt
- 1 tsp dried mixed herbs
- 1 tsp ground black pepper

For the chips (fries)
- 600g (1lb 5oz) Maris Piper potatoes, peeled or unpeeled, cut into chips 5mm (¼in thick)
- 3 tbsp vegetable oil
- 2 tbsp gluten-free plain (all-purpose) flour or cornflour (cornstarch) – if making in the air fryer
- 1 tsp salt
- ½ tsp black pepper
- 1 tsp mild chilli powder
- ½ tsp mild curry powder

To serve
- 100g (3½oz) mayonnaise
- 1 tsp wholegrain mustard
- Small handful of spring onion (scallion) greens, finely chopped

Place the beef joint on a board and generously spray/drizzle with oil. Rub with the salt, then with the mixed herbs and pepper.

To cook in an air fryer, add the chopped potatoes and oil to a bowl and mix until well coated. Next add the flour, salt, pepper, chilli powder and curry powder. Mix until the flour disappears, ensuring no chips are stuck together.

Heat the air fryer to 200°C (400°F) and lightly spray the base of the air fryer basket or crisping tray with oil.

Place the beef joint in the air fryer and cook for 20 minutes, flipping it halfway. Reduce the temperature to 180°C (350°F) and air fry for 27–30 minutes, or longer if you prefer it well done. Remove to a plate and allow to rest for 10–15 minutes before removing any string and using a sharp knife to cut it into thin slices or shavings – it should be a little pink in the middle.

While the beef is resting, heat the air fryer to 200°C (400°F). Place the chips in the air fryer and air fry for 15–22 minutes until browned at the edges and crisp, turning over halfway and separating any that are stuck together.

To cook in an oven, preheat the oven to 180°C fan/200°C (400°F). Place the prepared beef in a roasting tin and roast in the oven for 35–40 minutes, or 5–10 minutes longer if you prefer it more well done. Rest then slice as described opposite.

Around 10 minutes before the beef is done, fill a large saucepan with boiling water and place over a medium heat. Once the water is bubbling again, carefully add the chopped potatoes and boil for 3–4 minutes, then drain. While the beef is resting, preheat the oven to 220°C fan/240°C (460°F).

Transfer the chips to a large baking tray, drizzle with the oil and scatter over the salt, pepper, chilli powder and curry powder (no need to add the flour if making chips in the oven) then turn the chips a few times until well coated. Cook in the oven for 15–16 minutes, turning them after 8–10 minutes, or until golden brown at the edges and fluffy in the middle.

To serve, combine the mayonnaise and mustard in a small dish. Portion up the chips and top with roast beef slices/shavings and spring onion greens.

CRACKLING ROAST PORK

Serves 4–5

Prep 5 mins

Air Fryer 50–60 mins or
Oven 1 hour 40 mins

DF **LF**

F Serve with FODMAP-friendly sides.

❄ Once cooled, slice and store in airtight containers for up to 3 months. Allow the pork slices to fully defrost in the fridge, then air fry at 180°C (350°F) for 5–7 minutes. Check the internal temperature with a digital food thermometer against those given on page 255.

This recipe is the perfect example of how air fryers are capable of so much more than just cooking chips. I've honestly never had such outrageously crispy pork crackling with so little input or effort from myself, with the pork hiding underneath still remaining so succulent and juicy. If your oven is especially crammed when making a roast dinner, employing the use of your air fryer for one component of your roast can make life so much easier, although I have included oven temperatures and timings for this recipe too!

- 1–1.5kg (2lb 3oz–3lb 5oz) boneless pork loin joint, skin on
- 2 tsp fennel seeds, crushed, or dried mixed herbs
- 1½ tbsp salt
- 1 tsp ground black pepper
- 2 tbsp vegetable oil

Remove any string tying the pork loin together and pat dry using kitchen paper. Score the rind with a sharp knife in a criss-cross pattern. Make sure you don't cut too far through!

Mix the crushed fennel seeds or dried mixed herbs with the salt and pepper. Spread all over the skin and the meat itself, rubbing into every crevice. Brush the pork lightly all over with oil.

To cook in an air fryer, heat the air fryer to 180°C (350°F). Place the pork in the air fryer with the rind facing up and cook for 50–60 minutes, until the crackling is golden and crisp.

To cook in an oven, preheat the oven to 220°C fan/240°C (475°F). Place the prepared pork in a roasting tin and roast for 35–40 minutes.

After 40 minutes, lower the heat to 160°C fan/180°C (350°F) and roast for 50 minutes to 1 hour.

Remove to a wooden serving board and allow to rest for 10 minutes before slicing with a sharp knife. You may have to turn the pork upside down to carve it as the crackling is very crunchy!

Optionally serve with apple sauce, roasted veggies, steamed broccoli and gluten-free gravy.

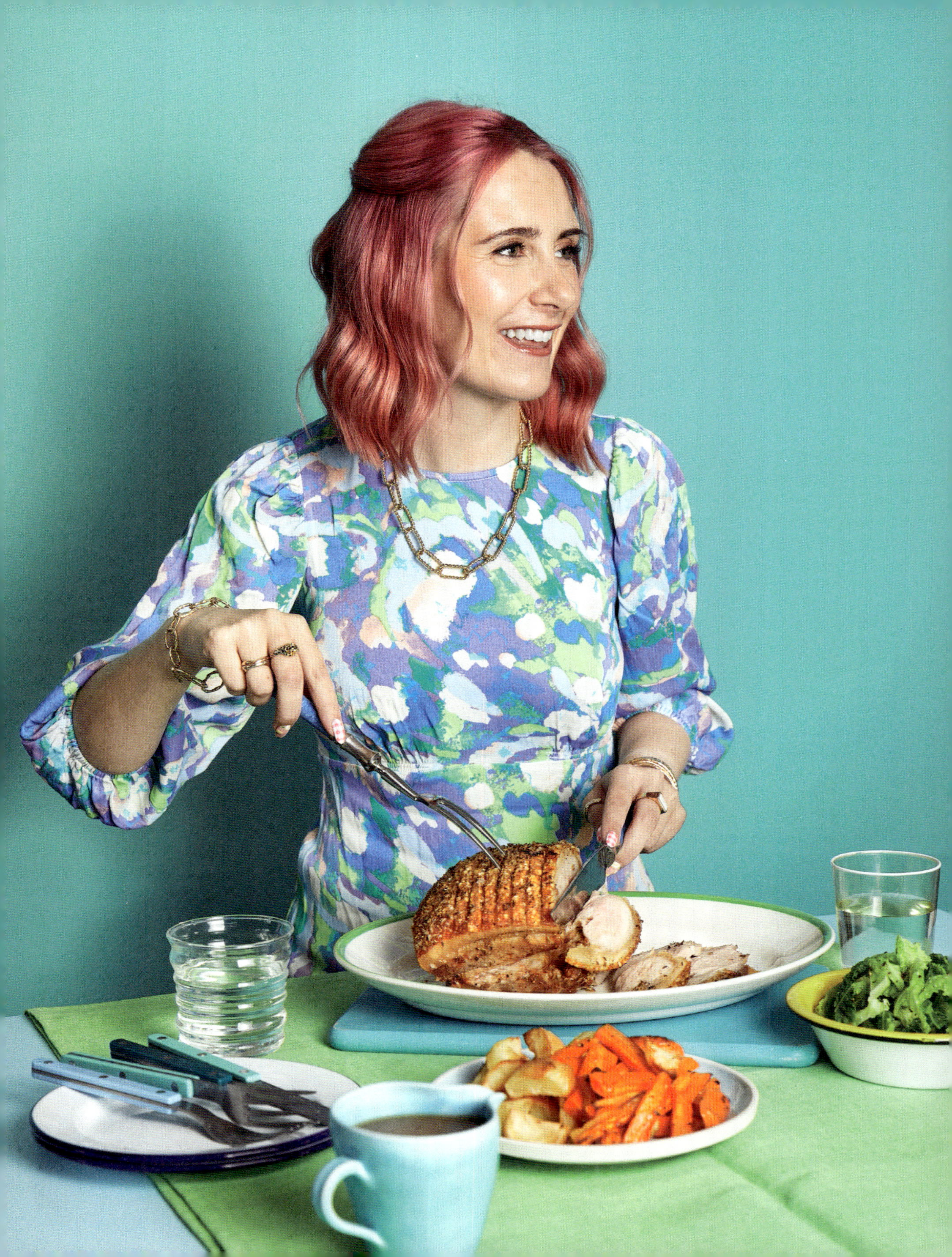

VEG PEEL CRISPS

These are quite often branded as 'fancy crisps' and usually have the price to match! But the inclusion of this recipe isn't just because you'll save money by making these instead of buying them, it's because they're almost free if you save your leftover peelings! They actually make a great little appetizer when friends and family are round for dinner and, for some reason, people are really impressed when you tell them you made them yourself!

Serves 3–4

Prep 5 mins

Air Fryer 10 mins or
Oven 25 mins

(DF) (LF) (F) (V) (VE)

- 400g (14oz) root vegetable peelings (such as potatoes, sweet potatoes, carrots, parsnips etc.), washed and dried
- 3 tbsp vegetable oil
- 1 tsp salt
- ½ tsp ground black pepper
- 1 tsp dried mixed herbs

Add the peelings to a large bowl, then add the oil, salt, pepper and mixed herbs. Toss until everything is evenly coated.

To cook in an air fryer, heat the air fryer to 200°C (400°F). Place the coated peelings in the air fryer basket, making sure you don't overfill it as this will affect the crispy finish. Air fry for 8–10 minutes or until golden brown and crisp, giving them a shake halfway through.

To cook in an oven, preheat the oven to 200°C fan/220°C (425°F). Coat the peelings as directed above, then spread out on a large baking tray and bake in the oven for 20–25 minutes until crisp and golden brown, turning them halfway.

Enjoy as a snack or as a topper on your favourite meals.

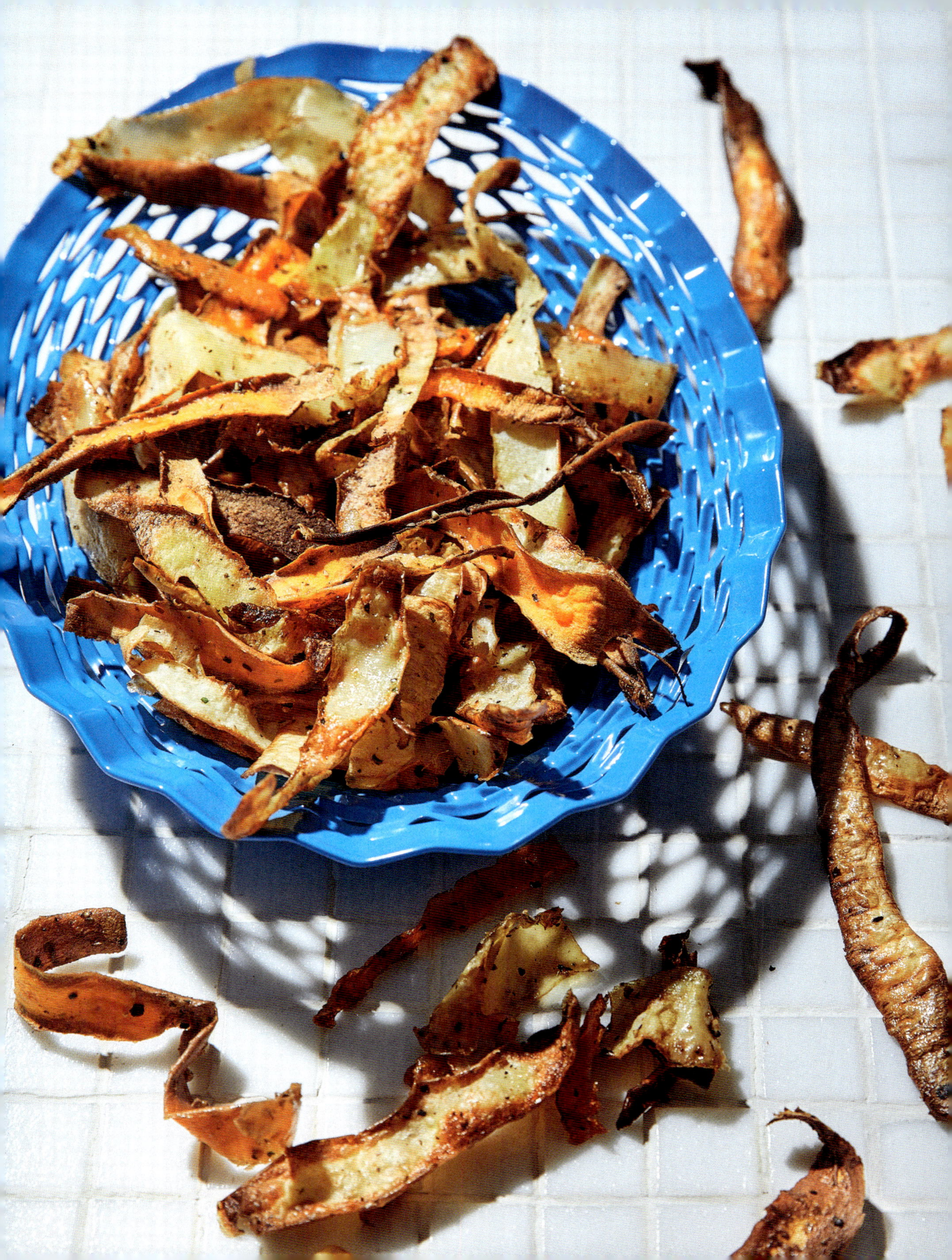

SAVVY STREET FOOD

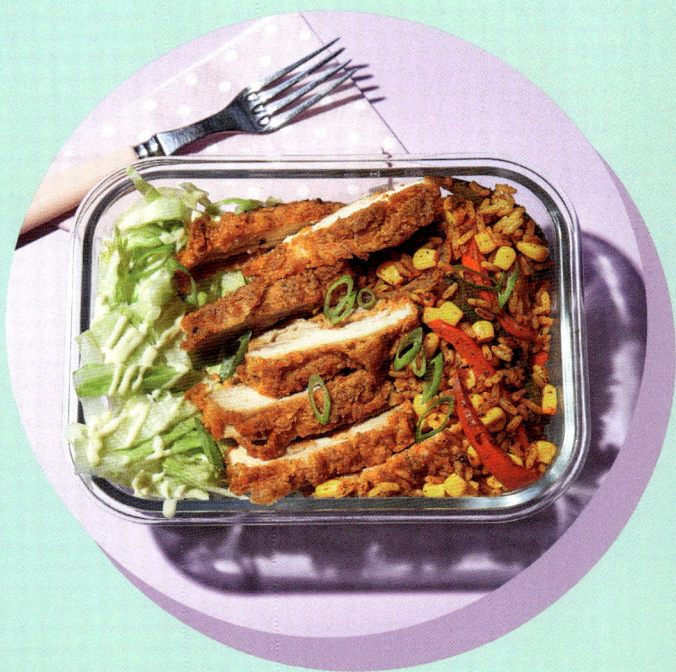

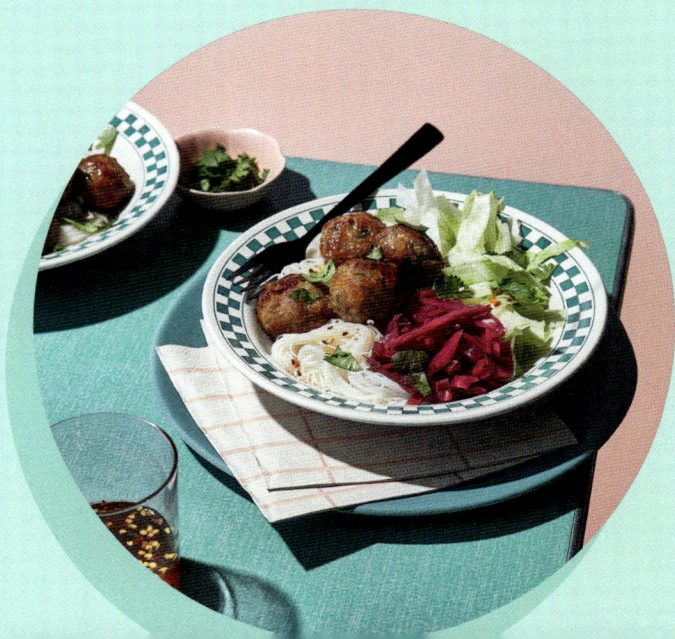

Say hello to the home of budget-friendly fakeaway favourites, street food and fast food where everything is gluten-free; that home being this chapter and, from now on, your own kitchen!

Though street food and fast food have a reputation for being rather costly, in reality most takeaway restaurants and street-food vendors are some of the best examples of how you can economize the balance of costlier ingredients with affordable ones to keep costs down. So in actual fact, if you made the exact same dish at home, you'd probably find it to be incredibly affordable!

But, perhaps most admirable of all, not only are vendors able to nail that balance of delicious dishes with down-to-earth costs, they're also able to whip them up in next to no time and bust the long queues they attract.

And it's exactly that essence that I've bottled in this chapter: an eclectic mix of different cuisines from around the world (and familiar favourites from closer to home) with the perfect harmony of affordability and maximum flavour, made as quickly and as simply as possible. So expect to see an exciting chapter of 'as fast as possible' recipes, each utilizing the magic of easily accessible, affordable store-cupboard ingredients to transform both costlier (yet essential!) and bargain ingredients into meals to remember.

But though it's safe to say that choosing to cook *almost anything* at home over ordering a takeaway will save you money, as these recipes also nail that harmony of costlier ingredients balanced with extremely affordable ones, they'll also be even cheaper to make versus just cooking *anything* at home. So in effect, by using this chapter, you're saving twice!

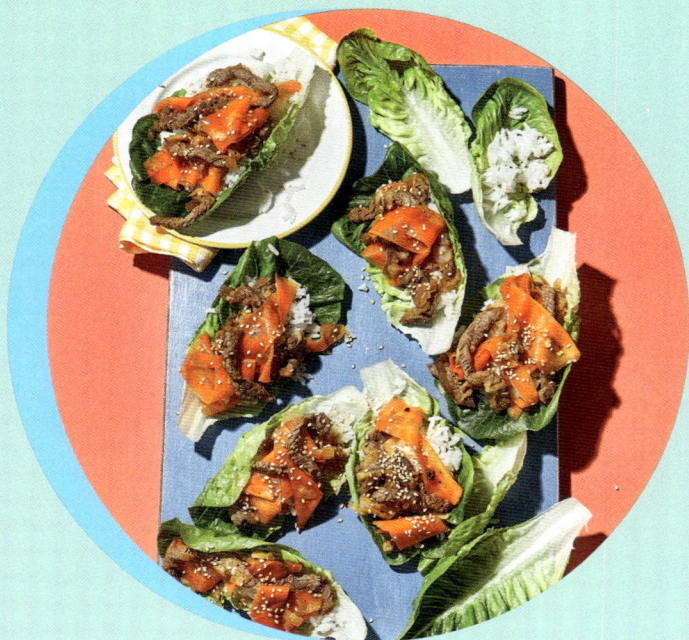

SMASH BURGER MAC 'N' CHEESE

This recipe combines two of my favourite fast food orders into one creamy, cheesy pasta dish with tinges of mustard, ketchup and burger sauce, packed with smash-burger-style beef. Higher-fat-percentage minced (ground) beef is usually incredibly affordable compared to lean and is actually commonly used to make burger patties due to its more intense flavour. However, if you'd prefer to keep things a little leaner while still keeping it affordable, simply drain the liquid that comes out of the beef while frying it, then continue with the recipe as directed.

Serves 3
Prep 5 mins
Hob 25 mins

DF Use dairy-free milk and dairy-free cheese.

LL Use lactose-free milk.

F Use asafoetida instead of onion powder, lactose-free milk, and serve with low FODMAP relish.

V Use a gluten-free and veggie alternative to mince.

VE Combine the dairy-free and veggie advice.

❄ See freezing and defrosting guidance for pasta dishes on page 28.

TIP
If you struggle to find gluten-free dried macaroni, feel free to use gluten-free penne, fusilli or even orzo.

- 300g (10½oz) gluten-free dried macaroni
- Vegetable oil spray
- 500g (1lb 2oz) minced (ground) beef, ideally 20% fat
- ½ tbsp smoked paprika
- ½ tbsp onion powder or asafoetida
- ½ tsp salt
- 1 tsp ground black pepper
- 3 small gherkins, finely diced
- 1½ tbsp cornflour (cornstarch) or potato starch
- 2 tbsp Dijon mustard
- 300ml (1¼ cups) milk
- 150g (5½oz) mature Cheddar, grated
- 1 tbsp tomato purée (paste)
- Small handful of chives, finely chopped (optional)

To serve
- ½ iceberg lettuce, shredded
- 6–8 tbsp tomato or chilli relish

Cook the macaroni in a pan of boiling, salted water according to the packet instructions, then drain.

Meanwhile, spray the base of a large pot that has a lid with oil and place over a medium heat. Once hot, add the beef – it should make a nice sizzling sound. Flatten with the back of a wooden spoon or spatula until it's all flat and even, like one huge burger. Fry until browned on the underside, then break up and flip to the uncooked side. Once both sides are browned, add the smoked paprika, onion powder or asafoetida, salt and pepper, then fry until fragrant.

Add the gherkins, cornflour or potato starch and mustard, then stir in and fry for a further 2–3 minutes. Add the milk and allow to simmer for 3–4 minutes until thickened a little, then stir in the grated cheese and tomato purée.

Add the drained macaroni and stir in until well coated. Scatter with the chives, if using, and serve alongside shredded lettuce and dollops of relish.

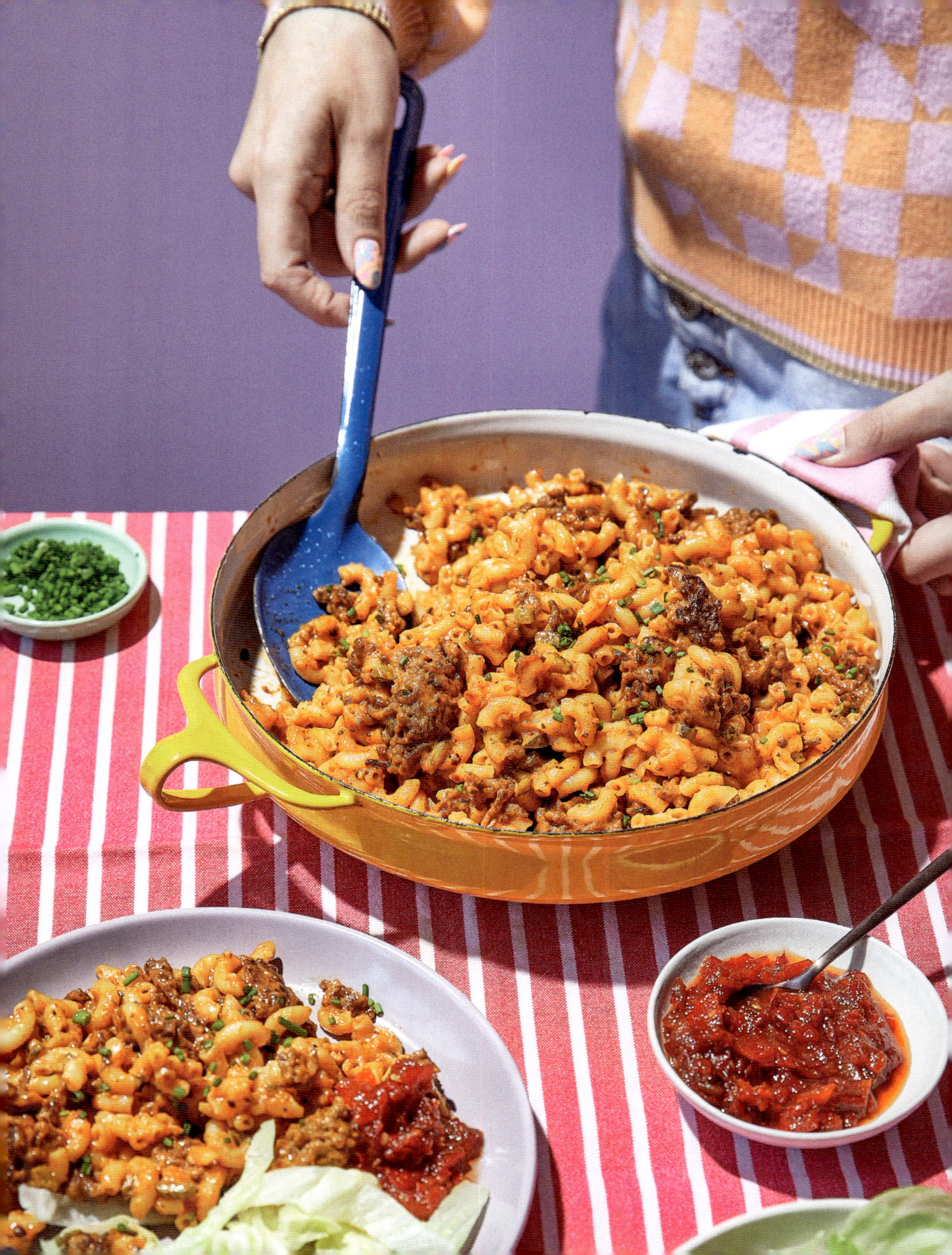

CHICKEN ZINGER RICEBOX

With a hearty portion of spicy rice and crispy chicken you'd swear was deep-fried, this recipe is far cheaper and quicker to throw together than waiting for a certain fast food outlet to come to their senses and serve a gluten-free version. Bonus points if you actually serve yours in a box somehow too! I've provided guidance on how to shallow fry the chicken on the hob for those without an air fryer, but due to the large amount of extra oil required, the air fryer will always be the most cost-effective way to make this one. Ideally cook the rice ahead of time.

Serves 4

Prep 10 mins

Hob only 40 mins or
Hob + Air Fryer 30 mins

DF **LF**

V Use 400–500g (14–17½oz) firm tofu instead of chicken thighs, cut into wide slices 1cm (½in) thick, and skip coating them in beaten egg (and the second coating of flour).

VE See veggie advice and use vegan-friendly mayonnaise.

❄ Once cooled, store the chicken and rice in separate airtight containers and freeze for up to 2–3 months. Allow the chicken to defrost completely in the fridge, then reheat in the air fryer for 6–8 minutes at 200°C (400°F) until crisp. Check the internal temperature with a digital food thermometer against those given on page 255. For advice on reheating the rice from frozen, see the freezing and defrosting guidance for risotto and rice dishes on page 28.

- 600ml (2½ cups) water
- 300g (1⅔ cups) long-grain rice
- 2 large eggs
- 600g (1lb 5oz) skinless, boneless chicken thighs
- Vegetable oil spray (for air frying) or vegetable oil (for shallow frying)

For the spicy coating

- 150g (1 cup plus 2 tbsp) gluten-free plain (all-purpose) flour
- 2 tsp gluten-free baking powder
- 1 tsp salt or celery salt

- 1 tbsp smoked paprika
- ½ tsp ground ginger
- 1½ tsp cayenne pepper or ground black pepper
- 1 tsp onion powder (optional)
- 1 tsp garlic powder (optional)

For the spicy rice

- 400g (14oz) frozen sliced (bell) peppers
- 1 tbsp garlic paste (optional)
- 2 tbsp smoked paprika
- 1 tbsp dried mixed herbs

- 1½ tsp cayenne pepper or ground black pepper
- 1 tsp ground turmeric
- 1½ tsp salt
- 300g (10½oz) frozen or canned sweetcorn (drained weight)

To serve

- ½ iceberg lettuce, roughly chopped
- 4 drizzles of mayonnaise, ideally from a squirty bottle
- Large handful of spring onion (scallion) greens, thinly sliced on the diagonal

To prepare the rice, add the water to a medium saucepan and bring to a rapid boil. Add the rice, pop the lid on and turn the heat down to low. Allow the rice to cook for 20 minutes, then take off the heat. Remove the lid and allow to cool for as long as you can (ideally allow to cool completely and store covered in the fridge until you need it) for the best rice texture.

Meanwhile, add all the spicy coating ingredients to a medium bowl and mix until well combined.

Crack the eggs into a small bowl and beat with a fork. Take the chicken and dredge in the spicy flour until well coated. Next, dip into the beaten egg bowl until coated. Finally, roll the chicken around in the spicy flour once more, squeezing and compacting it to the chicken, until well covered with no eggy patches showing.

To cook the chicken in the air fryer, heat the air fryer to 200°C (400°F) and generously spray the base of the air fryer basket or crisping tray with oil. If you have an air fryer with 2 drawers, use both. Place the coated chicken in the air fryer basket and spray generously with oil until the floury patches disappear. Make sure the chicken pieces are touching as little as possible then air fry for 15–16 minutes until the coating is crisp and golden, turning them over halfway and spraying lightly with oil. Allow to rest for 5–10 minutes in the air fryer with the drawer open.

continued overleaf

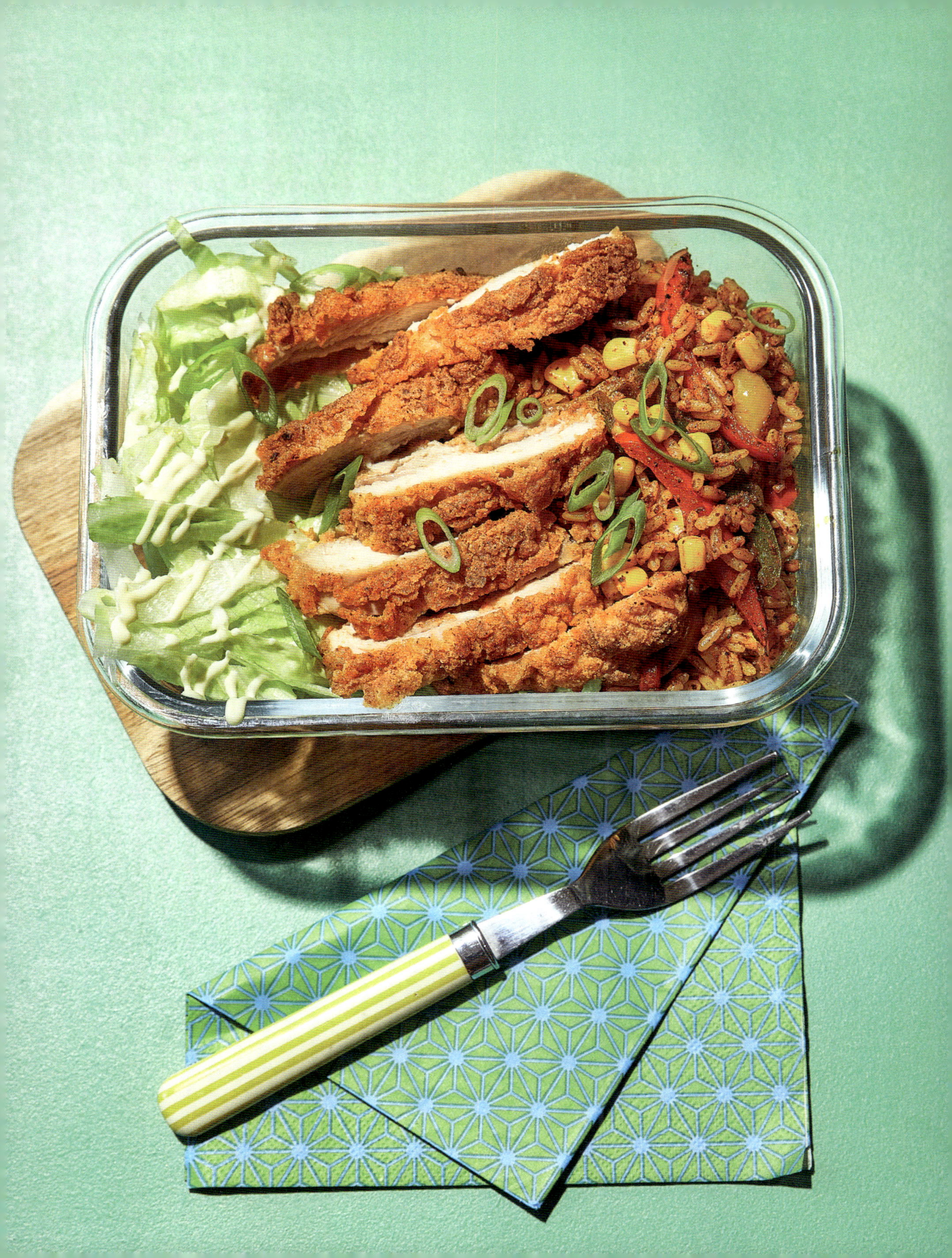

To cook the chicken on the hob, add enough oil to a large frying pan so it is around 1cm (½in) deep. Place over a medium heat for 7–10 minutes or until it reaches 180°C (350°F). If you don't have a digital food thermometer to check the temperature, you can use the wooden spoon-handle test: place the handle in the oil and observe the oil around it – if bubbles form around the wood and rise up, then it's ready. Line a large plate with kitchen paper, ready for later.

Take the coated chicken and carefully lower it into the hot oil using a pair of small tongs – it should sizzle nicely. Cook for 11–12 minutes, turning halfway, or until the crispy coating starts to turn golden. Remove with a slotted spoon and place on the plate lined with kitchen paper. Allow to rest for 5–10 minutes, ideally on a wire rack. Repeat with any coated chicken pieces that wouldn't fit into the pan.

Meanwhile, prepare the rice. Lightly spray the base of a large wok or frying pan with oil and place over a medium-high heat. Once hot, add the frozen peppers and fry until softened and any water released has mostly evaporated. Add the garlic paste, if using, smoked paprika, dried herbs, cayenne or black pepper, turmeric and salt, then stir in and fry until fragrant. Add the cooked rice, spray well with oil and stir fry for 2 minutes until it's all well coated. Add the sweetcorn and continue to stir fry for another 2 minutes.

To serve, portion up the rice, leaving space for the lettuce. Drizzle a little mayo over the lettuce leaves. Use a sharp knife to slice each coated chicken piece into strips, then place on top of the rice and garnish with spring onion greens.

TIPS

For a proper deep-fried finish on the chicken when cooking them in the air fryer, don't be afraid to be generous when spraying the chicken fillets with oil – spray them until it looks like the flour has vanished and you can actually see the chicken beneath. Conversely, if you want to use as little oil as possible, simply spray until there are no more white patches of flour visible; dry patches of flour will never turn golden and burn, so make sure you spray just enough oil to prevent that!

See my microwave sweet and sour chicken recipe on page 128 for guidance on how to cook the rice in the microwave – use the measurements for rice and boiling water given here.

TURKISH-STYLE LAHMACUN

Makes 4
Prep 15 mins
Hob + Air Fryer 25 mins or
Hob + Oven 30 mins

Sometimes referred to as 'Turkish pizza', this topped flatbread is commonly spread with a delicious spiced tomato, red pepper and herb lamb or beef topping (though I'll be going with beef as the more economical choice!). Using my speedy flatbread recipe not only makes this gluten-free, but means you don't need to wait around for hours for yeasted dough to prove. If you've never tried this before, then you absolutely need to – it's something I can't ever imagine easily finding gluten-free in my entire lifetime!

DF Use a thick dairy-free yoghurt.

LF Use lactose-free Greek yoghurt.

F Use lactose-free Greek yoghurt, no more than 200g (7oz) jarred red (bell) pepper and no more than 180g (6½oz) cherry tomatoes. Use leek (green parts only) instead of onion and omit the tomato purée.

V Use 400g (14oz) firm tofu, blitzed in a food processor until coarse or finely chopped, instead of beef.

VE Combine dairy-free and veggie advice.

❄ Store in airtight containers and freeze for up to 2–3 months; reheat in the air fryer from frozen at 200°C (400°F) for 5–6 minutes.

TIP

In this recipe and throughout the rest of this book, you'll notice that herby garnishes are often labelled as optional. This is purely because they are usually for visual appeal of the final dish rather than being an absolute essential ingredient. As this book prioritizes lowering the total cost of each dish per portion, I've made sure to always let you know when something is optional and not mandatory, but also ensured you know how to give a dish that perfect finishing touch when you really need to impress.

- Vegetable oil spray
- 100g (3½oz) frozen chopped onion **or** ½ medium leek, finely chopped
- 300g (10½oz) jarred roasted red (bell) peppers, cut into 1cm (½in) slices
- 250g (9oz) cherry tomatoes, halved
- 1 tbsp tomato purée (paste)
- 500g (1lb 2oz) minced (ground) beef (20% fat)
- 1 tbsp cornflour or potato starch
- 15g (½oz) jarred jalapeños, finely chopped
- 1½ tbsp smoked paprika
- 1 tbsp dried mixed herbs

- 1 tbsp ground cumin or mild curry powder
- ½ tsp ground allspice
- ½ tsp ground cinnamon
- ½ tsp salt
- ¼ tsp ground black pepper

For the flatbread

- 200g (1½ cups) gluten-free self-raising flour, plus extra for dusting
- 75g (⅓ cup) Greek yoghurt or thick natural yoghurt
- 110ml (½ cup minus 2 tsp) water
- 1 tbsp dried mint or dried mixed herbs
- 1 tsp salt
- ½ tsp ground black pepper

For the herby yoghurt drizzle

- 125g (generous ½ cup) Greek yoghurt or thick natural yoghurt
- 1 tbsp dried mint or dried mixed herbs
- Grated zest of ½ lemon
- Pinch each of salt and ground black pepper
- 3–5 tbsp water

To serve

- 1 little gem lettuce, shredded
- Small handful of coriander (cilantro) leaves, roughly chopped (optional)

Spray the base of a large pot that has a lid with oil and place over a medium heat. Once hot, add the onion or leek and red pepper and fry until softened. Add the cherry tomatoes (cut side down) and place the lid on top. Allow to cook for 3–4 minutes or until you can easily squish them with a wooden spoon.

Remove the lid and stir in the tomato purée until it disappears, then push everything to the sides of the pan, leaving as much space in the middle as possible, and spray the pan with oil.

Add the beef and break up, fry until browned on one side, then turn over and fry until nearly browned all over. Stir in the cornflour or potato starch, which will help absorb all the flavour.

Add in the jalapeños, smoked paprika, mixed herbs, cumin or curry powder, allspice, cinnamon, salt and pepper, then mix everything up. Fry for a further 4–5 minutes, then remove from the heat.

continued overleaf

Add all the flatbread ingredients to a large bowl and mix thoroughly using a spatula to ensure there are no hidden clumps of yoghurt-coated flour. As it starts to come together, use your hands to bring it together into a slightly sticky ball. Allow to rest and hydrate for 10 minutes.

Knead the dough briefly in the bowl until smooth and combined but still a little sticky and loose. Divide into 4 equal portions. Transfer one portion of the dough to a medium sheet of lightly floured non-stick baking parchment and cover the others.

Using floured hands, gradually push the dough down into a circle. Use a rolling pin to roll it out further into a round 2–3mm (⅛in) thick if cooking in the oven, or into the shape of your air fryer drawer if a circle won't fit. Ensure it's not thicker or thinner in certain areas and keep lightly re-flouring your hands/rolling pin whenever it starts to stick to them. Use your fingers to gently push in the edges all around the perimeter to neaten them. Repeat with the remaining 3 portions of dough so you have 4 flatbreads on individual sheets of parchment.

To cook in an oven, preheat the oven to 200°C fan/220°C (425°F) and have ready 2 large baking trays. Using the parchment to lift them, transfer 2 flatbreads to each tray. Spray well with oil, especially the edges, or they can remain very pale.

Place both trays in the oven on the upper and middle shelves and bake for 4–5 minutes, then remove from the oven and spread a quarter of the beef on top of each base in a thin layer that covers the entire flatbread, ensuring there are no gaps and going right up to the edges.

Return to the oven for 10 minutes – if you sprayed enough oil on the edges, they should be a little golden on the very edge.

To cook in an air fryer, heat the air fryer to 200°C (400°F). Using the parchment to lift them, transfer as many flatbreads that can fit in your air fryer (in a 2-drawer air fryer, I fit in one per drawer). Spray well with oil, especially the edges.

Air fry for 3 minutes, then spread a quarter of the beef on top of each base in a thin layer that covers the entire flatbread, ensuring there are no gaps and going right up to the edges. Return to the air fryer for 6–7 minutes – if you sprayed enough oil on the edges, they should be a little golden on the very edge. Remove from the air fryer using a spatula and repeat to cook any remaining flatbreads.

Meanwhile, mix together the herby yoghurt drizzle ingredients in a small bowl. Once the flatbreads are done, drizzle some of the yoghurt mixture over each and scatter over the lettuce and coriander, if using. Optionally fold in half to serve.

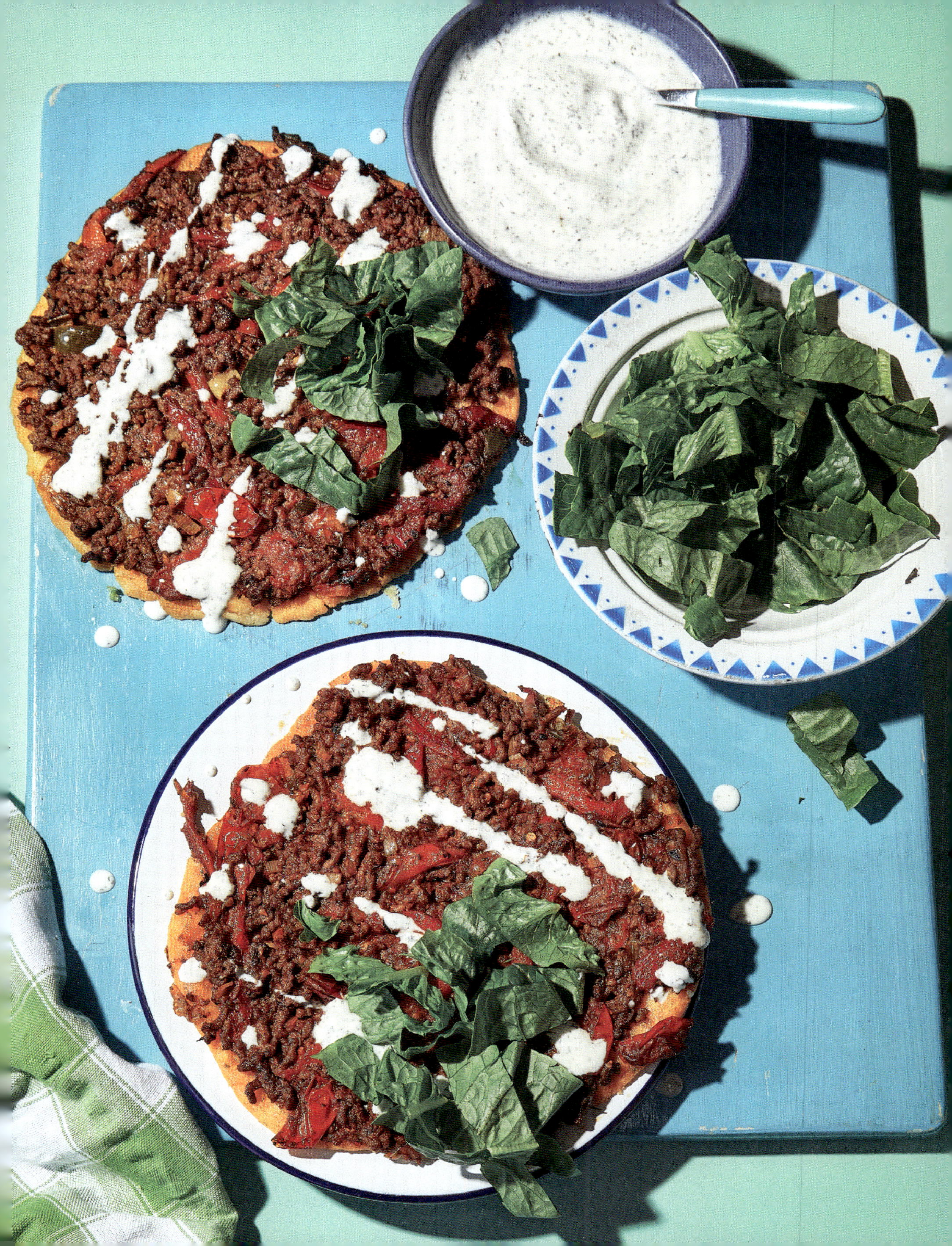

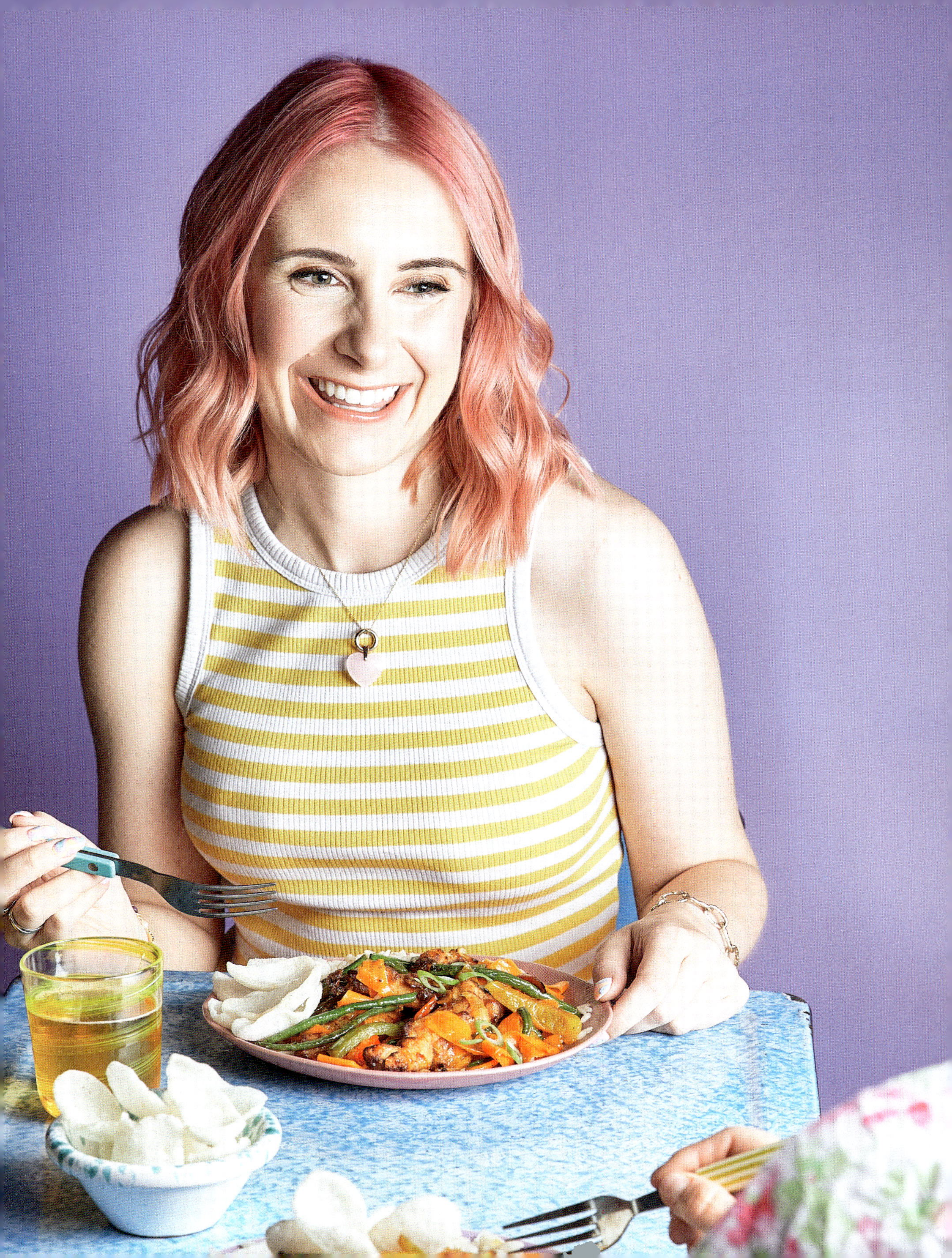

STICKY HONEY CRISPY CHICKEN

If there's one thing that I learned from my Japanese-style karaage chicken recipe (see page 64), it's that while chicken in a crispy coating is never not mind-blowing, chicken that's been marinated and *then* given a crispy coating, is even better. And if there's anything that this book is all about, it's maximum flavour at minimal cost! I often make this as a quick fakeaway served with rice and gluten-free prawn crackers.

Serves 4–5

Prep 5 mins + 15 mins marinating

Hob + Air Fryer 20 mins or
Hob only 25 mins

DF **LF**

F Use light brown sugar/maple syrup instead of honey and all green peppers instead of mixed colours.

V Use 400g (14oz) firm tofu instead of chicken, marinating, coating and cooking in the same way as directed to cook the chicken.

VE See veggie advice and use maple syrup instead of honey.

❄ Ideally store the crispy chicken separately from the sauce, or it will lose its crispy coating. Freeze in airtight containers for up to 2–3 months. If stored separately, allow both to defrost completely in the fridge, then reheat the chicken in the air fryer for 5–6 minutes at 200°C (400°F). Check the internal temperature with a digital food thermometer against those given on page 255. Reheat the sauce in the microwave (covered) for 1–2 minutes at full power.

TIP

Double frying the chicken is the key to getting the crispest results! Whether you cook the chicken in the air fryer or in a pan, ensure you follow the final step, and thank me later.

- Vegetable oil spray (for air frying), or vegetable oil (for pan frying)
- 3 medium carrots, pared into ribbons using a swivel peeler
- 250g (9oz) frozen sliced red, green and yellow (bell) peppers
- 180g (6½oz) frozen green beans
- Small handful of spring onion (scallion) greens, thinly sliced on the diagonal, to serve

For the crispy chicken
- 400–500g (14–17½oz) chicken breast fillets, cut into 5mm (¼in) strips
- 2 tbsp gluten-free soy sauce
- 1 tbsp rice wine vinegar
- 1 tbsp ginger paste
- ½ tsp Chinese five spice
- ¼ teaspoon ground black pepper
- ¼ tsp salt

- 70g (generous ½ cup) gluten-free plain (all-purpose) flour

For the sauce
- 1 tbsp ginger paste
- 4 tbsp honey
- 2 tbsp rice wine vinegar
- ¼ tsp salt
- ¼ tsp ground black pepper
- 6 tbsp water
- 1 tsp gluten-free plain (all-purpose) flour

Add all the crispy chicken ingredients (except the flour) to a large bowl, mix well, cover and marinate for 15 minutes to overnight in the fridge.

When ready to cook, spread the flour out on a large dinner plate and have another empty plate ready. Coat each piece of chicken in the flour, squeezing and compacting it to the chicken, then place onto the empty plate. Repeat until all the chicken is coated.

To cook in an air fryer, heat the air fryer to 200°C (400°F) and spray the basket or crisping tray with oil. If you have an air fryer with 2 drawers, use both. Place as many of the chicken pieces in the air fryer as will comfortably fit without touching, then spray with oil until no white floury patches remain. Air fry for 9 minutes, turning the pieces over halfway and spraying any remaining floury patches with oil once turned. Allow to cool for 5–10 minutes with the drawer open, then air fry for another 2–3 minutes. This makes the coating extra crispy!

To pan-fry the chicken, add 6–7 tablespoons of oil to the base of a large frying pan and place over a medium heat. Once hot, add the chicken and fry for 8–9 minutes, turning halfway, then remove to a dinner plate lined with kitchen paper to drain. Return to the pan just before putting them in the sauce and fry once more for 2 minutes on each side, then allow to drain briefly on kitchen paper again.

Meanwhile, lightly spray the base and sides of a large wok with oil and place over a high heat. Add the carrot ribbons and fry until softened, then add the frozen peppers and green beans and continue to fry until softened and any moisture released has mostly evaporated.

For the sauce, combine the ingredients in a small dish and mix well until free of any lumps.

Add the sauce mixture to the wok and allow it to bubble until it reduces to a sticky consistency. Add the crispy chicken, scatter with spring onion greens and serve immediately.

2-FOR-1 THIN + CRISPY TRAYBAKE PIZZA

Makes 2 large rectangular pizzas
(each pizza serves 2)
Prep 15 mins
Oven 15 mins

In the past, I'd always make my pizza dough using equal measurements of flour to Greek yoghurt, but recently I've started substituting more than half of the yoghurt measurement with water. Not only does this reduce the cost of that ingredient by half, but the water actually improves the texture of the pizza base by making it crustier. The '2-for-1' part of this recipe means making two large pizzas at once – if you won't be eating both now, simply freeze one to enjoy later with zero effort required!

DF Use a thick dairy-free yoghurt and dairy-free cheese.

LL Use lactose-free Greek yoghurt.

F Use lactose-free Greek yoghurt and a low FODMAP BBQ sauce, if using, and use FODMAP-friendly toppings.

V Use veggie-friendly toppings.

VE See dairy-free advice and use vegan-friendly toppings.

❄ With the topped, uncooked and covered pizza(s) on baking trays, store in the freezer for 2–3 months. Cook from frozen at 240°C fan/260°C (500°F) for 16–18 minutes. If already cooked, store the sliced pizza in airtight containers and freeze for up to 2–3 months; reheat in the air fryer from frozen at 200°C fan/220°C (425°F) for 5–6 minutes.

TIPS

The key to a crispy base is to first of all ensure the dough is rolled as thinly as possible, as instructed opposite. Secondly, don't overload each base with sauce and toppings, or this can make the base more 'bready' than crispy.

If using a different type of yoghurt that isn't quite as thick, simply add a little more flour to compensate.

For the base
- 440g (3⅓ cups) gluten-free self-raising flour, plus extra for dusting
- 200g (1 cup minus 1 tbsp) Greek yoghurt or thick natural yoghurt
- 160ml (⅔ cup) water
- 2 tbsp dried mixed herbs (optional)
- 2 tsp salt

For the pizza sauce
- 200ml (generous ¾ cup) passata (sieved tomatoes)
- 3 tsp dried mixed herbs
- 4 tbsp gluten-free BBQ sauce (optional; for a BBQ base)
- Pinch each of salt and ground black pepper

To finish
- Toppings of your choice, such as pepperoni, tuna, thinly sliced (bell) pepper, ham and pineapple
- Large handful of grated mozzarella
- Small handful of basil leaves, roughly chopped (optional)

Preheat the oven to 240°C fan/260°C (500°F) or as hot as it will go. Prepare 2 large baking trays and 2 sheets of baking parchment larger than the trays.

Add the flour, yoghurt (give it a good stir before using), water, mixed herbs, if using, and salt to a large bowl. Mix well using a spatula to ensure there are no hidden clumps of yoghurt-coated flour. As it comes together, use your hands to bring it together into a slightly sticky ball. Knead the dough briefly in the bowl until smooth and no longer sticky.

Transfer the dough to the baking parchment and cut it in half. Return one half to the bowl and cover. Lightly flour a rolling pin. Roll out the dough to a large rectangle 2–3mm (⅛in) thick and around the same size as your baking tray – ensure it's even and not thicker or thinner in certain areas. Re-flour the rolling pin as needed.

Create a crust by folding the dough over at the edges by 1cm (½in), then gently press it down. Repeat with the other half of the dough so you have 2 pizza bases on parchment.

Combine the ingredients for the pizza sauce in a bowl, then spread it over both bases, right up to the crust. Add your toppings, then scatter over the mozzarella. Use the parchment to lift and slide them onto the baking trays.

If enjoying both pizzas now, bake both for 12–15 minutes, or until the cheese is golden, ensuring you keep an eye on them for the last 5 minutes. Remove from the oven and use the parchment to lift the pizzas onto a flat surface, then cut into 12 small or 4 large slices. Finish with basil, if using, and serve.

If only enjoying one pizza now, cook as directed above. Cover the uncooked pizza in cling film (plastic wrap) and follow the instructions in the freezer key.

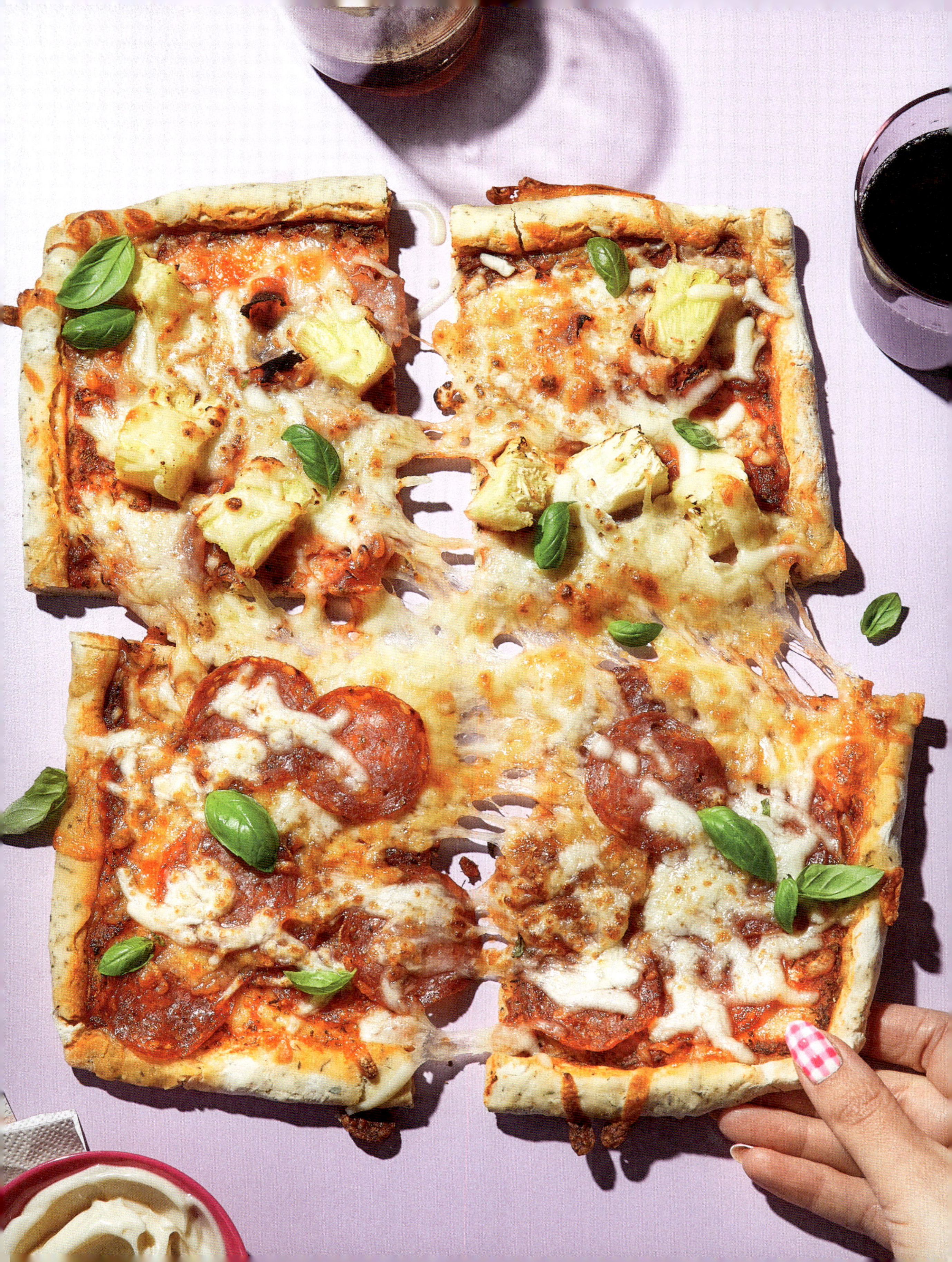

CRISPY CHILLI TOFU OR PORK

While this fakeaway favourite is commonly served with beef in a sweet chilli-style sauce, there are several reasons to mix things up a little and try it with tofu or pork. Firstly, it's up to 70% cheaper than using the sirloin steaks I'd normally use! Secondly, if you've been craving a meat-free version, or simply just fancy something new and exciting, then tofu or pork make great alternatives to beef in this recipe – it's not just because they're cheaper. However, if you still just really want crispy chilli beef regardless of all of the above, you can always attempt this recipe using 395g (14oz) thin-cut beef steaks. Serve with rice and gluten-free prawn crackers.

Serves 3

Prep 5 mins

Hob + Air Fryer 20 mins or **Hob only** 20 mins

DF **LF**

F
Use pork instead of tofu, omit the garlic paste or use ½ tbsp garlic-infused oil instead and use light brown sugar/maple syrup instead of honey. Use no more than 225g (8oz) green (bell) pepper instead of mixed colours.

V
Use tofu instead of pork.

VE
See veggie advice and use light brown sugar instead of honey.

❄
Ideally store the tofu or pork separately from the sauce, or it will lose its crispy coating. Freeze in airtight containers for up to 2–3 months. If stored separately, allow both to defrost completely in the fridge, then reheat the tofu or pork in the air fryer for 5–6 minutes at 200°C (400°F). Check the internal temperature with a digital food thermometer against those given on page 255. Reheat the sauce in the microwave (covered) for 4–5 minutes at full power.

- Vegetable oil spray (for air frying), or vegetable oil (for pan frying)
- 3 medium carrots, pared into ribbons using a swivel peeler
- 400g (14oz) frozen sliced red, green and yellow (bell) peppers
- 100g (¾ cup) gluten-free plain (all-purpose) flour
- 2 tsp salt
- 400g (14oz) firm tofu, cut into 1.5cm (⅔in) cubes **or** 480g (1lb 1oz) pork loin steaks, sliced into very thin strips

For the sauce
- 200ml (generous ¾ cup) pineapple or orange juice
- 8 tbsp rice wine vinegar
- 8 tbsp honey
- 2 tbsp gluten-free soy sauce
- 1 tsp garlic paste (optional)
- 2 tsp dried chilli flakes
- 4 tbsp cornflour (cornstarch) or potato starch mixed with 6 tbsp water

Lightly spray the base and sides of a large wok with oil and place over a high heat. Once hot, add the carrots and stir fry until softened, then add the peppers and continue to stir fry until any water released by the vegetables has mostly evaporated.

Add all the sauce ingredients except the cornflour or potato starch slurry to the wok and bring to the boil. Lower the heat and wait a couple of minutes before adding the cornflour or potato starch slurry, while stirring, and continue to simmer for 3–5 minutes until thickened. Keep warm over a low heat until the tofu or pork is ready.

Place the flour and salt in a large bowl and mix to combine. Add the tofu cubes or pork strips to the bowl and toss until well coated.

To cook the tofu or pork in the air fryer, heat the air fryer to 200°C (400°F). Generously spray the base of the air fryer basket or crisping tray with oil. If you have an air fryer with 2 drawers, you'll likely need to employ both, so grease both if necessary.

Place as many tofu or pork pieces as will fit in the air fryer basket without touching and generously spray with oil, ensuring any white floury patches disappear. Air fry for 7–8 minutes, turning over halfway and spraying any remaining floury patches with oil once turned. Optionally allow to cool for 5–10 minutes with the drawer open, then air fry for another 2–3 minutes. This makes the coating even crisper!

To cook the tofu or pork on the hob, add 6–7 tablespoons of oil to the base of a large frying pan and place over a medium heat. Once hot, add the tofu or pork and fry for 7–8 minutes, turning halfway, then remove to a dinner plate lined with kitchen paper to drain. Return to the pan just before putting them into the sauce, and fry once more for 2 minutes on each side, then allow to drain briefly on kitchen paper again.

Add the cooked tofu or pork to the sauce in the wok and serve immediately while still crispy.

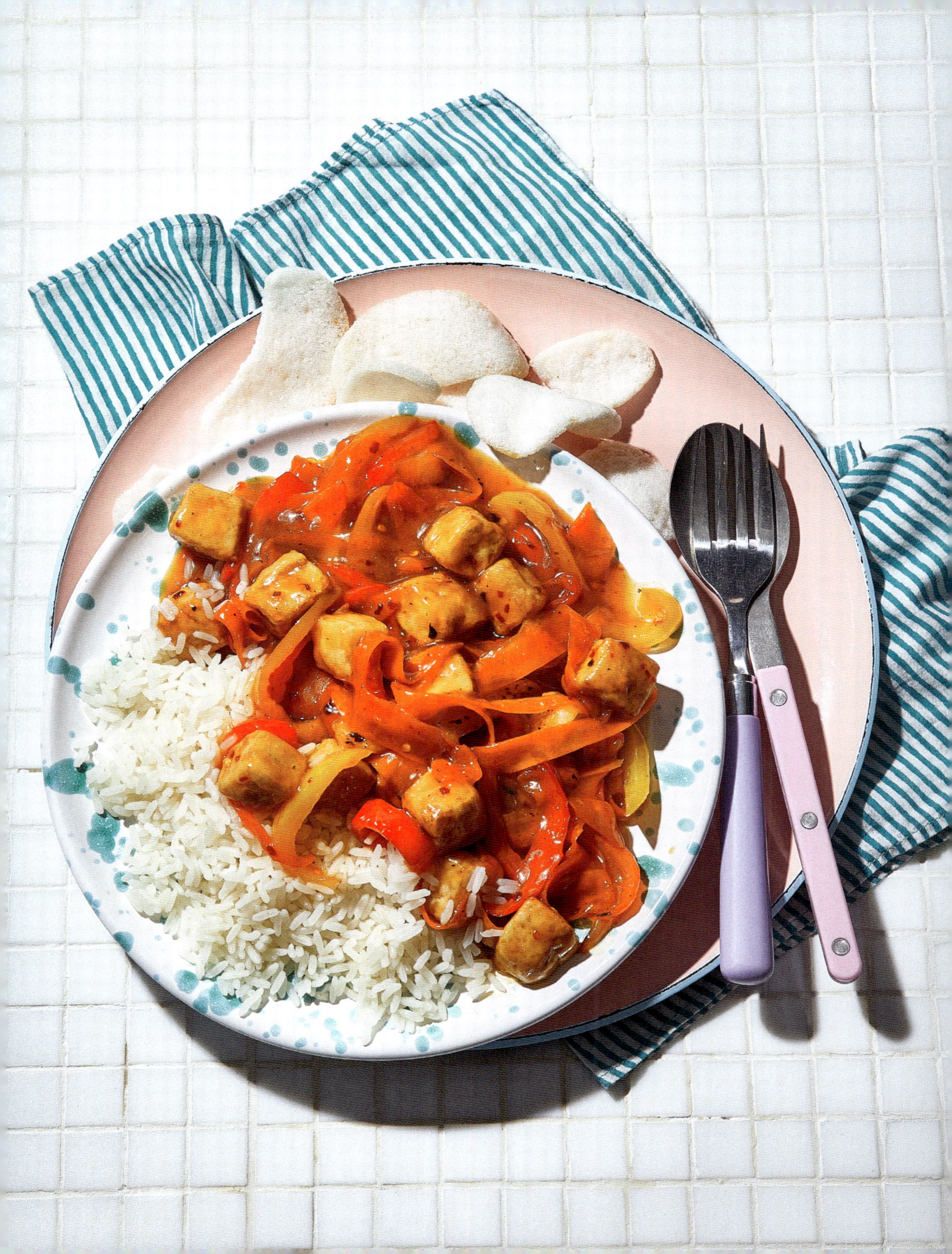

MARK'S 'HIGH FIVE' BRAISED PORK

When I smell the aroma of this wafting about the house as Mark is cooking, I know that dinner is going to be next level! This traditional-style Chinese pork dish features super-tender pork that's been braised for a melt-in-the-mouth texture in a sweet, sour and savoury five-spice coating. The addition of boiled eggs and veg brings an extra dimension to this dish, plus you probably won't be surprised to learn that pork belly is an excellent, cost-effective ingredient. If you're curious about the origin of the 'high five' nickname, Mark attributes it to the measurements for most of the ingredients (plus the inclusion of five spice!) which helps him to remember it so he doesn't need to look at a recipe to make it. However, I'm not sure I could personally remember everything off the top of my head like he can! Serve with jasmine rice.

Serves 5

Prep 15 mins

Hob only 1 hour or
Hob + Air Fryer 1 hour

DF **LF**

F Use light brown sugar instead of honey. Use leek (green parts only) instead of onion. Use 1 tbsp garlic-infused olive oil instead of garlic paste. Use 4 medium carrots, pared into ribbons using a swivel peeler, instead of mushrooms. Use low FODMAP stock.

❄ See freezing and defrosting guidance for soups, stews and curries on page 28.

- 5 large eggs
- 5 tbsp gluten-free soy sauce
- 1½ tbsp cornflour (cornstarch) or potato starch
- 5 tbsp honey
- 5 tbsp rice wine vinegar
- 1 tbsp Chinese five spice
- ½ tsp ground black pepper

- Vegetable oil spray
- 500g (1lb 2oz) pork belly, thinly sliced
- 100g (3½oz) frozen chopped onion **or** ½ medium leek, finely chopped
- 1 tsp garlic paste (optional)
- 500g (1lb 2oz) frozen sliced mushrooms

- 500ml (generous 2 cups) gluten-free ham or vegetable stock
- 150g (5½oz) frozen green beans
- Small handful of spring onion (scallion) greens, thinly sliced on the diagonal, to serve

Cook the eggs in a pan of boiling water for 7–8 minutes. (Alternatively, heat the air fryer to 150°C/300°F, place the eggs in the air fryer and cook for 10 minutes.) Remove and allow to cool until cool enough to handle, then peel them and set aside.

Meanwhile, in a small dish, combine the soy sauce and cornflour or potato starch until smooth, then stir in the honey, vinegar, five spice and pepper. Set aside.

Spray the base of a large pot that has a lid with oil and place over a medium-high heat. Once hot, add the pork and stir fry until liquid is released, then continue to fry until the water has evaporated and the pork is starting to brown.

Add the onion or leek and continue to stir fry until softened. Add the garlic paste, if using, and the frozen mushrooms. Once the mushrooms have softened and any water released has mostly evaporated, pour in the soy sauce mixture and allow it to bubble excitedly until reduced a little and starting to look a little sticky. At this point, add the stock and bring to the boil.

Reduce the heat to low and simmer for 45–50 minutes until thickened, adding the green beans and eggs for the final 15 minutes.

Remove the eggs, halve them, then add them to each plate when serving. Scatter the spring onion greens on top.

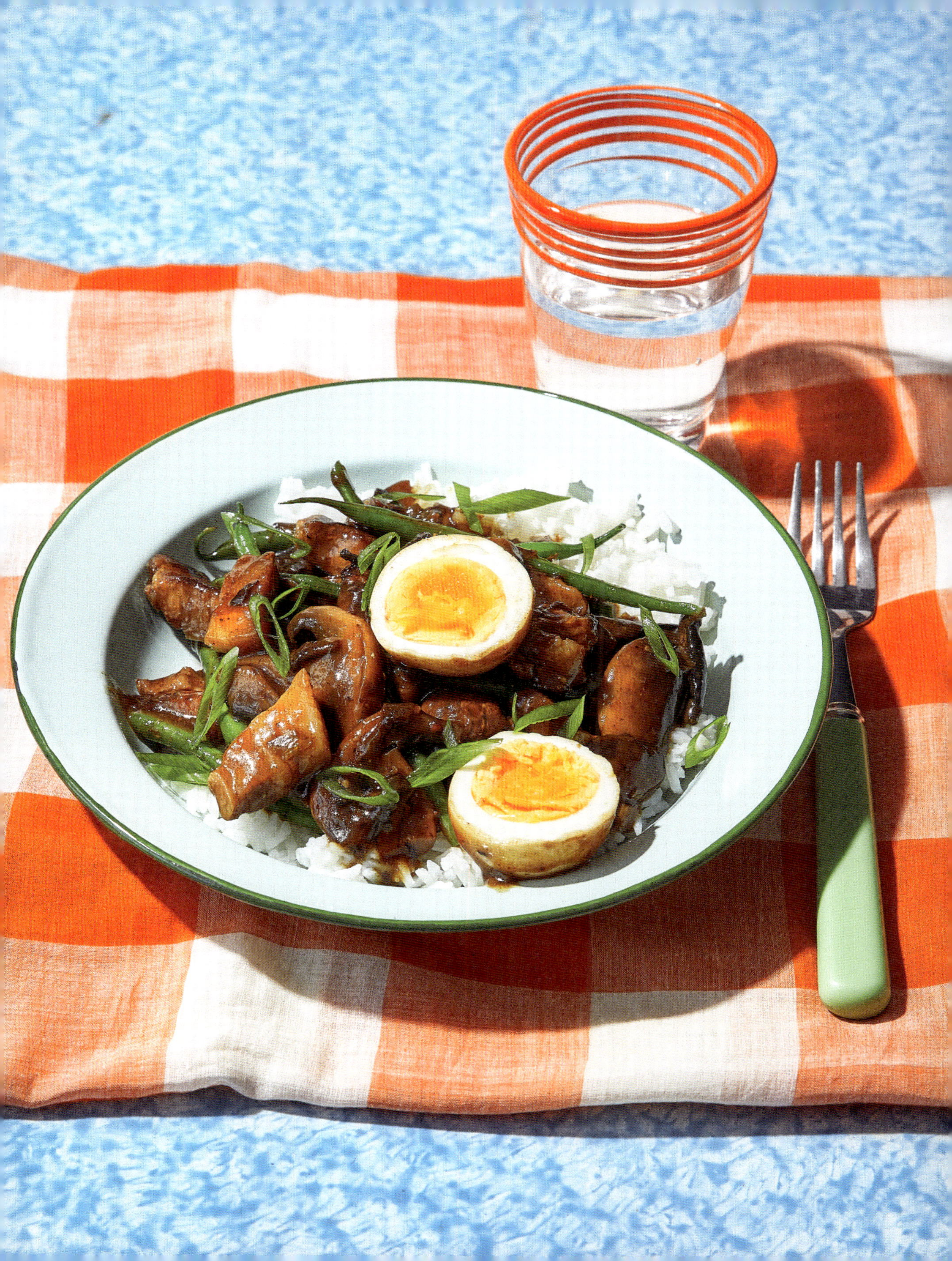

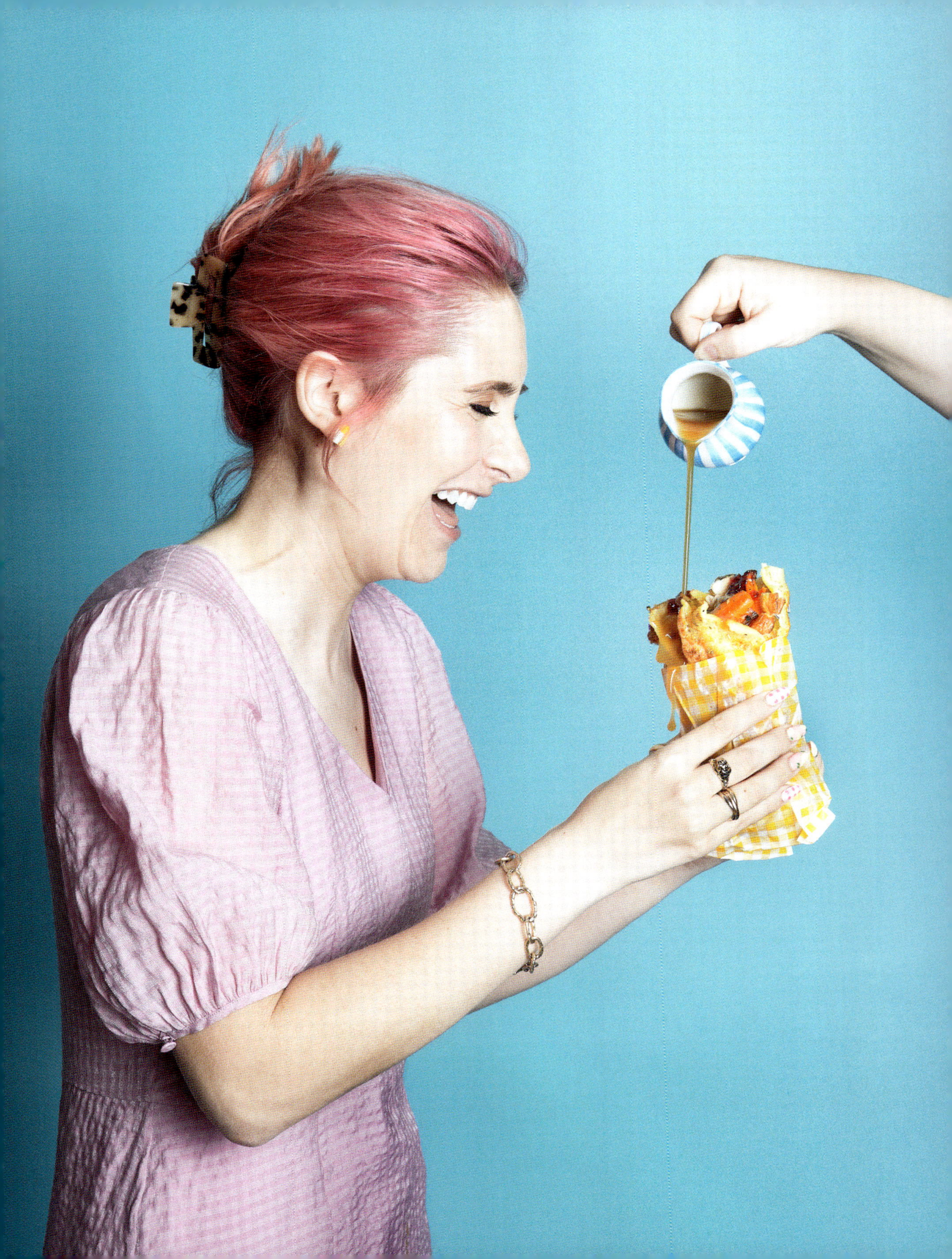

YORKSHIRE PUDDING WRAP

Makes 4
Prep 15 mins
Oven 1 hour 20 mins

DF Use dairy-free milk.

LF Use lactose-free milk.

V Swap the chicken for 500g (1lb 2oz) frozen cubed butternut squash. Use whatever gluten-free veggie-friendly stuffing you can get your hands on instead of making the pork stuffing, and use gluten-free vegetable gravy.

F Use lactose-free milk, use no more than 12g (¼oz) of apple sauce for the stuffing and serve with FODMAP-friendly gravy. Omit the cranberry sauce.

TIP

Although this recipe is intended for making Yorkshire pudding wraps with a roast dinner filling, if you'd rather you can very easily serve this up as a traditional roast dinner too. It might just be the easiest, simplest and most budget-friendly roast dinner you've ever made!

Believe it or not, one of the most popular street food options at most food markets I frequent is this unlikely contender: the contents of a roast dinner rolled up in a Yorkshire pud! But as creating a full roast dinner with chicken, potatoes, veg, stuffing and Yorkshire puds at home can be quite a mission (not forgetting the washing up afterwards), you'll be pleased to know I've infinitely streamlined the process especially for this recipe. All it now involves is making two massive Yorkshire puds in two rectangular roasting tins, then I've turned the rest of the filling effectively into two traybakes of chicken, potatoes and carrots, along with the stuffing in a separate tin. These quantities are much too big to stand a chance of fitting into your air fryer all at once (like they can in the oven) and you'd end up having to make everything separately, which is why this remains an oven-exclusive recipe!

For the Yorkshire pudding wraps

- 4 tbsp vegetable oil, plus oil spray
- 200g (1⅔ cups) cornflour (cornstarch) or tapioca starch
- 6 medium eggs
- 300ml (1¼ cups) milk
- 2 pinches of salt
- 3 tsp dried or fresh rosemary (optional)

For the roasted veg

- 1kg (2lb 3oz) Maris Piper potatoes, peeled and cut into 2cm (¾in) chunks
- 6 medium carrots, peeled and cut into sticks 1cm (½in) thick and 5cm (2in) long

- 1 tsp salt
- ½ tsp ground black pepper

For the chicken

- 6 skin-on, bone-in chicken thighs
- 1 tbsp dried sage or mixed herbs
- ½ tsp salt
- ½ tsp ground black pepper
- ½ tbsp vegetable oil

For the stuffing

- 500g (1lb 2oz) minced (ground) pork (20% fat)
- 3 tbsp apple sauce
- 4 tbsp cornflour (cornstarch)
- 1 tbsp dried sage

- ½ tsp salt
- Pinch of ground black pepper
- Small handful of spring onion (scallion) greens, roughly chopped

To serve

- Enough gluten-free gravy granules to make 400ml (1⅔ cups) chicken or vegetable gravy (or use homemade chicken gravy from page 163)
- 4–8 tbsp cranberry sauce

To make the Yorkshire pudding wraps, preheat the oven to 200°C fan/ 220°C (425°F) and arrange the shelves so that there's equal space between them. Grab 2 rectangular roasting tins (pans), about 23 x 33cm (9 x 13in) and 5cm (2in) deep, and add 2 tablespoons of vegetable oil to each. Place in the oven for 10–12 minutes until very hot.

While the oil is heating, add the cornflour or tapioca starch and the eggs to a large bowl and whisk together until smooth, then add half of the milk and whisk until free of lumps. Whisk in the remaining milk, the salt and rosemary, if using.

continued overleaf

Remove the roasting tins from the oven and quickly pour half of the batter into each one – it should sizzle a little. Immediately return to the oven. Cook for 20–22 minutes until browned, crispy and miraculously increased in size. Never open the oven during cooking to check on it, as this will cause it to instantly deflate! Remove the Yorkshire puddings to a wire rack.

To make the roasted veg and chicken, spread the potatoes and carrots out in the same two roasting tins. Spray well with oil, then season both with the salt and pepper. Turn everything over a few times until the veg is evenly coated in the oil and seasoning, then spray all over with oil once more.

To a large (cleaned) bowl, add the chicken thighs, sage or mixed herbs, salt, pepper and oil, then briefly mix until well coated. Make space in the roasting tins for the chicken, then add 3 thighs to each tin (or just lay them on top if there's not much space). Roast for 10 minutes.

To make the pork stuffing, lightly spray a 23cm (9in) square (or round if you don't have a square one) baking tin (pan) with oil.

In the large bowl (no need to clean it again this time) mix all the stuffing ingredients well with a wooden spoon until smooth. Transfer to the baking tin and press down with the back of the wooden spoon into a flat, even layer.

Once the chicken and veg has been in for 10 minutes, place the stuffing tin in the oven and roast everything for a further 45 minutes or until the chicken is golden brown, turning the veg and chicken halfway. While waiting, mix up the gluten-free gravy granules in a jug (pitcher) according to the packet instructions and have ready the cranberry sauce. Once everything is cooked, allow the chicken to rest for 5–10 minutes.

To construct the wraps, while the chicken is resting, cut both Yorkshire puddings across in half using a pizza cutter to create 2 squares, then transfer to a board and roll flat with a rolling pin. As the puds have likely almost cooled completely by now, place in the oven for 5 minutes on the shelf racks to warm up again, then switch off the oven and keep them warm while you prepare the filling.

Transfer the rested chicken to the board and shred with 2 forks until you've removed all the meat from the bone. If you have guests, it can be fun to plate up the chicken, carrots, roast potatoes and stuffing, along with the jug of gluten-free gravy, a small dish of cranberry sauce and a pile of the warm Yorkshire pudding wraps, and allow them to create their own filled Yorkshire pudding wraps.

Otherwise, simply lay each Yorkshire pudding wrap flat on a plate, fill with chicken, carrots, roast potatoes and stuffing, drizzle on the gravy and dollop on the cranberry sauce. Fold the bottom of the Yorkshire pudding upwards so it overlaps the filling by around an inch, then fold over the left and right sides of the wrap and turn over so it's resting on the plate seam side down. Repeat until you've made 4 in total, then serve.

MANGO CHUTNEY STICKY CHICKEN DRUMSTICKS
WITH PILAF RICE

Serves 4

Prep 10 mins

Hob + Oven 35 mins or
Hob + Air Fryer 30 mins

It couldn't be easier to transform an ever affordable pack of chicken drumsticks into sweet and sticky, curried chicken that tastes like it was flame grilled right on the BBQ. Best of all, when served with a minty or herby yoghurt dip and speedy pilaf-style rice on the side, this is a budget-friendly, all-in-one fakeaway meal that comes together surprisingly fast.

DF Use a dairy-free 'buttery' margarine and a thick dairy-free yoghurt instead of Greek yoghurt.

LF Use a lactose-free 'buttery' margarine and lactose-free Greek yoghurt.

F See lactose-free advice; brush with maple syrup instead of mango chutney (no need to add the water); use leek (green parts only) instead of onion; use all green (bell) peppers instead of mixed colours; and use no more than 28g (1oz) of sultanas.

❄ Once cooled, store the chicken and rice in separate airtight containers and freeze for up to 2–3 months. Allow the chicken to defrost completely in the fridge, then reheat in the air fryer for 8–10 minutes at 200°C (400°F). Check the internal temperature with a digital food thermometer against those given on page 255. For advice on reheating the rice from frozen, see the freezing and defrosting guidance for risotto and rice dishes on page 28.

- 1kg (2lb 3oz) chicken drumsticks
- 1 tbsp smoked paprika
- 2 tbsp mild curry powder
- 1 tsp ground turmeric
- ½ tsp cayenne pepper
- 1 tsp salt
- 1 tbsp ginger paste
- 200g (1 cup minus 1 tbsp) Greek or natural yoghurt
- Vegetable oil spray
- 2 tbsp mango chutney mixed with 1 tbsp water

For the rice
- 2 tbsp 'buttery' margarine

- 100g (3½oz) frozen chopped onion **or** ½ medium leek, finely chopped
- 300g (10½oz) frozen sliced red, green and yellow (bell) peppers
- ½ tsp ground cinnamon
- 1 tsp mild curry powder
- 1 tsp ground turmeric
- ½ tsp ground black pepper
- 1 tsp salt
- 300g (1⅔ cups) basmati or long-grain rice
- 800ml (3⅓ cups) boiling water

- 200g (7oz) frozen green beans
- 50g (1¾oz) sultanas (golden raisins), roughly chopped (optional)
- 2 tbsp flaked (slivered) almonds, toasted (optional)

For the yoghurt dip
- 125g (generous ½ cup) Greek or natural yoghurt
- 1 tbsp dried mint or dried mixed herbs
- Grated zest of ½ lemon
- Pinch each of salt and ground black pepper
- 2–3 tbsp water

Add the drumsticks, smoked paprika, curry powder, turmeric, cayenne pepper, salt, ginger paste and yoghurt to a large bowl and mix well until well combined and the chicken is coated.

To cook in an oven, preheat the oven to 200°C fan/220°C (425°F). Set a grill (broiler) pan wire rack over a large baking tray lined with foil and generously spray the rack with oil. Place the drumsticks on the rack, spaced apart so they're not touching,

then bake in the oven for 35 minutes, turning them over halfway with a pair of tongs (give them a wiggle to loosen them before lifting) and spraying both sides with oil. Once done, brush both sides with the mango chutney and water mixture and turn the oven down to 120°C fan/140°C (285°F). Keep them warm in the oven until the rice is done.

continued overleaf

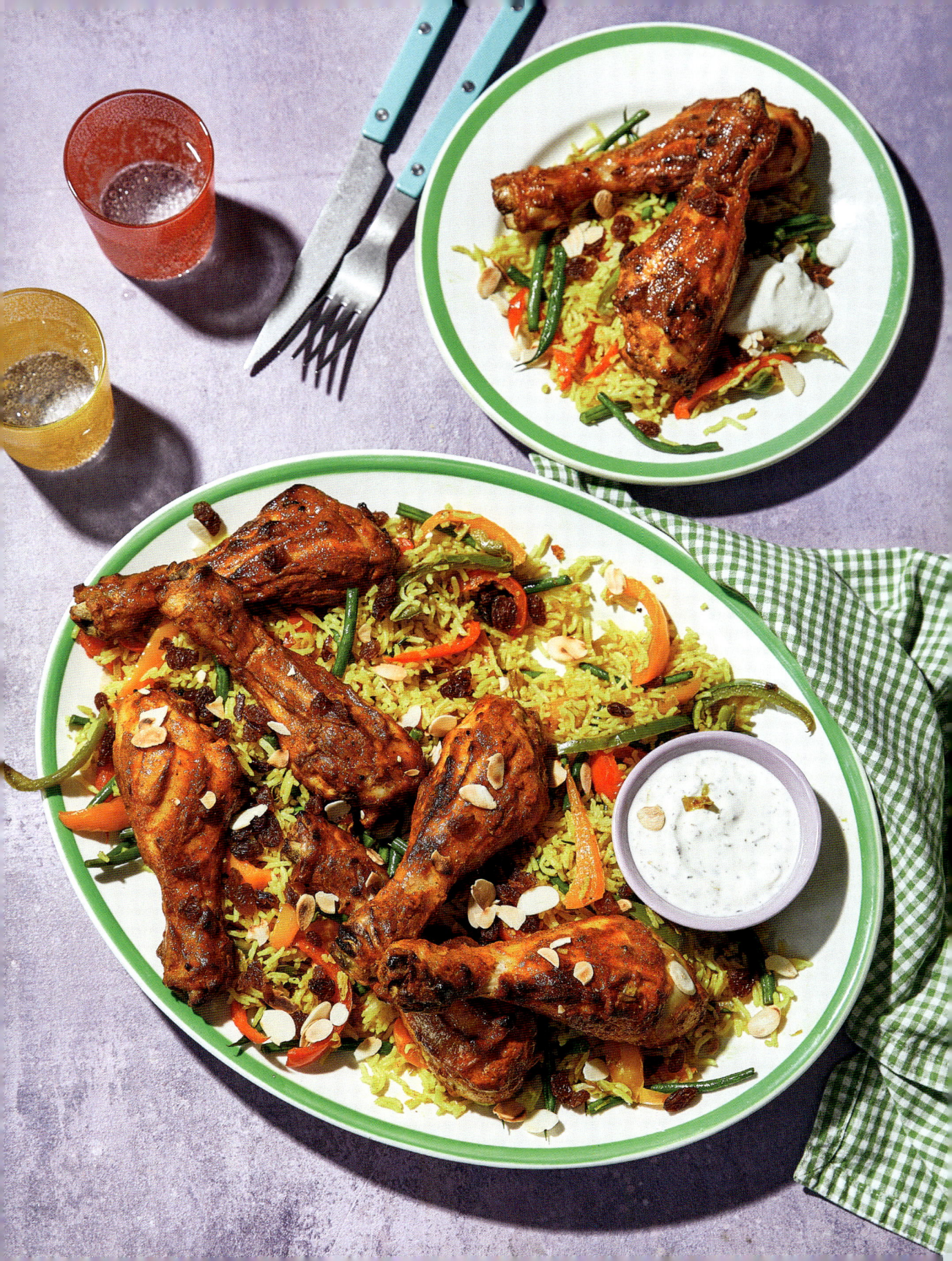

To cook in an air fryer, heat the air fryer to 200°C (400°F). Generously spray the base of the air fryer basket or crisping tray with oil. If you have an air fryer with 2 drawers, you'll likely need to employ both, so grease both if necessary. Place as many drumsticks as will fit in the air fryer basket without touching and air fry for 18–20 minutes, turning them over halfway and spraying lightly with oil on both sides.

Once done, brush both sides with the mango chutney and water mixture and keep warm in the (closed) air fryer until the rice is cooked.

Meanwhile, for the rice, place a large pot that has a lid over a medium heat and add the margarine. Once melted, add the onion or leek and fry until the onion is browned or the leek has lightly browned in places.

Add the frozen peppers and turn the heat to high. Fry until water is released and the peppers have softened, then add all the spices, the salt and the rice. Stir in and fry until fragrant for around 2–3 minutes.

Add the boiling water and frozen green beans and stir. Pop the lid on and simmer for 20–25 minutes or until the rice is cooked. Meanwhile, mix together the ingredients for the yoghurt dipping sauce in a small bowl.

Scatter the sultanas and flaked almonds, if using, over the rice and serve the rice alongside the chicken with dollops of the dipping sauce.

MARK'S MONGOLIAN BEEF STIR FRY

Serves 3–4

Prep 5 mins

Hob 20 mins

Mark's transformation of this Chinese-American takeout favourite from a stand-alone dish into an all-in-one complete meal is one that regularly features on our meal plans. With everything enveloped in a sticky honey, soy and ginger coating, this truly is a fast food fakeaway at its very best! Mongolian beef is commonly made with costly cuts of steak, but by using minced (ground) beef and turning it into a full-on stir fry (an extremely cost effective dish!), Mark's recipe is as thrifty as it is flavourful.

DF **LF**

F Use light brown sugar instead of honey, all green (bell) peppers instead of mixed colours, and 1 tbsp garlic-infused oil instead of garlic paste.

V Swap the chicken for 400g (14oz) firm tofu, prepared and cooked as in the crispy chilli tofu recipe on page 98.

VE See veggie advice and use light brown sugar instead of honey.

❄ Once cooled, store in airtight containers for up to 2–3 months. Allow to defrost completely in the fridge, then reheat in the air fryer for 8–9 minutes at 200°C (400°F), turning them over two or three times during cooking.

TIP

It can be hard to stir fry in larger quantities, so if you're not tossing the contents of your wok like a professional chef, simply use two wooden spatulas to keep turning everything over constantly. This is important to stop the bottom from burning and also to ensure everything cooks evenly!

- 300g (10½oz) dried ribbon rice noodles
- 4 tbsp gluten-free soy sauce
- 1 tbsp cornflour (cornstarch) or potato starch
- 4 tbsp honey
- 100ml (generous ⅓ cup) water
- 2 tbsp vegetable oil, plus oil spray

- ½ tsp salt
- ¼ tsp ground black pepper
- 2 medium carrots, pared into ribbons using a swivel peeler
- 250g (9oz) frozen sliced red, green and yellow (bell) peppers
- 500g (1lb 2oz) minced (ground) beef

- 1 tbsp jarred jalapeños, finely chopped
- 1 tbsp ginger paste
- 1 tsp garlic paste (optional)
- 150g (5½oz) beansprouts
- Small handful of spring onion (scallion) greens, thinly sliced on the diagonal

Prepare the rice noodles according to the packet instructions – I simply place mine in a saucepan of just-boiled water for 4–5 minutes, drain and set aside.

Add the soy sauce and cornflour or potato starch to a small dish and combine until smooth. Stir in the honey, water, oil, salt and pepper, and set aside.

Lightly spray the base and sides of a large wok with oil and place over a high heat. Once hot, add the carrot ribbons and stir fry until softened, then add the peppers and continue to stir fry until any water released has mostly evaporated. Add the beef and stir fry until browned, then add the jalapeños, ginger paste and garlic paste, if using. Stir well to coat everything.

Pour in the soy sauce mixture (stir briefly before adding) and allow it to bubble excitedly until reduced a little and starting to look a little sticky. At this point, add the drained noodles and stir fry for 2–3 minutes until the noodles are well coated and everything is evenly dispersed. Stir in the beansprouts.

At this point, everything is essentially done but due to the volume of food, it can still be quite wet. To finish off the dish, use the high heat of the wok to continue to stir fry for 5–6 minutes until you get a little extra char on everything and the coating starts to look a little shiny and sticky.

Garnish with the sliced spring onion greens and serve.

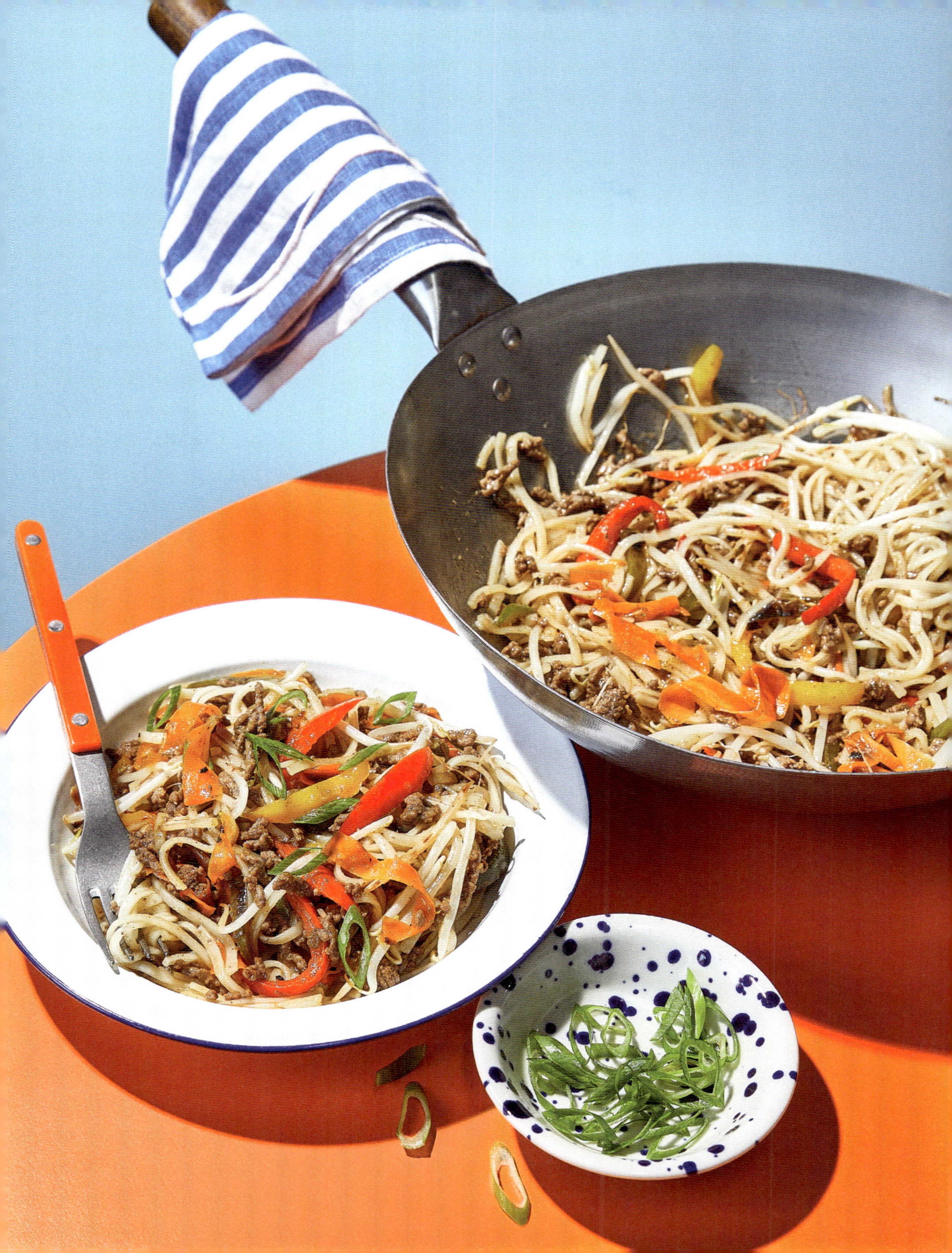

GOAN-STYLE FISH CURRY

This fish curry is inspired by a rather famous dish from Goa in India; however, the first time I experienced it was at Glastonbury festival after queuing for hours at an extremely popular curry van! And it's exactly that version that I aimed to recreate in this recipe, featuring a creamy, coconut curry sauce with so much depth of flavour, packed with flaky white fish and crisp, roasted broccoli and cauliflower. The price of frozen white fish (usually pollock, which is commonly used in fish fingers here in the UK) is astoundingly low compared to buying fresh fillets of cod, so make sure you take advantage of that by using it in this recipe. Serve with rice and gluten-free naan.

Serves 3–4

Prep 5 mins

Hob + Oven 35 mins or
Hob + Air Fryer 25 mins

DF **LF**

V Swap the fish for 2 x 400g (14oz) cans of drained chickpeas.

VE See veggie advice.

❄ See freezing and defrosting guidance for soups, stews and curries on page 28.

TIPS

This recipe uses a few different pastes: chilli, tamarind and ginger. All of these can be found in supermarkets in the world food section (usually the cheapest place to find them) or near the spices or Asian cooking ingredients. You'll usually find them in jars, and if you always store them in the fridge and use a clean spoon to portion them out, they'll last for a very long time! The bigger the jar, the better value it'll be.

The size of frozen broccoli and cauliflower florets can vary, meaning smaller florets can overcook while large florets remain uncooked in the middle. To combat this, you can allow them to defrost at room temperature, then chop down to more consistent sizes.

- Vegetable oil spray
- 300g (10½oz) frozen cauliflower florets
- 300g (10½oz) frozen broccoli florets
- 100g (3½oz) frozen chopped onion or ½ medium leek, finely chopped
- 1 x 400g (14oz) can of coconut milk
- 520g (1lb 2oz) frozen white fish fillets
- Small handful of coriander (cilantro) leaves, roughly chopped, to serve (optional)

For the curry paste
- 1 tsp chilli paste **or** ½ tsp dried chilli flakes
- 1 tsp tamarind paste
- 1 tbsp ginger paste
- 1 tbsp tomato purée (paste)
- 1 tsp ground turmeric
- 1 tsp mild curry powder
- ½ tsp ground black pepper
- 1 tsp salt

Combine the curry paste ingredients in a small dish and set aside.

To cook the cauliflower and broccoli in an oven, preheat the oven to 200°C fan/220°C (425°F). Spray a large baking tray with vegetable oil. Add the frozen cauliflower and broccoli florets to the tray, spray all over with oil and bake in the oven for 30–35 minutes, turning them over halfway, until lightly blackened in places and fork-tender.

To cook the cauliflower and broccoli in an air fryer, heat the air fryer to 200°C (400°F). Add the cauliflower and broccoli florets to the air fryer (making sure they're touching as little as possible) and spray generously with oil, then air fry for 20 minutes until browned at the edges and fork-tender, shaking them halfway (or 3 or 4 times if particularly piled up).

Meanwhile, spray the base of a large pot that has a lid with oil and place over a medium heat. Once hot, add the onion or leek and fry until the onion is browned or the leek has softened. Add the curry paste and fry for 30 seconds or until fragrant, then add a third of the coconut milk and stir well. Bring to a rapid bubble before stirring in the rest of the coconut milk. Add the frozen fish, pop the lid on and reduce the heat to low–medium for around 10 minutes, or until the fish is cooked through.

Remove the lid and break the fish fillets into bite-sized chunks. Take off the heat and optionally allow to cool for 10 minutes – it will thicken more as it cools. Stir in the roasted or air fried veg just before serving.

Sprinkle the coriander over to serve, if using.

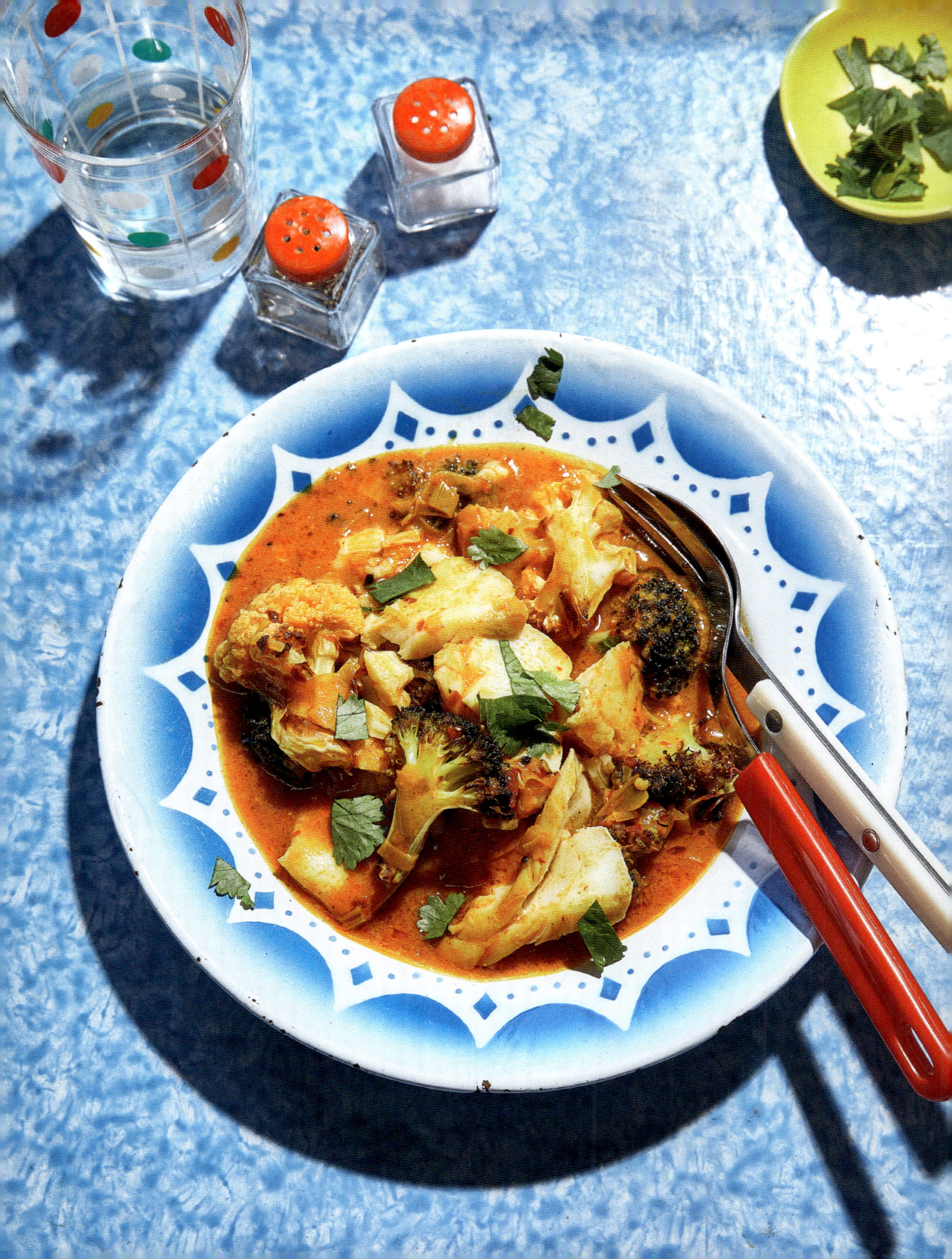

SCRAMBLED EGG SCALLION PANCAKE

Makes 2

Prep 5 mins

Hob 15 mins

Here's my gluten-free take on this popular Asian street food favourite that's perfect for lunch or a light, speedy supper: crisp spring onion pancakes folded and filled with omelette and cheese, dipped in sweet chilli sauce. Despite the inherent humble, affordable ingredients, every bite is bursting with flavour, and the dish can be whipped up in around 15 minutes.

V

DF Use squares of dairy-free cheese that melt well.

LL Use mature Cheddar instead of American-style cheese.

F See low lactose advice and use low FODMAP sweet chilli sauce.

For the pancakes
- 100g (¾ cup) gluten-free plain (all-purpose) flour
- 2 large eggs
- 180ml (¾ cup) water
- 1 tsp Chinese five spice
- 2 pinches of salt

- 2 small handfuls of spring onion (scallion) greens, sliced on the diagonal
- Vegetable oil spray
- 2 slices of American-style cheese or 80g (2¾oz) mature Cheddar, grated

For the omelettes
- 4 eggs
- 2 pinches of salt

For the dipping sauce
- 4 tbsp sweet chilli sauce (ensure gluten-free)
- ½ tsp gluten-free soy sauce

For the pancakes, add the flour and eggs to a large bowl and whisk together until smooth. Whisk in almost all the water – the consistency should be just a little thicker than water, so if you're already there, don't add any more; if it's still looking a bit on the thick side, add the rest of the water. Stir in the five spice, salt and spring onion greens.

Place a medium frying pan or crêpe pan over a medium heat and spray generously with oil. Once hot, pour half the batter into the centre of the pan. Lift the pan and use a circular tilting motion to help the batter spread as much as possible.

Fry for 3–4 minutes or until the edges are starting to look cooked, then flip and cook for a further 1–2 minutes. Remove from the pan to a plate, spray the pan again with oil and repeat for the second pancake.

Spray the pan once more and beat 2 of the omelette eggs in a small bowl, then add a pinch of salt. Add the beaten eggs to the pan – they should immediately start sizzling – and very gently stir for the first 20 seconds. Allow to fry for 1 minute, then lay a pancake on top and gently press down with the back of a spatula. Fry for 2–4 minutes or until golden brown on the bottom, then flip and place the cheese on one side of the omelette. Fry for a further 1–2 minutes, then fold shut like a book. Lift out onto a plate and repeat for the second omelette and pancake.

In a small dish, combine the sweet chilli sauce and soy sauce, then serve with the pancakes.

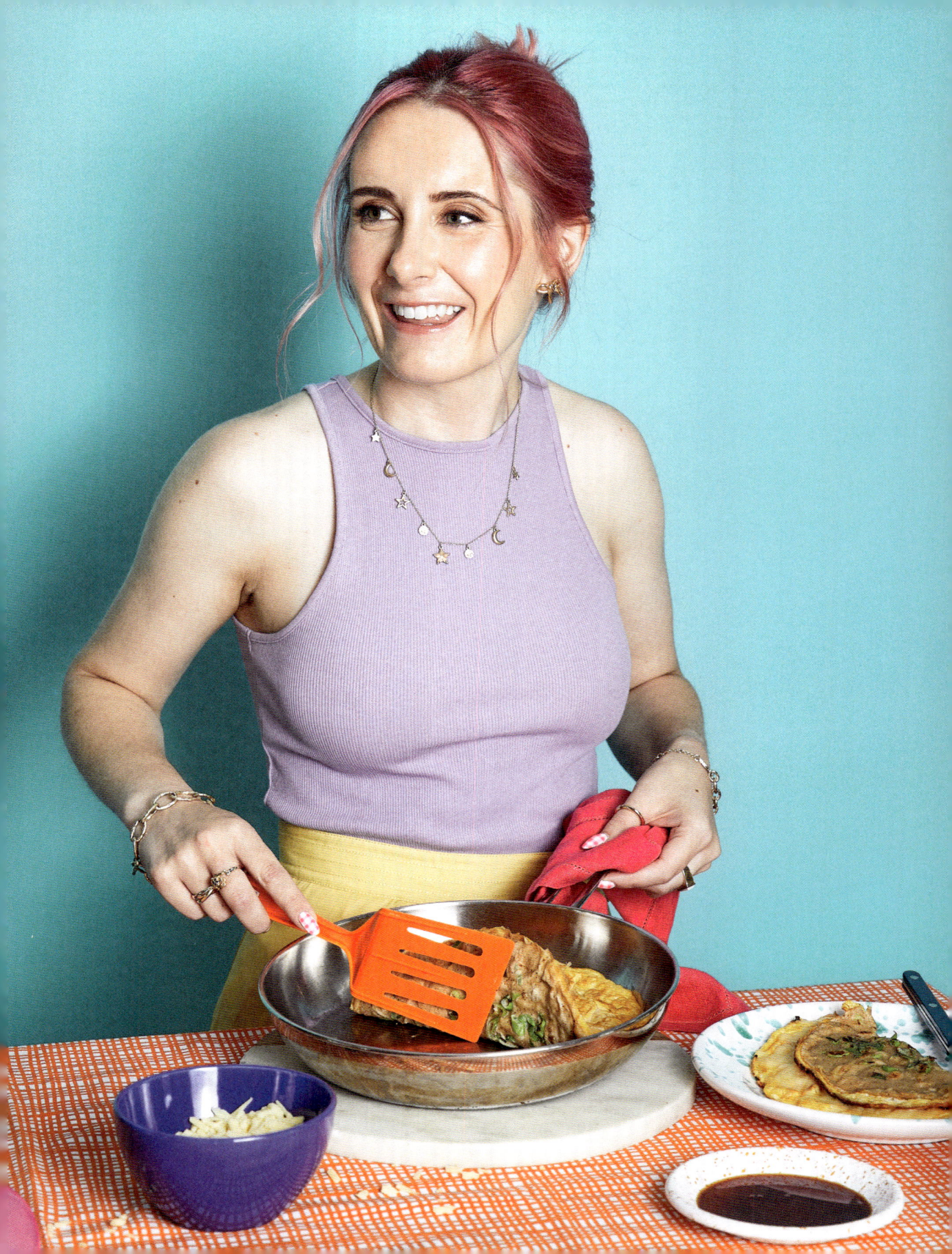

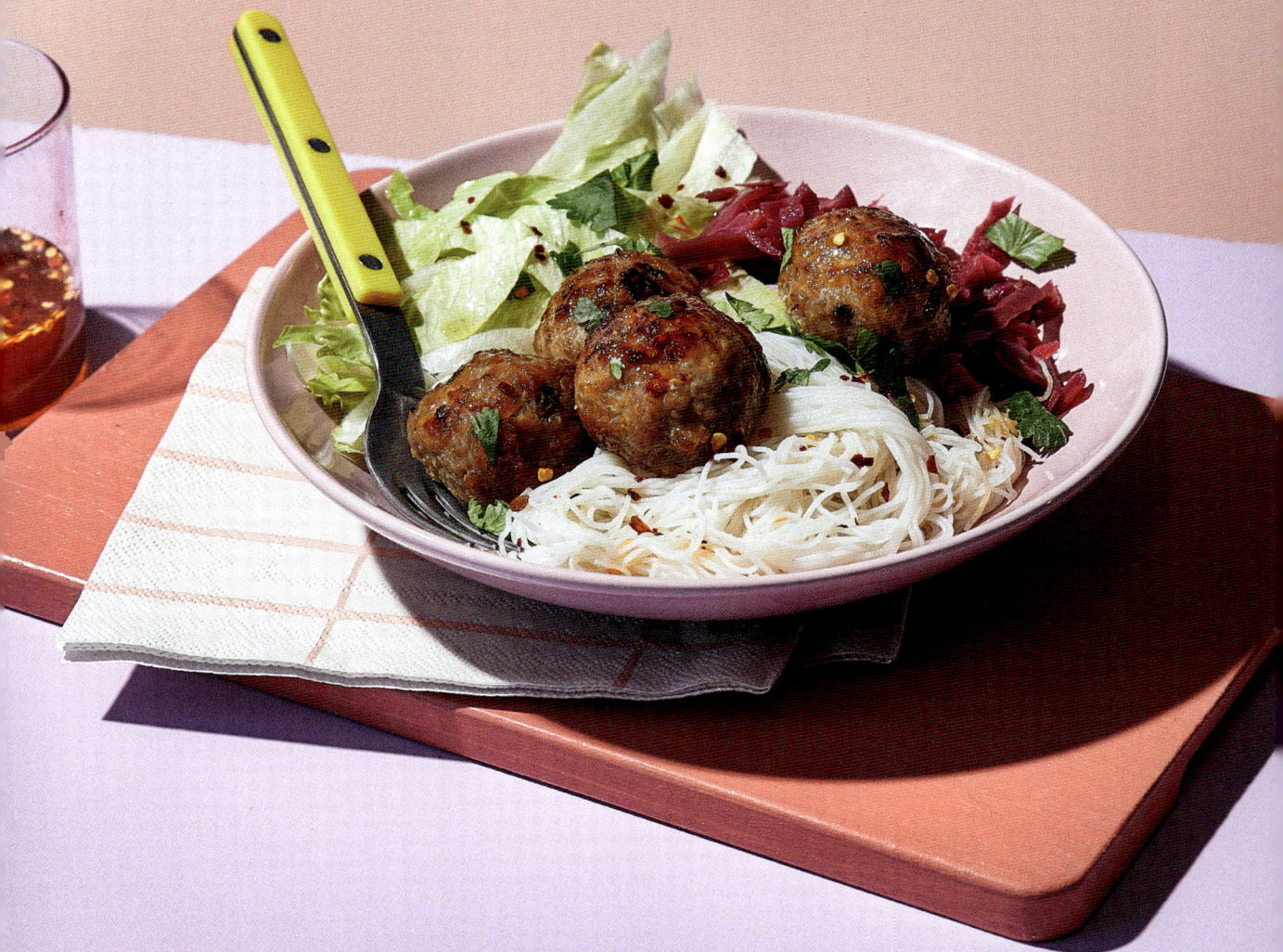

VIETNAMESE-STYLE MEATBALLS (BÚN CHẢ)

Serves 4

Prep 10 mins

Oven 25 mins or
Air Fryer 15 mins

Though I'm yet to visit Vietnam, we've been lucky enough to have lots of wonderful Vietnamese restaurants open in London over the last two decades or so. And I'm sure you won't be surprised to hear that I've always been a frequent visitor, as so many of my favourite dishes are served with rice noodles! Sadly, I can't always visit London when I specifically crave these seriously addictive ginger and lemongrass pork meatballs, so that's where this recipe comes in! Minced (ground) pork is usually on par with the price of the cheapest beef and for the rest of the magic, you'll mostly need store-cupboard, budget-friendly ingredients.

DF **LF**

F Use maple syrup instead of honey.

❄ Once cooled, store the meatballs and noodles in separate airtight containers and freeze for up to 2–3 months. Allow both to defrost completely in the fridge, then reheat the meatballs in the air fryer for 7–9 minutes at 200°C (400°F), turning them over once during cooking. Reheat the noodles in the microwave (covered) for 2–4 minutes at full power, turning everything over halfway.

For the meatballs
- 500g (1lb 2oz) minced (ground) pork
- 1½ tbsp fish sauce
- 2 tbsp honey or light brown sugar
- 1 tsp ginger paste
- 1½ tsp lemongrass paste
- 2 tbsp cornflour (cornstarch) or potato starch
- Small handful of spring onion (scallion) greens, thinly sliced

- ½ tsp salt
- ½ tsp ground black pepper
- Vegetable oil spray

For the nước chấm dressing
- 5 tbsp honey
- 6 tbsp fish sauce
- 3 tbsp rice wine vinegar
- Juice of 1 lime
- 1½ tsp chilli paste or ¾ tsp dried chilli flakes
- 4 tbsp water

To serve
- 300–400g (10½–14oz) dried vermicelli rice noodles
- ½ iceberg lettuce, shredded
- 6–8 tbsp pickled red cabbage
- Small handful of coriander (cilantro) leaves, roughly chopped (optional)

TIP

While lemongrass paste used to be easily available in small jars in all supermarkets, as of late it has become a little trickier to find. If you can't find it in your local supermarket, feel free to use fresh lemongrass (with two of the outer layers peeled off and then finely grated) – you'll find it in the fresh veg section – or substitute it for the zest of 1 small lemon.

Add all the meatball ingredients except the oil to a large bowl and mix well until everything is evenly dispersed. Roll into ping-pong-sized balls (about 35g/1¼oz each, making 16 meatballs).

To cook the meatballs in an oven, preheat the oven to 180°C fan/200°C (400°F). Spray a large baking sheet with oil. Place the meatballs on the baking sheet and bake for 20–25 minutes, or until golden brown, turning them over halfway.

To cook the meatballs in an air fryer, heat the air fryer to 190°C (375°F). Generously spray the base of the air fryer basket or crisping tray with oil. If you have an air fryer with 2 drawers, grease both. Place as many meatballs as will fit in the air fryer basket(s) without touching and generously spray with oil. Air fry for 12–15 minutes until crisp and golden brown, turning them over halfway.

Meanwhile, combine the dressing ingredients in a bowl, then divide between 4 small serving bowls, ready for serving. Cook the noodles according to the packet instructions (I simply place mine in a pan of just-boiled water for 4–5 minutes) then drain and keep warm.

Serve up the rice noodles alongside a handful of shredded lettuce, pickled red cabbage, 4 meatballs per person and a scattering of coriander, if using. Serve alongside the portioned dressing, which should be poured over the dish just before serving.

KOREAN-STYLE BULGOGI BEEF OR PORK

This deeply flavourful Korean-inspired dish traditionally features super-thin slices of tender, sticky beef that are bursting with umami flavour. However, in case you didn't notice, the price of any beef steak in supermarkets is quite shocking when you consider how little you're usually getting. So, because of that, I often use thin-cut beef steaks, which nets you a generous amount for a reasonable price. Or, for a change that's a third cheaper than beef, pork loin steaks work extremely well too – and you get more in the packet!

Serves 3

Prep 10 mins + 15 mins marinating

Hob 10 mins

DF **LF**

F
Use light brown sugar instead of honey, apple instead of pear, and swap the garlic paste for ½ tbsp garlic-infused oil. Use leeks (green parts only) instead of onion.

❄
Once cooled, store the beef filling in airtight containers and freeze for up to 2–3 months. Allow to defrost completely in the fridge, then reheat in the microwave (covered) for 4–5 minutes at full power. Check internal temperature with a digital food thermometer against those given on page 255.

- 395g (14oz) thin-cut beef steaks **or** 480g (1lb 1oz) pork loin steaks, cut into 3mm (⅛in) slices
- Vegetable oil spray
- 100g (3½oz) frozen chopped onion **or** ½ medium leek, finely chopped
- 2 medium carrots, pared into ribbons using a swivel peeler
- 2 tbsp toasted sesame seeds, plus a little extra to serve
- 1–2 little gem lettuce, leaves separated or shredded

For the marinade
- 4 tbsp gluten-free soy sauce
- 2 tbsp honey
- 1 tbsp rice wine vinegar
- ½ red apple or pear, grated
- ½ tsp ginger paste
- ½ tsp garlic paste (optional)
- Small handful of spring onions (scallions), green parts only, finely sliced
- ½ tsp ground black pepper

In a large bowl, combine all the marinade ingredients. Add the slices of beef or pork, cover and marinate in the fridge for anywhere from 15 minutes to 12 hours.

Lightly spray the base and sides of a large wok with oil and place over a high heat. Once hot, add the onion or leek and fry until softened. Add the carrot ribbons and stir fry until softened, then add the beef or pork and all of the marinade. Stir fry for 3–5 minutes until the beef or pork is cooked through, but don't overdo it. Stir through the sesame seeds.

Serve with rice alongside shredded lettuce, or fill the lettuce leaves with the bulgogi and enjoy as wraps. Scatter the extra sesame seeds on top.

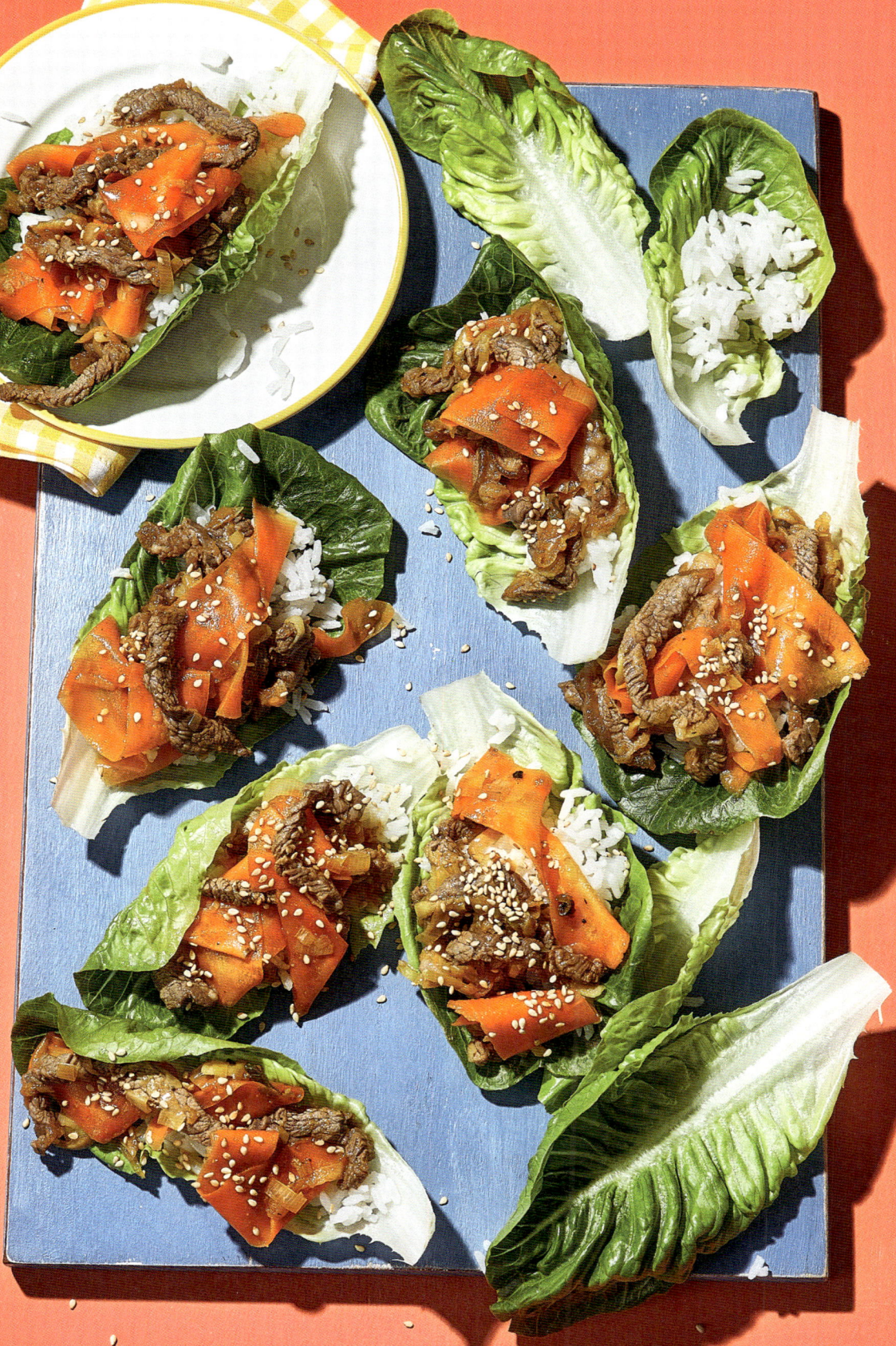

VIETNAMESE-STYLE GINGER CHICKEN (GÀ KHO GỪNG)

Serves 4

Prep 5 mins

Air Fryer 18 mins or
Hob 25 mins

This dish isn't commonly made with cabbage or carrot, but these affordable ingredients help to make it go further and ensure it's more of a full meal; doing things this way means I don't have to prepare veg separately to serve with it. As an unexpected result, the cabbage is now one of my favourite parts of this dish!

DF **LF**

F Omit the garlic paste or use ½ tbsp garlic-infused oil instead, use light brown sugar/maple syrup instead of honey, and serve no more than 40g (1½oz) cabbage per person. Use leeks (green parts only) instead of onion.

❄ Once cooled, store in airtight containers for up to 2–3 months. Allow to defrost completely in the fridge, then reheat in the air fryer for 8–9 minutes at 200°C (400°F), turning them over halfway during cooking.

- 3 tbsp fish sauce
- 3 tbsp honey
- 1 tsp cornflour (cornstarch) or potato starch
- Vegetable oil spray
- 400–500g (14–17oz) skinless, boneless chicken thighs or breast, cut into 5mm (¼in) strips
- ½ tsp salt
- ¼ tsp ground black pepper
- 3 medium carrots, pared into ribbons using a swivel peeler
- 100g (3½oz) frozen chopped onion **or** ½ medium leek, finely chopped
- 1 tsp garlic paste (optional)
- 2 tsp ginger paste
- 300g (10½oz) green cabbage, such as Savoy or sweetheart, shredded
- 300–400g (10½–14oz) dried vermicelli rice noodles

To serve
- Handful of spring onion (scallion) greens, thinly sliced on the diagonal
- ½ cucumber, thinly sliced into rounds

In a small dish, combine the fish sauce, honey and cornflour or potato starch, then set aside.

To cook in the air fryer, heat the air fryer to 200°C (400°F) and spray the base (basket or crisping tray removed) with oil. If you have an air fryer with 2 drawers, use both. Place as many chicken strips as will fit in the air fryer without touching, spray with oil and season with the salt and pepper. Air fry thighs for 5–6 minutes or breast for 3–4 minutes until sealed on both sides.

Add the carrot ribbons, onion or leek, garlic paste, if using, and ginger paste to the air fryer, then add the cabbage and stir in well. Air fry for a further 8 minutes before adding the sauce mixture and mixing everything well to coat. Air fry for a final 2–3 minutes until the sauce is sticky and no longer wet.

To cook on the hob, spray a wok with oil and place over a medium heat. Once hot, add the chicken. Fry thighs for 10–12 minutes or breast for 5–6

minutes, turning them halfway, until golden brown and cooked through, then remove to a plate and set aside.

Re-spray the wok with oil and place over a high heat. Once hot, add the onion or leek and fry until softened. Add the carrot ribbons and fry until softened, then add the garlic paste, if using, and ginger paste, and stir fry until everything is well coated.

Add the shredded cabbage and stir fry for 3–4 minutes. Once softened, make a well in the middle of the wok and pour in the sauce mixture. Bring to the boil and allow to bubble until it thickens into a sticky sauce. Return the chicken and stir fry for 2–3 minutes until everything is well coated.

Meanwhile, cook the rice noodles according to the packet instructions, then drain and keep warm.

Sprinkle the chicken with spring onion greens and serve with the rice noodles and sliced cucumber.

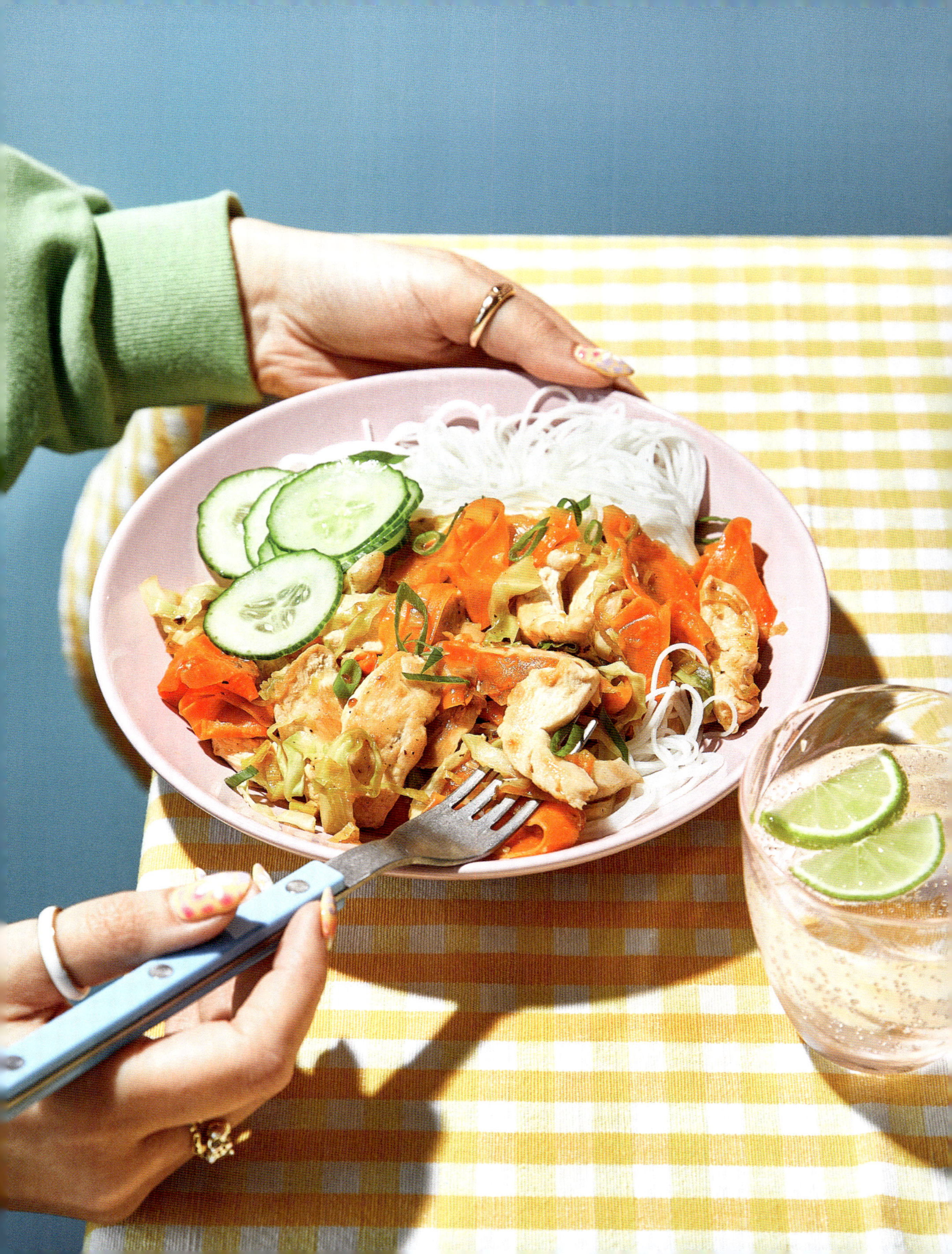

SPEEDY SUPPERS

Out in the wild world we live in, things like skipping the queue, speeding things up and cutting corners usually come at a premium. And at home, the prospect of magically conjuring up a last-minute dinner out of thin air at short notice can often end in a costly takeaway (not forgetting the sneaky extra charges restaurants like to hand us for the 'pleasure' of being gluten-free).

But never fear! At home in your own kitchen, with this chapter to hand, you can still have your dinner and eat it as quickly as possible, all while saving money. In fact, I've even thrown in some of my favourite 15-minute budget-friendly meals and speedy pasta dishes too!

This chapter is the polar opposite of the Big Batch Slow Cooking chapter, which allows you to economize by buying larger quantities of ingredients at cheaper prices while purposefully making too much food, so the extras can be stored as no-extra-effort ready meals so you can even enjoy days off cooking. Those pre-made meals would sure come in extra handy in last-minute situations like I'm describing here, huh?

Yet, as I am an actual real, non-perfect human with a hectic life, despite my best intentions there will always be situations where I have absolutely nothing prepared in the case of a last-minute dinner emergency. And in those situations, I don't even have the option of a takeaway because due to my intolerance to onion and garlic, there is nowhere I can order anything anyway!

So, obviously, I don't just sulk and starve; the recipes in this chapter are the ones I turn to and – *poof *– all my dinner dilemmas are solved. And, like I said at the start, in your own kitchen, there's no reason that a last-minute 'ASAP dinner' should break the bank or be any less mouth-watering than one that took hours and hours to cook. And if you're wondering how these quick meals could possibly be budget-friendly without the benefits that the Big Batch Slow Cooking chapter provides, here's how: humble, cost-effective ingredients combined with big, bold store-cupboard-sourced flavours and a dash of keeping things super simple.

So here are my best 'break in case of emergency' recipes that can all be made in about 30 minutes or less. Don't forget to check out the Savvy Street Food chapter which has lots of 30-minute-or-under recipes mixed into it too.

GREEN GODDESS CHICKEN
WITH BUTTER RICE

After discovering Green Goddess dressing on social media, I quickly realized that this heavenly herby concoction not only tasted as good as it looked, but also that absolutely nobody can agree on what goes in it. After deciding to turn it from a dressing into a fully fledged chicken and rice dish, I settled on my own concoction of herbs, honey, Greek yoghurt, lemon and a little heat from jalapeños. When paired with my buttery, lemon chicken-infused rice, you can very quickly make a budget-friendly meal fit for any gluten-free deity! Serve alongside a side salad or cherry tomatoes (prepared as in my 'Marry Me' chicken pasta recipe on page 166).

Serves 3–4

Prep 5 mins

Hob + Air Fryer/Grill (broiler) 25 mins

DF Use a dairy-free 'buttery' margarine and a thick dairy-free yoghurt instead of Greek yoghurt.

LL Use lactose-free Greek yoghurt.

F See lactose-free advice and use a low FODMAP stock cube, light brown sugar instead of honey, and garlic-infused oil instead of garlic paste.

❄ Once cooled, store the chicken and rice in separate airtight containers and freeze the chicken for up to 2–3 months. Allow the chicken to defrost completely in the fridge, then reheat in the air fryer for 8–9 minutes at 200°C (400°F). Check internal temperature with a digital food thermometer against those given on page 255. For the rice, see freezing and defrosting guidance for risotto and rice dishes on page 28.

- 35g (1¼oz) parsley, including stalks
- 20g (¾oz) chives
- 30g (1oz) basil, including stalks
- 15g (½oz) jarred jalapeños
- 200g (scant 1 cup) Greek yoghurt
- 1 tbsp honey
- Grated zest and juice of ½ lemon
- 1 tsp garlic paste or 1 tbsp garlic-infused oil

- 1 tsp salt
- ½ tsp ground black pepper
- 600g (1lb 5oz) skinless, boneless chicken thighs
- Vegetable oil spray, for air frying

For the rice
- 4 tbsp butter
- 600ml (2½ cups) gluten-free chicken stock (see page 163 for homemade, or made using 1 stock cube)

- Grated zest and juice of 1 lemon
- 1½ tbsp dried mixed herbs
- ¾ tsp salt
- ¾ tsp ground black pepper
- 300g (1⅔ cups) long-grain rice

To prepare the rice, add the butter to a large saucepan or pot that has a lid, and place over a medium-high heat. Once melted, add the stock, lemon zest and juice, mixed herbs, salt and pepper and bring to the boil. Once rapidly boiling, add the rice, pop the lid on and turn the heat down to low. Allow the rice to cook for 20 minutes, then turn off the heat and keep warm with the lid on until the chicken is ready.

Meanwhile, prepare the chicken. Add the herbs (keep back a little parsley, to garnish), jalapeños, yoghurt, honey, lemon zest and juice, garlic, salt and pepper to a large bowl. Mix briefly and blend until smooth using a stick blender. Add the chicken thighs and stir in until well coated.

To cook in an air fryer, heat the air fryer to 200°C (400°F). Generously spray the base of the air fryer basket or crisping tray with oil. If you have an air fryer with 2 drawers, you'll likely need to employ both, so grease both if necessary. Add the chicken to the air fryer, making sure the pieces are touching as little as possible. Air fry for 17–18 minutes or until the chicken is golden brown in places, turning them over after about 12 minutes.

To cook under a grill (broiler), set the grill to high. Place the marinated chicken thighs on the wire rack of a grill pan, ensuring the pan underneath is lined with foil. Grill until the coating is completely dry and a little blackened in places, then flip and repeat. This should take 7–8 minutes each side, depending on how hot your grill gets.

Allow to rest for 5 minutes before transferring to a chopping board and slicing into strips.

To serve, spread the rice over the base of each plate, followed by the chicken, and scatter over the reserved parsley.

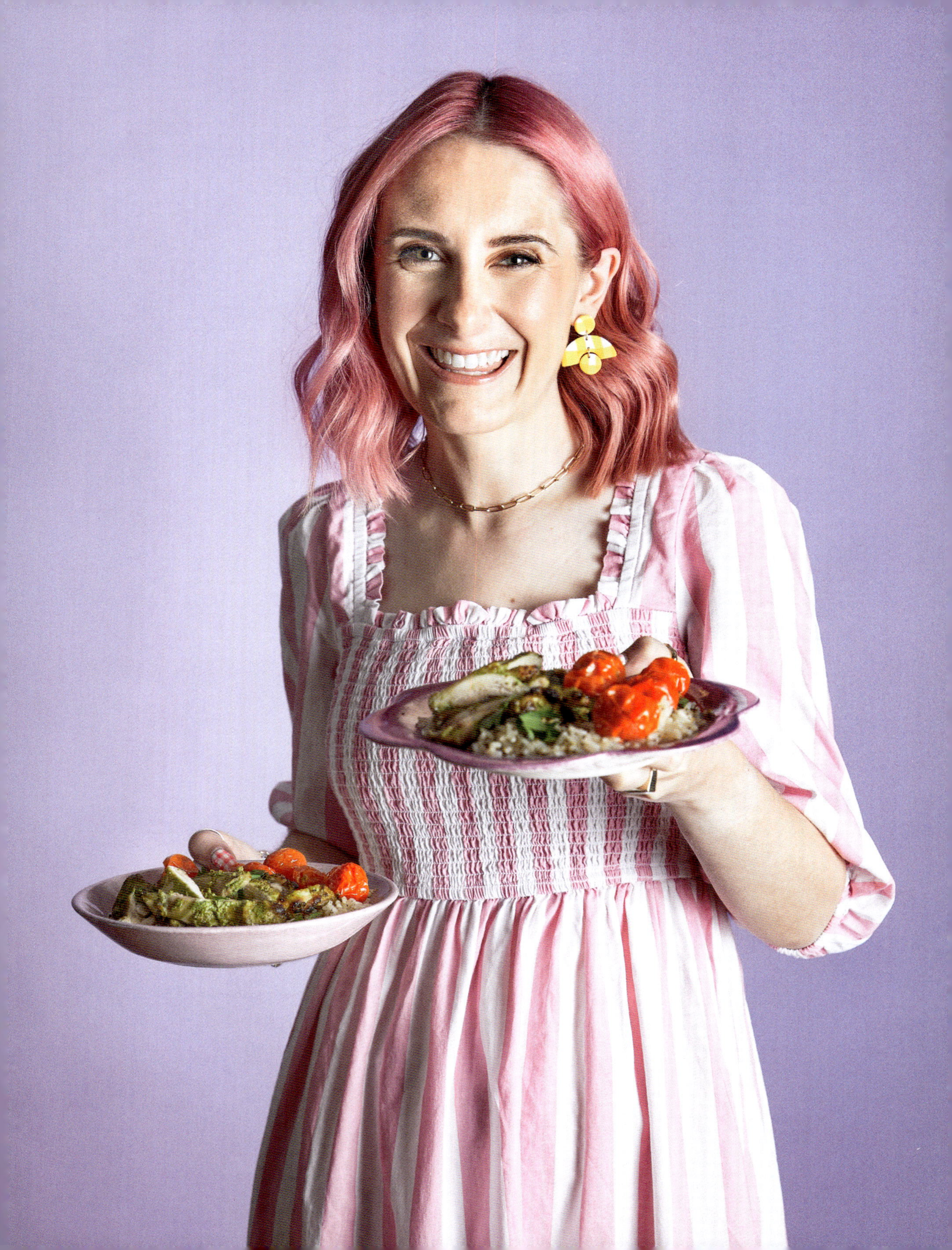

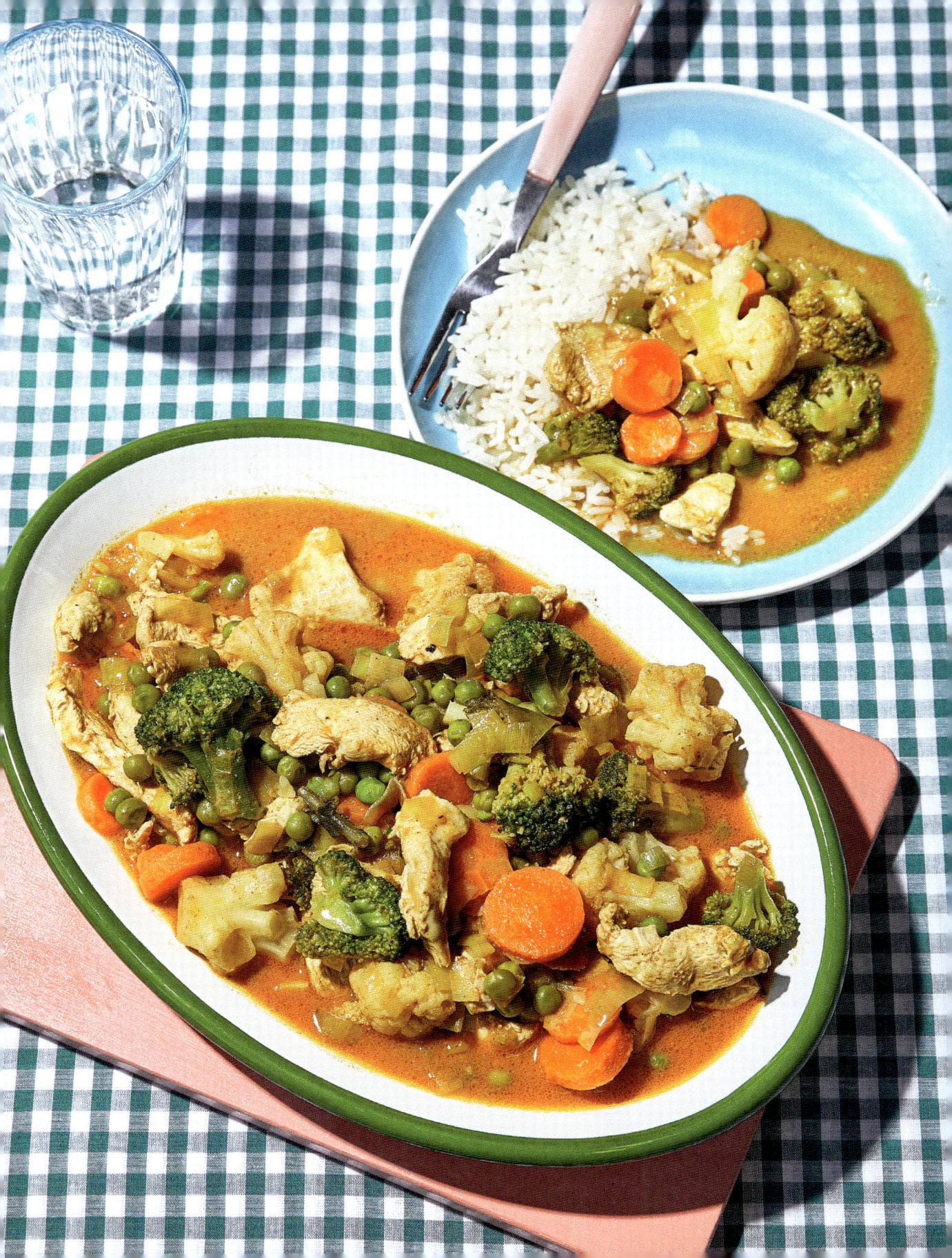

15-MINUTE COCONUT CURRY IN A HURRY

Serves 2–3

Prep 2 mins

Hob 14 mins

DF **LF**

V If adding optional additions, use either butter beans or chickpeas.

VE See veggie advice.

✳ See freezing and defrosting guidance for soups, stews and curries on page 28.

Despite our best intentions and planning, you never know when you'll be caught out with dinner looming and very few ingredients in the fridge. But that doesn't change the fact that you still need a last-minute meal that doesn't involve the hefty cost of a takeaway! And that's exactly where this curry in a hurry fits into my life. With a creamy coconut curry sauce that's packed with veg and realistic optional extras that you might have left over or in the cupboard/ freezer, this versatile curry is as delectable as it is useful when you're in a pinch. Serve with rice.

- Vegetable oil spray
- 100g (3½oz) frozen chopped onion or ½ medium leek, finely chopped
- 2 tbsp mild curry powder
- ½ tsp salt
- ¼ tsp ground black pepper
- 500g (1lb 2oz) frozen mixed veg (such as carrots, cauliflower, green beans and peas)

- 250ml (1 cup) gluten-free vegetable stock
- 1 x 400g (14oz) can of coconut milk
- 1 tbsp tomato purée (paste)

Optional additions, choose one of:

- 2 skinless, boneless chicken breasts, thinly sliced

- 3–4 skinless, boneless chicken thighs
- 250g (9oz) frozen white fish fillets
- 1 x 400g (14oz) can of butter (lima) beans, drained
- 1 x 400g (14oz) can of chickpeas, drained

Spray the base of a large pot that has a lid with oil and place over a medium heat. Once hot, add the onion or leek, curry powder, salt and pepper, then fry until fragrant.

Add the frozen mixed veg, the stock, coconut milk and tomato purée to the pan and stir to combine. At this point, add one of the optional additions, if using. Turn the heat up to high and bring to the boil, then turn the heat to medium and keep the pot bubbling for around 10 minutes or until it's thickened up a little.

Once the curry has reduced and thickened, take off the heat and optionally allow to cool for 10 minutes – it will thicken more as it cools.

TOMATO AND SCRAMBLED EGG STIR FRY (西红柿炒鸡蛋)

Serves 2
Prep 2 mins
Hob 18 mins

DF **LF** **V**

I had to include the Chinese characters for this dish in the title as otherwise I feel like most people would look at this humble recipe and think it was something basic I just made up in a rush! In reality, this is our version of a traditional Chinese dish which, while being incredibly affordable by nature, tastes like a million quid. All of the ingredients combine to make a sweet, sour, savoury and mildly spicy sauce with soft, perfectly broken down tomatoes – and the omelette shows up late to the party to soak up all that wonderful flavour. Best of all, you can make it in around 20 minutes! Serve with rice.

- Vegetable oil spray
- 4 large eggs, beaten with ½ tsp salt
- 500g (1lb 2oz) medium tomatoes, cut into wedges
- 1 tsp ginger paste
- 2 tbsp honey
- 2 tbsp gluten-free soy sauce
- 1 tsp tomato purée (paste)
- ¼ tsp dried chilli flakes
- Small handful of spring onion (scallion) greens, sliced on the diagonal

Lightly spray the base and sides of a large wok with oil and place over a high heat. Once hot, add the beaten eggs – it should immediately start sizzling – and very gently stir for the first 20 seconds, then allow to fry for 4–5 minutes or until golden brown on the bottom. Flip and fry for a further 1–2 minutes, then slide the omelette out onto a plate and set aside.

Remove the wok from the heat and carefully wipe with kitchen paper, then respray with oil and allow to reheat for 30 seconds or so. Add the tomatoes and stir fry for 1 minute, then stir in the ginger paste and drizzle over the honey and soy sauce. Allow to sit in the wok until liquid is released from the tomatoes, then turn down the heat a little, ensuring it's still gently bubbling.

Allow to simmer for around 10 minutes or until the tomatoes are looking nicely softened and broken down, then stir in the tomato purée and chilli flakes. Continue to simmer until the liquid has thickened, then add the omelette back to the wok. Stir fry well, breaking the omelette up, until it is all coated, then scatter over the spring onion greens.

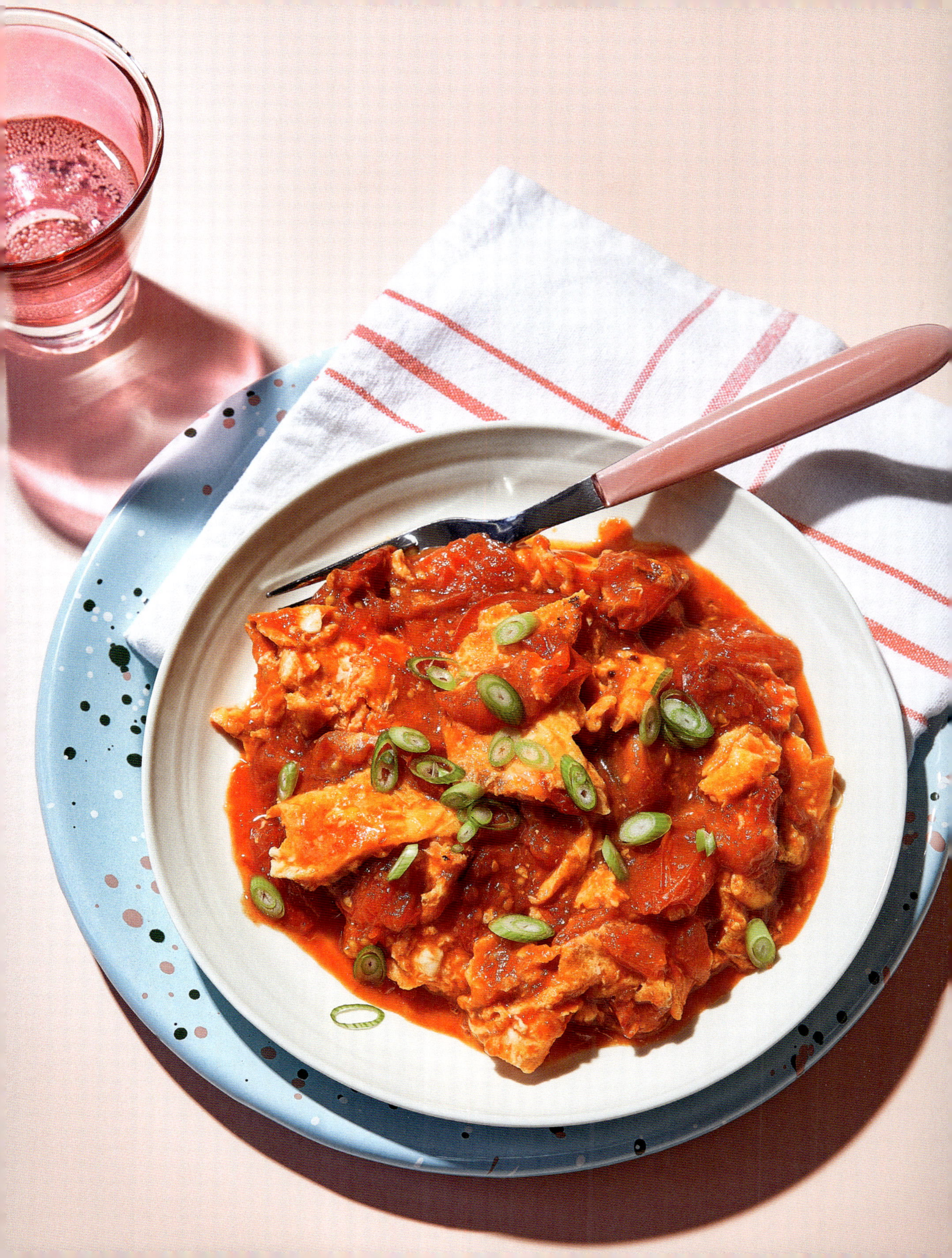

MICROWAVE SWEET + SOUR CHICKEN

Serves 2

Prep 2 mins

Microwave 12–13 mins
(+ 30–35 mins for the rice; optional)

Yep, you read that right, a delicious takeaway favourite made entirely in your microwave, yet nobody would ever notice the difference! The chicken comes out especially tender and the sauce thickens like magic. We've also made rice in the microwave like this for years and I'm so glad I found an excuse to share it here in my seventh book; it'll save you tons of money if you're in the habit of using packets of microwave rice, and is completely hands off (turn to page 14 if you're interested to know how much packets of microwavable rice are costing you!).

DF **LF**

F Omit the garlic paste or use ½ tbsp garlic-infused oil instead. Use light brown sugar/maple syrup instead of honey. Use no more than 150g (5½oz) green (bell) peppers instead of mixed colours. Use orange juice instead of pineapple juice.

❄ See freezing and defrosting guidance for soups, stews and curries on page 28 – it'll work for this perfectly! Freeze the rice and sweet and sour separately.

- 200g (7oz) frozen sliced red, green and yellow (bell) peppers
- 2 skinless, boneless chicken breasts, thinly sliced
- 4 canned pineapple rings
- Handful of spring onion (scallion) greens, thinly sliced on the diagonal

For the rice (optional)
- 1 mug of long-grain rice
- 2 mugs of boiling water

For the sauce
- 110ml (scant ½ cup) pineapple or orange juice
- 4 tbsp rice wine vinegar
- 4 tbsp honey

- 1 tbsp gluten-free soy sauce
- 2 tbsp cornflour (cornstarch) or potato starch
- ½ tsp garlic paste (optional)
- ½ tsp ginger paste
- ¼ tsp Chinese five spice

TIPS

Although this recipe doesn't use a weight measurement for the rice or boiling water, the ratio still remains the same when weighing out your rice. So take any measurement of rice, then double it: that's how much boiling water you'd add – 200g (7oz) of rice would require 400ml (14fl oz) of boiling water, for example.

Mark's mum has used the same glass Pyrex casserole dish with a lid for the past two decades to make rice like this. You can find them in most supermarkets, and certainly online. Microwaving the rice at too high a temperature will result in the water overflowing out of the pot, so between low and medium (180W in my microwave) is the sweet spot.

If you're making the rice, do this first. Add the rice and boiling water to a microwave-proof glass dish that has a lid, place the lid on and microwave on low–medium power (180W – definitely NOT full power!) for 30–35 minutes. Don't open the lid at any point. Once cooked, set aside and keep warm.

Place the sauce ingredients in a medium microwavable plastic bowl and stir to combine. Add the peppers, chicken and pineapple rings and push them below the surface of the sauce.

Loosely cover with a plate and microwave on full power (1000W or as close to yours will do) for 10 minutes, stirring halfway. Then remove the plate and microwave for 2–3 minutes or until the sauce is nicely thickened. If the sauce is thickened, then the chicken is definitely cooked!

Scatter the spring onion greens on top and serve with rice.

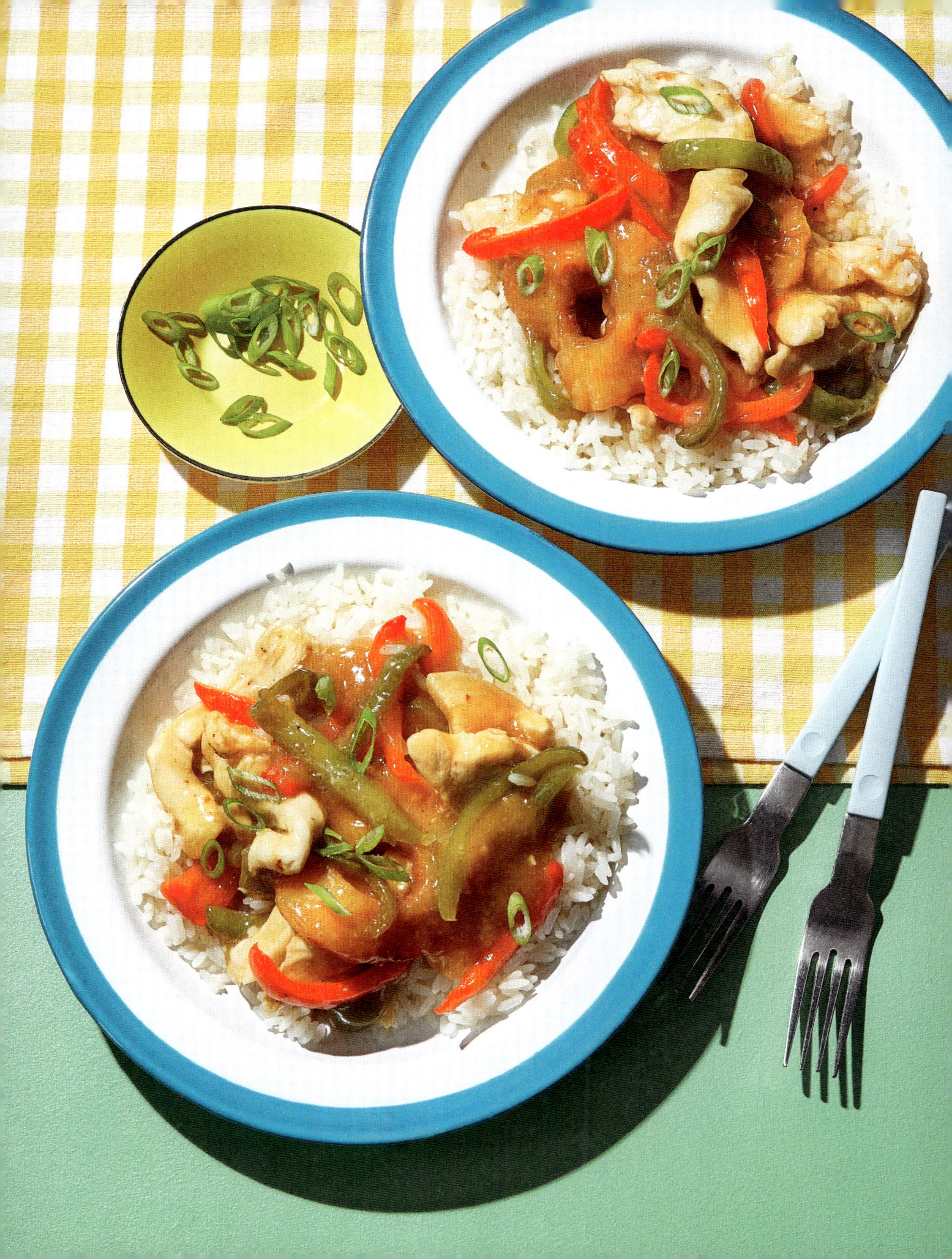

SUPER INSTANT NOODLES 2.0

Serves 2
Prep 2 mins
Hob 10 mins

Due to all the overwhelmingly positive comments I've received on part one of this recipe which was first published in my fourth book, *Quick + Easy Gluten Free*, it's back with three brand-new variations. Needless to say, these are extremely budget-friendly and can come in handy for a last-minute dinner, lunch or snack.

- 2 nests of dried vermicelli or ribbon rice noodles (100g/3½oz in total)
- 300ml (1¼ cups) boiling water

For BBQ beef flavour
- 1 gluten-free beef stock cube
- Pinch of ground black pepper
- ½ tsp dried mixed herbs
- 1 tbsp gluten-free BBQ sauce

For bacon flavour
- 1 gluten-free ham stock cube
- Pinch of ground black pepper
- ½ tsp dried mixed herbs
- ½ tsp honey

For southern-fried chicken flavour
- 1 gluten-free chicken stock cube
- Pinch of ground cumin
- ¼ tsp smoked paprika
- Pinch of dried chilli flakes
- 1 tsp dried mixed herbs

DF **LF**

F Use a low FODMAP stock cube and FODMAP-friendly BBQ sauce, if using. Use light brown sugar instead of honey, if using.

V Use a gluten-free veggie/vegan stock cube for all the variations, and add ¼ tsp smoked paprika to the 'bacon' noodles for an extra smoky flavour.

VE See veggie advice and use light brown sugar instead of honey.

❄ Once cooled, freeze in airtight containers for 2–3 months. Defrost in the fridge, then reheat in the microwave for 3–5 minutes until piping hot.

TIP

There's no need for any salt here! Stock cubes usually have more than enough. If your stock cubes are particularly salty, consider using ¾ cube instead of a whole one. Half a teaspoon of honey (or any type of sugar) can help to offset the saltiness if you found this out too late!

Add the noodles and boiling water to a large saucepan, crumble in the relevant stock cube for your chosen variation, place over a medium heat and bring to the boil. Once boiling, give the noodles a stir so they don't clump, then add the remaining ingredients for your chosen variation. Reduce the heat to low and simmer for around 3–4 minutes or until all the moisture has gone.

Take off the heat and allow to stand in the saucepan for 1 minute. This will allow the noodles to magically dry out a little and be perfect to eat – straight from the pan if you must!

How to take your instant noodles to the next level:

I'm a huge fan of remixing these humble instant noodles into more substantial meals, so here's a little inspiration and guidance on how I do so for each variation. Feel free to use these ideas exactly as I've given opposite, or use them to inspire your own additions. Bear in mind that these additions aren't factored into the dietary key at the top of the page, so use your own judgement here depending on your own dietary requirements!

- **To make beef and roasted broccoli noodles (pictured):** Air fry 200g (7oz) frozen broccoli florets (spray well with oil first) at 200°C (400°F) for 10–15 minutes – make sure they're touching as little as possible in the basket. Turn over halfway or shake 3–4 times if particularly piled up. Add to the **BBQ beef flavour** noodles once they're done.

- **To make crispy bacon noodles with peas:** Air fry 3 rashers of smoked back bacon (lightly grease the basket by spraying well with oil first) at 200°C (400°F) for 7–8 minutes until super crisp, then finely chop. Microwave 200g (7oz) frozen peas in a medium bowl with 2 tbsp water added, covered with a plate, for 4–5 minutes, stirring halfway; drain and stir into the **bacon flavour** noodles along with the bacon.

- **To add leftover chicken to the southern-fried chicken noodles:** Reheat 150g (5½oz) leftover, cooked shredded chicken (see recipe on page 163 to make your own 'leftovers') in the air fryer at 200°C (400°F) for 3–4 minutes, until piping hot. Add the chicken to the **southern-fried chicken flavour** noodles and optionally scatter over a small handful of finely chopped chives.

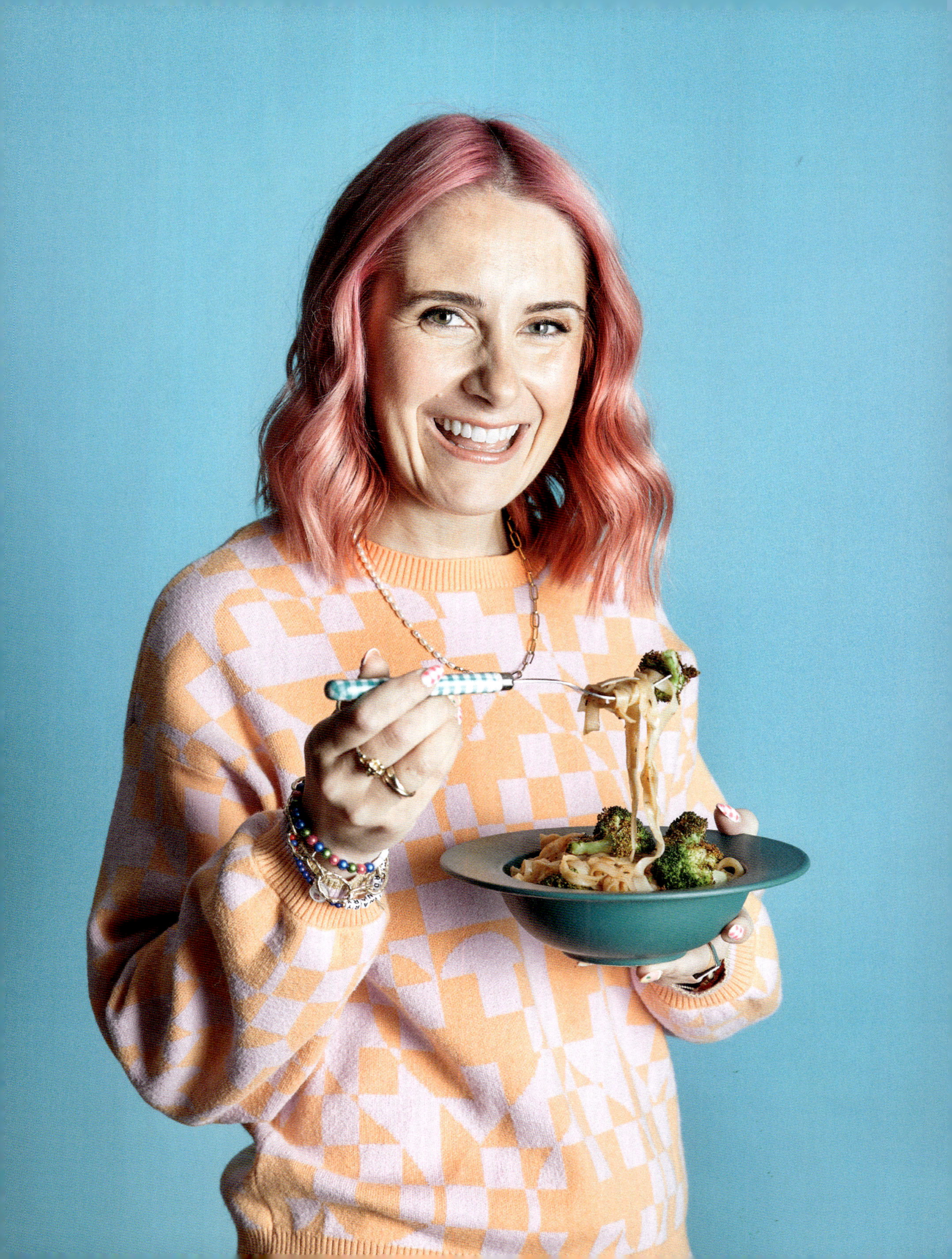

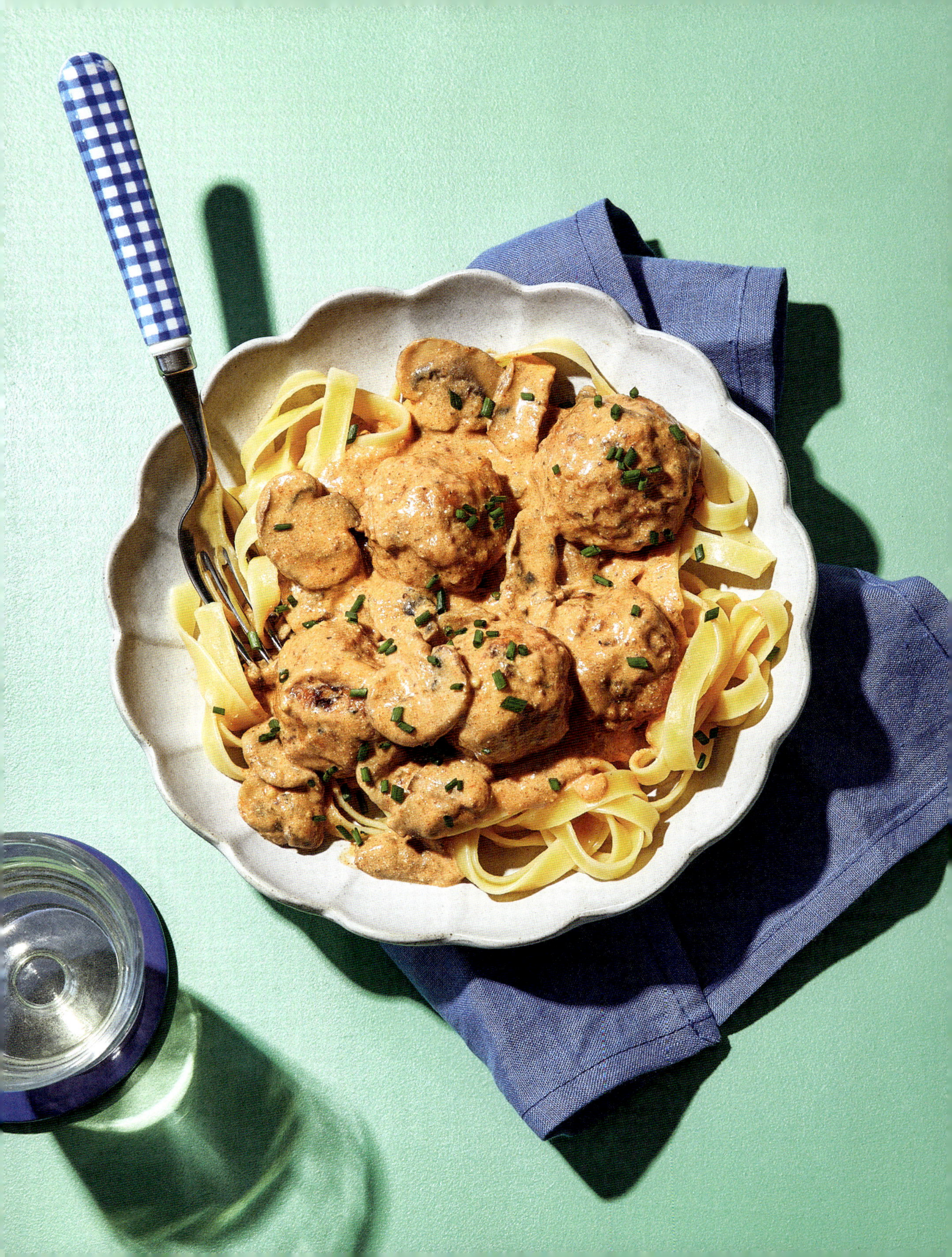

MEATBALL STROGANOFF

Serves 3–4

Prep 5 mins

Hob + Oven 30 mins or
Hob + Air Fryer 25 mins

A good stroganoff is something I absolutely can't resist and there's nothing else out there quite like it. There's something about that creamy sauce, tinged with smoked paprika, tomato purée and mustard that marries together in the pot. I make my stroganoff with meatballs, alternating between using minced (ground) turkey or beef to keep things fresh. Serve with mashed potato, pasta or rice.

DF Use a dairy-free 'buttery' margarine and dairy-free cream cheese.

LF Use a lactose-free 'buttery' margarine and lactose-free cream cheese.

F See lactose-free advice and use leek (green parts only) instead of onion; swap the mushrooms for 4 medium carrots, sliced into 5mm (¼in) rounds and boiled until fork-tender; and use ½ low FODMAP stock cube.

❄ See freezing and defrosting guidance for soups, stews and curries on page 28.

- 2 tbsp 'buttery' margarine
- 100g (3½oz) frozen chopped onion **or** ½ medium leek, finely chopped
- 500g (1lb 2oz) frozen sliced mushrooms
- 1 tbsp cornflour (cornstarch) or potato starch
- 1½ tsp smoked paprika
- 2 tsp wholegrain or Dijon mustard

- ½ tbsp tomato purée (paste)
- 300ml (1¼ cups) gluten-free vegetable stock (made with ½ stock cube)
- ¼ tsp salt
- ¼ tsp ground black pepper
- 90g (scant ½ cup) sour cream **or** 120g (½ cup) cream cheese
- Small handful of chives, finely chopped

For the meatballs
- 500g (1lb 2oz) minced (ground) turkey thigh or beef
- 1 large egg
- ½ tsp salt
- ½ tsp ground black pepper
- 5–7 tbsp cornflour (cornstarch) or potato starch
- Vegetable oil spray

TIPS

If you're not super-precious about what your meatballs look like, you can always use an ice-cream scoop to portion out the meat mixture. Once you've scooped a portion of meat mixture, press the ice cream scoop up against the side of the bowl to compress it into the scoop a bit. Not only will this method keep each meatball to a uniform size and weight, it's also quicker and far less messy too!

Extremely lazy and can't even be fussed to make meatballs? Simply leave the onion or leek in the pan, then add the mince and cook until sealed/browned. Add the mushrooms and flour, then skip the meatball making/cooking steps and proceed with the rest of the recipe. I won't judge you for it, promise!

Add the margarine to a large pot that has a lid and place over a medium-high heat. Once melted, add the onion or leek and fry until browned. Transfer to a large bowl.

Add the frozen mushrooms to the pot, immediately followed by the cornflour or potato starch, then stir well until the flour disappears. Fry until softened and/or until water is released and mostly evaporated. Turn the heat down to low to keep them warm while you make the meatballs.

Add the turkey, egg, salt, pepper and 5 tablespoons of cornflour or potato starch to the onion or leek in the large bowl. Mix well until everything is evenly dispersed and the mixture looks smooth. If it still looks wet, add the extra cornflour or potato starch. Roll into ping-pong-sized balls (about 40g/1¾oz each, making 16 meatballs).

To cook the meatballs in an oven, preheat the oven to 200°C fan/220°C (425°F). Spray a large baking sheet

with oil. Place the meatballs on the baking sheet and bake in the oven for 20 minutes or until golden brown.

To cook the meatballs in an air fryer, heat the air fryer to 190°C (375°F) and spray the basket or crisping tray with oil. If you have an air fryer with 2 drawers, use both. Place as many meatballs as will fit in the air fryer basket without touching and spray with oil. Air fry for 12–15 minutes until crisp and golden brown, turning them over halfway.

In the meantime, turn the heat back to medium-high and add the smoked paprika, mustard and tomato purée to the mushrooms, then mix in. Pour in the stock, add the salt and pepper and simmer for a few minutes until slightly thickened. Reduce the heat and stir in the sour cream or cream cheese, then allow to cook for a minute more before adding in the meatballs to finish.

Serve the meatballs and sauce garnished with chives.

ONE-POT CHICKEN ALFREDO

It's a speedy one-pot pasta dish to the rescue and, to be honest, whether it's a last-minute meal or not, I'm not sure I'd prefer anything else over tender chicken in a rich, velvety cheese sauce. Anything tinged by this creamy, cheesy Alfredo sauce tastes otherworldly, which is why I make the most of adding broccoli (who doesn't love cheese and broccoli?) which is a disappointingly uncommon vegetable in most chicken Alfredo recipes. Best of all, the addition of ever-affordable frozen broccoli makes the meal go further.

Serves 3
Prep 2 mins
Hob 25 mins

DF Use dairy-free milk, dairy-free cheese and dairy-free cream or cream cheese.

LL Use lactose-free milk and lactose-free cream or cream cheese.

F See low lactose advice and swap the frozen broccoli for 225g (8oz) fresh broccoli (heads only) and 2 medium carrots, sliced into 5mm (¼in) rounds and boiled until fork-tender. Use low FODMAP stock.

V Swap the chicken for 150g (5½oz) frozen green beans and 150g (5½oz) frozen peas (both added along with the frozen broccoli).

VE Combine dairy-free and veggie advice.

❄ See freezing and defrosting guidance for pasta dishes on page 28.

- Vegetable oil spray
- 2 skinless, boneless chicken breasts, cut into bite-sized chunks
- 1 tsp salt
- 500g (1lb 2oz) frozen broccoli florets
- 350ml (1½ cups) gluten-free chicken stock (see page 163 for homemade)
- 400ml (1⅔ cups) milk
- ½ tsp ground black pepper
- 300g (10½oz) gluten-free dried tagliatelle
- 70g (2½oz) mature Cheddar, grated
- 120ml (½ cup) double (heavy) cream **or** 100g (scant ½ cup) cream cheese
- Handful of parsley leaves, roughly chopped (optional)

Spray the base of a large pot that has a lid with oil and place over a medium heat. Once hot, add the chicken and salt and fry until almost sealed. Add the frozen broccoli and allow to defrost for 1–2 minutes before adding the stock, milk and pepper. Bring to the boil, then add the pasta and push below the surface of the liquid.

Reduce the heat to low–medium so it's gently bubbling, then pop the lid on for 10 minutes, stirring halfway and pushing the pasta below the liquid once again.

Remove the lid and allow to simmer for 5 more minutes or until the pasta is cooked and the sauce has thickened. Stir in the cheese and cream or cream cheese and simmer for a few more minutes until thickened to your liking.

Serve with a sprinkling of chopped fresh parsley, if using.

TIP

While this recipe instructs the use of gluten-free dried tagliatelle (and my smash burger mac 'n' cheese over on page 86 instructs the use of dried gluten-free macaroni) please remember that you can always use other shapes of dried pasta – such as penne or fusilli – instead. Not only are these pasta shapes easier to come by, but they'll often be cheaper too!

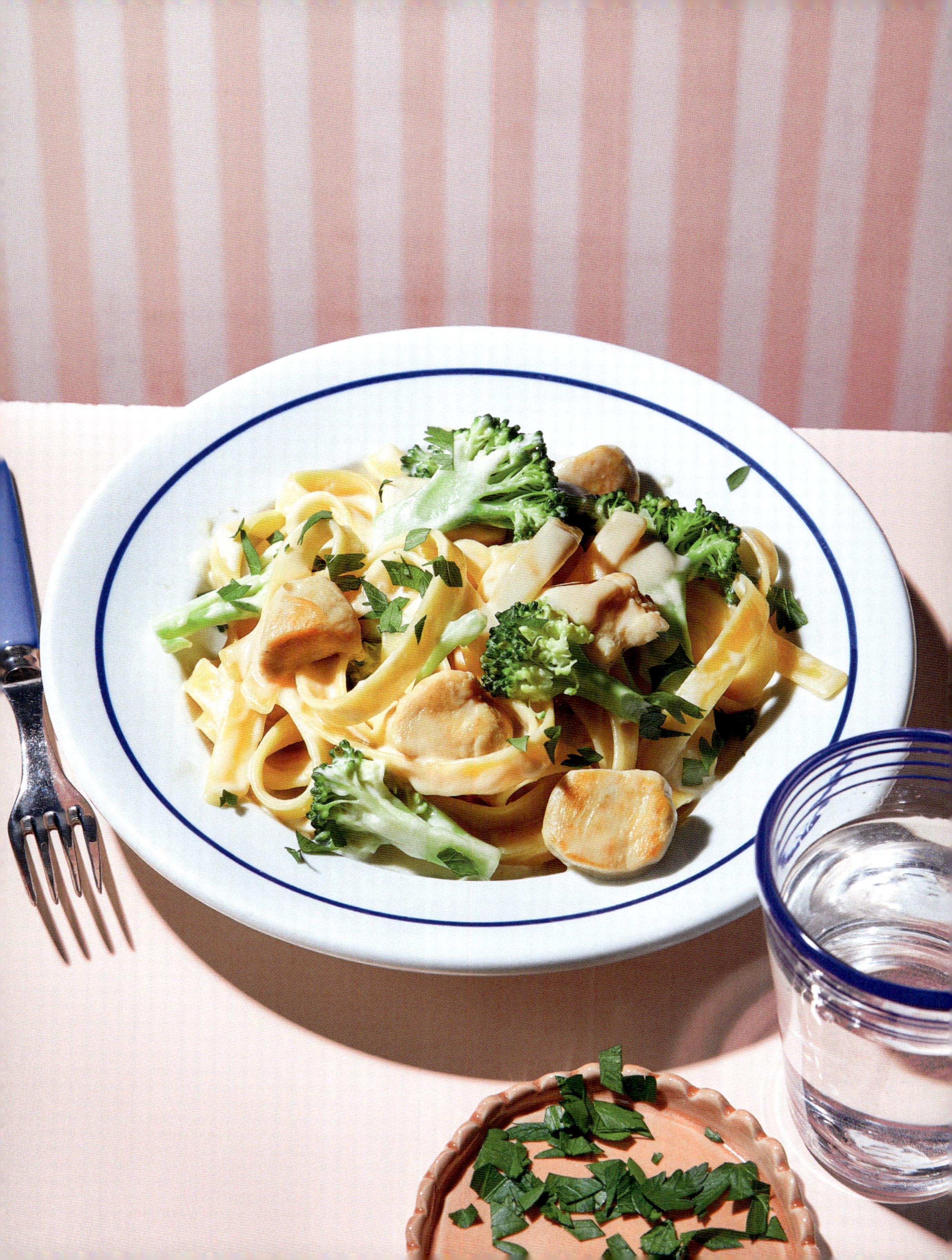

'BLG' SPAGHETTI

Serves 3

Prep 2 mins

Hob 20 mins

DF Use dairy-free cheese and dairy-free cream cheese.

LL Use lactose-free cream cheese.

F Use 1 tbsp garlic-infused oil instead of garlic paste, use ½ a low FODMAP stock cube, swap the frozen broccoli for 225g (8oz) fresh broccoli (heads only), use 225g (8oz) green (bell) pepper instead of mixed colours and use lactose-free cream cheese.

V Swap the bacon for 300g (10½oz) frozen mushrooms (fry until the water evaporates and the mushrooms soften) and use veggie/vegan-friendly stock.

VE Combine dairy-free and veggie advice.

❄ See freezing and defrosting guidance for pasta dishes on page 28.

While you're welcome to look at the photo and guess what BLG stands for, I can tell you already that it doesn't stand for 'Becky loves gluten'… it stands for bacon, lemon and garlic. I can't actually tolerate garlic myself, but see the FODMAP notes for my little sneaky work around, and whichever way you make it, this creamy, cheesy meal is guaranteed to be on the table in 30 minutes and loved by everyone. This recipe is a great example of how a harmony of affordable ingredients can easily offset the additional cost of buying gluten-free pasta, and then some!

- 300g (10½oz) gluten-free dried spaghetti
- Vegetable oil spray
- 10 rashers of smoked back bacon
- 250g (9oz) frozen broccoli florets
- 250g (9oz) frozen sliced red, green and yellow (bell) peppers

- 1 tbsp cornflour (cornstarch) or potato starch
- 1 tsp garlic paste
- 1 tbsp dried mixed herbs
- 250ml (1 cup) gluten-free ham or vegetable stock (made with ½ stock cube)
- ½ tsp salt

- ½ tsp ground black pepper
- 3–4 tbsp cream cheese
- Grated zest of 1 lemon and juice of ½
- 75g (2½oz) mature Cheddar, grated

Cook the spaghetti in a pan of boiling, salted water according to the packet instructions, then drain.

Meanwhile, spray the base of a large pan with oil and place over a high heat. Add the bacon and fry until crispy. Add the broccoli and mixed peppers and continue to fry until the peppers are softened. Add the cornflour or potato starch and stir in until it disappears, then stir in the garlic paste and mixed herbs.

Add the stock, salt and pepper and cream cheese. Turn down the heat to low–medium, stir briefly and simmer until slightly thickened. Add the lemon zest and juice and the drained spaghetti, then stir until the spaghetti is well coated. Continue to simmer until the sauce has thickened and coats everything nicely. Serve sprinkled with the grated cheese.

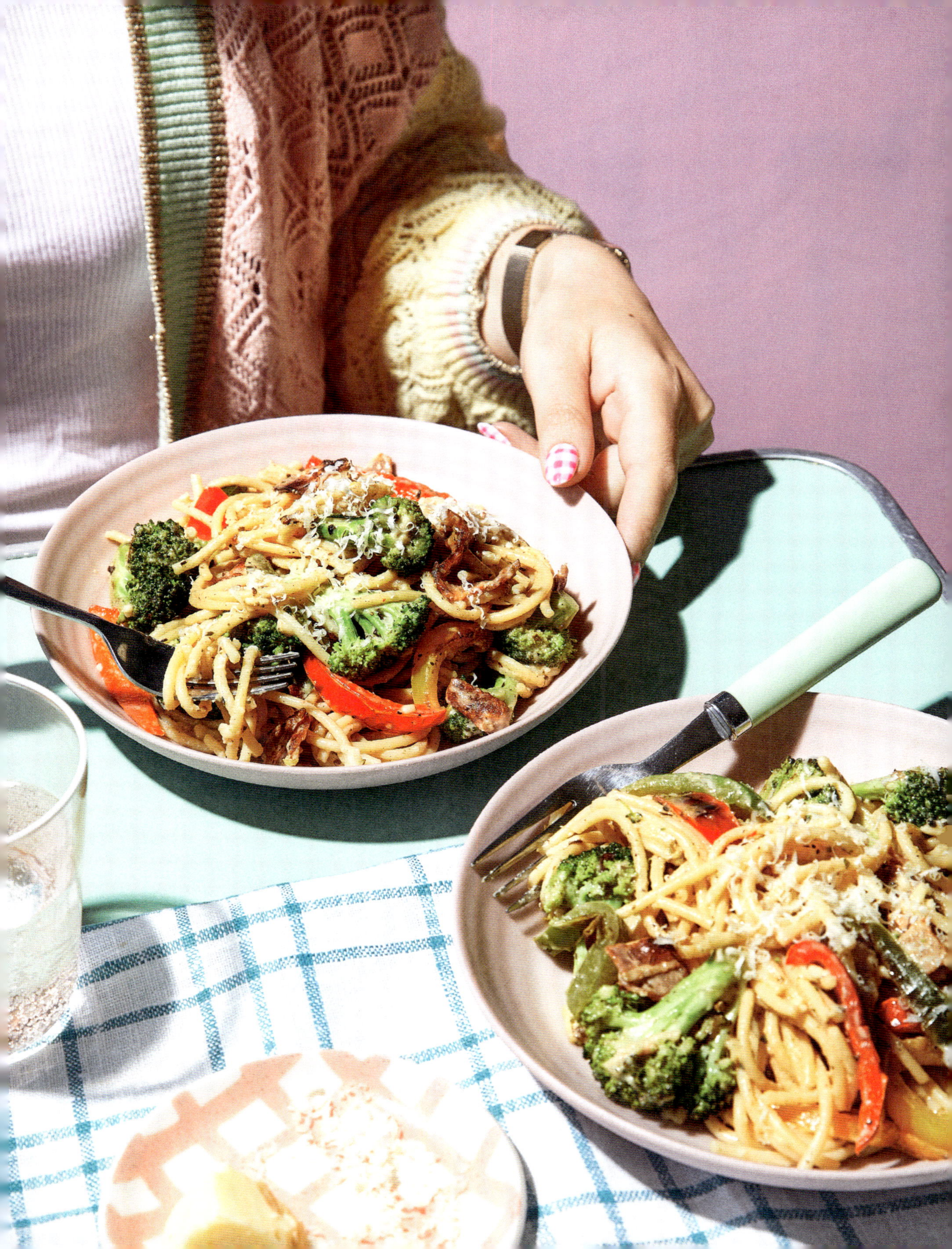

CREAMY SPAGHETTI AI FUNGHI

Serves 3
Prep 2 mins
Hob 20 mins

V

DF Use dairy-free cheese and dairy-free cream cheese.

LL Use lactose-free cream cheese.

VE See dairy-free advice.

❄ See freezing and defrosting guidance for pasta dishes on page 28.

This dinner ticks all the boxes: it's super-quick to make, uses budget-friendly ingredients, yet still tastes like you've poured your heart and soul into it. With a luxuriously creamy sauce with a kick of black pepper, tender mushrooms and a tang of extra-mature Cheddar, this meal is an all-round winner of a dinner that makes the cost advantages of cooking from scratch feel like a walk in the park. Serve with rocket (arugula).

- 300g (10½oz) gluten-free dried spaghetti
- Vegetable oil spray
- 500g (1lb 2oz) frozen sliced mushrooms
- 1 tbsp cornflour (cornstarch) or potato starch

- 225ml (scant 1 cup) gluten-free vegetable stock (made with ½ stock cube)
- ½ tsp salt
- ½ tsp ground black pepper

- 3 tbsp double (heavy) cream or cream cheese
- Handful of basil leaves, roughly chopped **or** ½ tbsp dried basil
- 50g (1¾oz) mature Cheddar, grated

Cook the spaghetti in a pan of boiling, salted water according to the packet instructions, then drain.

Meanwhile, spray the base of a large pan with oil and place over a medium heat. Add the sliced mushrooms and fry until softened and most of the water has evaporated. Add the cornflour or potato starch and stir in until it disappears.

Add the stock, salt, pepper and double cream or cream cheese. Turn down the heat to low–medium, stir briefly and simmer until slightly thickened.

Add the drained spaghetti and basil, then stir well and continue to simmer until the sauce has thickened.

Serve sprinkled with the grated cheese.

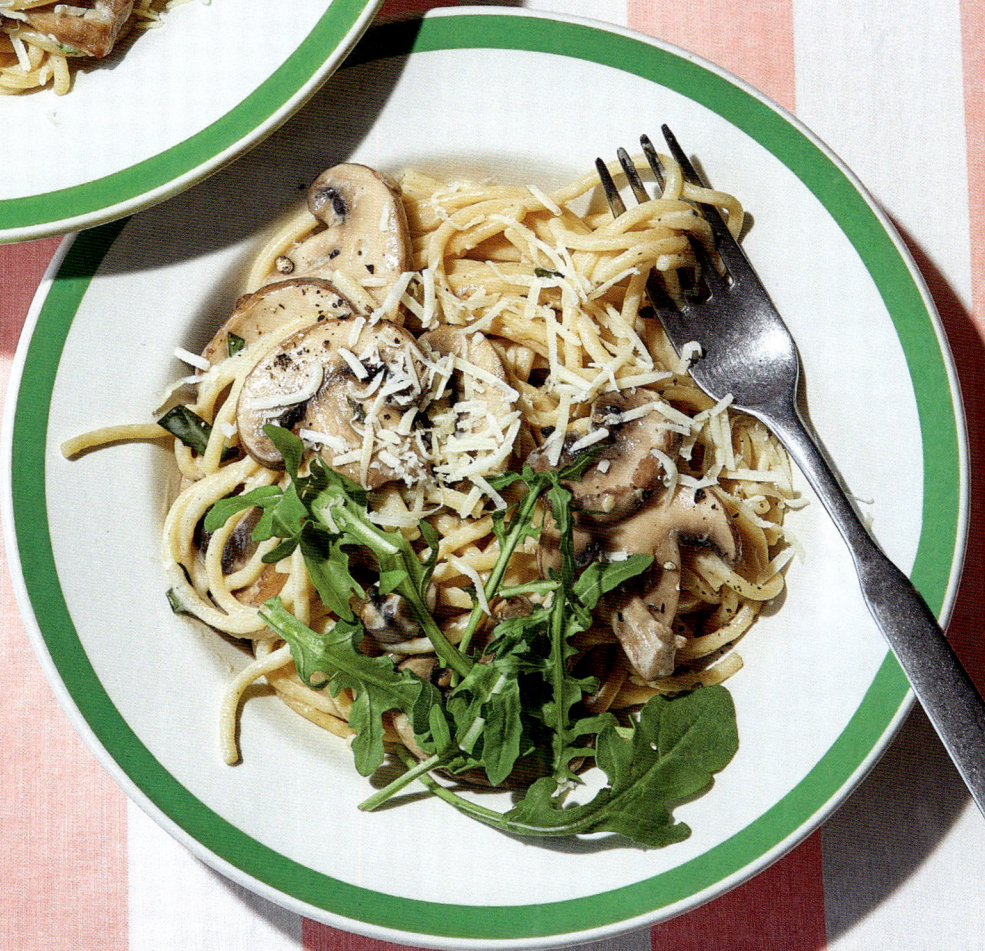

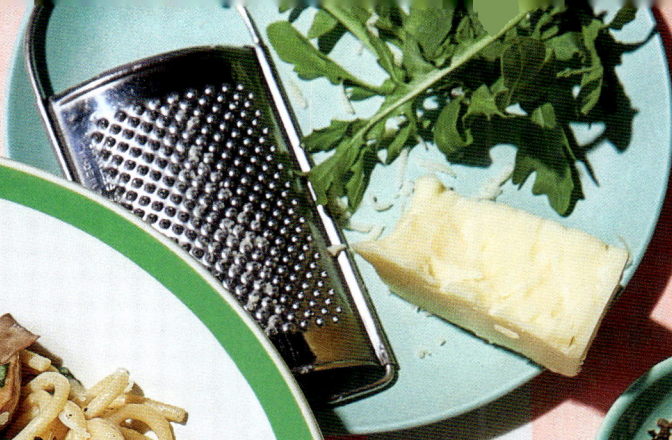

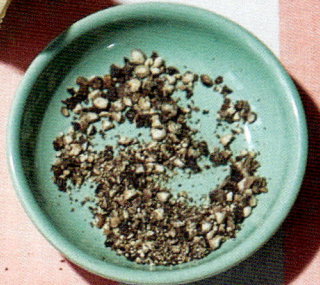

LOW-COST COMFORT FOOD

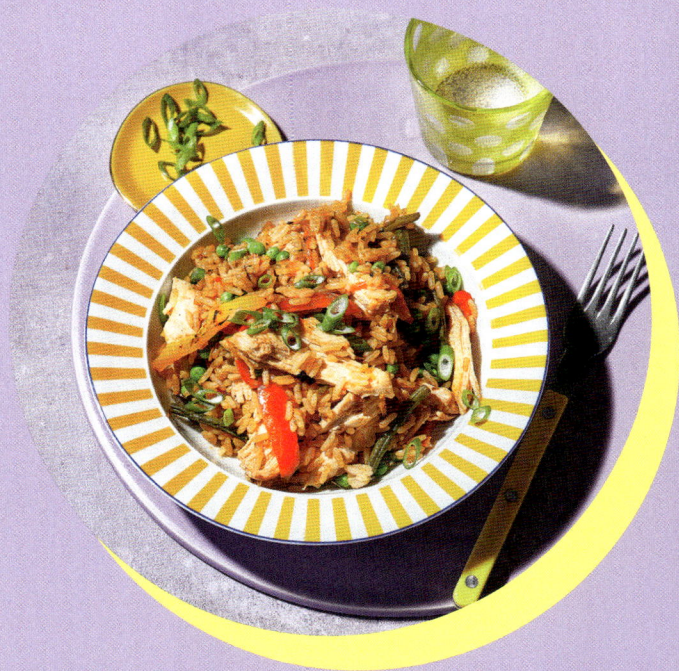

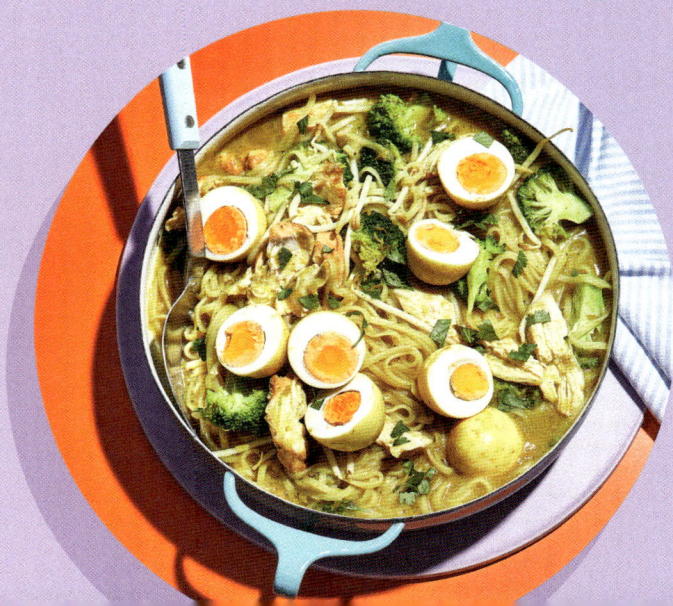

As you'll see in this chapter, I've been able to recreate some of my all-time personal favourites from past and present in a gluten-free form, while keeping the cost per person incredibly down to earth.

This chapter is an eclectic mix of taste, texture and cuisines, one-pot wonders, pasta/rice bakes and legendary veggie dishes that even meat eaters won't pass up, with new and exciting ways to cook and serve meat too. Yet even with a focus on cost-effective store-cupboard ingredients, paired with ever-economical veg and more affordable protein sources, this chapter aims to make comfort food accessible, affordable and awesome.

In this chapter you'll find a few more different spices used than in the Big Batch Slow Cooking chapter (but don't panic – my top 5 spices and seasonings first mentioned on page 24 still feature heavily here too). This is not only in the name of expanding our range of possibilities, but also to enable us to create our own spice blends on demand. Supermarket premixed spice blends bring convenience, but often at a cost. However, with a small set of spices, you'll learn how to make your own Lebanese-style spice blend on page 150, sticky Chinese-style blend on page 160, peri-peri spice blend on page 146 and more, at a noticeably reduced cost. See the savvy shopping tips on page 12 to ensure you get your spices for the best price to keep the costs of your spice blends as economical as possible.

Although the recipes in this chapter take longer to get onto plates than those in the Speedy Suppers chapter, you'll find that the actual prep time required is similar. Meaning that these recipes will take very little effort on your part and just require a longer cooking time. You'll often find that cooking time to be entirely 'hands off' too, meaning you can be anywhere else other than in the kitchen – just don't forget to set a timer!

CHEESE + TOMATO ARANCINI BAKE

Serves 4–5

Prep 10 mins

Hob + Oven 1 hour

V

DF Use a dairy-free 'buttery' margarine and dairy-free cheese instead of Cheddar and mozzarella.

LL Use a lactose-free 'buttery' margarine.

VE See dairy-free advice and use vegan-friendly stock.

❄ See freezing and defrosting guidance for risotto and rice dishes on page 28 (ensure you store leftovers with the breadcrumb layer facing up). Once defrosted, cook in the oven at 180°C fan/200°C (400°F) for 15 minutes or the air fryer at 200°C (400°F) for 8–10 minutes once more to crisp up the top.

TIP

If you don't have an ovenproof pot, once the rice has been briefly fried, you can instead transfer the contents of the pot to a large roasting dish (around 33 x 25cm/13 x 10in). Continue with the rest of the recipe as directed, tightly covering the roasting dish in foil instead of a lid, then removing as directed. See the photo opposite for the finished result!

If you've got a craving for crispy, cheesy, tomato and herb arancini but you either don't have enough leftover risotto to make them or simply don't fancy waiting a few hours for a cooked risotto to completely cool (and also lack the patience to then roll them into balls and coat them in breadcrumbs...), then this is the recipe for you. It's essentially one big baked risotto with crispy breadcrumbs on top that very much tastes like one big arancini! If you struggle to find gluten-free breadcrumbs in shops, very finely crushed gluten-free cornflakes work really well here too. Needless to say, this one is a veggie budget-wonder that no meat eaters will turn down! Serve with a side of rocket (arugula).

- 2 tbsp 'buttery' margarine
- 100g (3½oz) frozen chopped onion **or** ½ medium leek, finely chopped
- 400g (14oz) frozen mixed veg (such as carrots, cauliflower, green beans and peas)
- 300g (generous 1½ cups) risotto rice

- 500ml (generous 2 cups) passata (sieved tomatoes)
- 1 litre (generous 4 cups) gluten-free vegetable stock
- 1 tsp salt
- ½ tsp ground black pepper
- 1 tbsp dried mixed herbs
- 70g (2½oz) mature Cheddar, finely grated

For the breadcrumb topping

- 1 x 125g (4½oz) ball of mozzarella, cut into small chunks
- 70g (2½oz) gluten-free breadcrumbs
- Vegetable oil spray

Preheat the oven to 180°C fan/200°C (400°F).

Add the margarine to a large ovenproof pot that has a lid and place over a medium heat. Once melted, add the onion or leek and fry until the onion is browned or the leek has softened.

Add the frozen veg and, once defrosted a little, add the rice and stir well. Fry for 2–3 minutes before adding the passata, stock, salt, pepper and mixed herbs. Briefly stir, then pop the lid

on, transfer to the oven and bake for 25 minutes. Remove the lid, briefly stir and place back in the oven with the lid removed for 10 minutes.

Stir in the grated Cheddar until melted, then scatter the chopped mozzarella on top and pat down to form a flat layer. Sprinkle the breadcrumbs all over the top so that no risotto can be seen below and spray well with oil. Return to the oven for 15 minutes or until the breadcrumbs are golden and crisp.

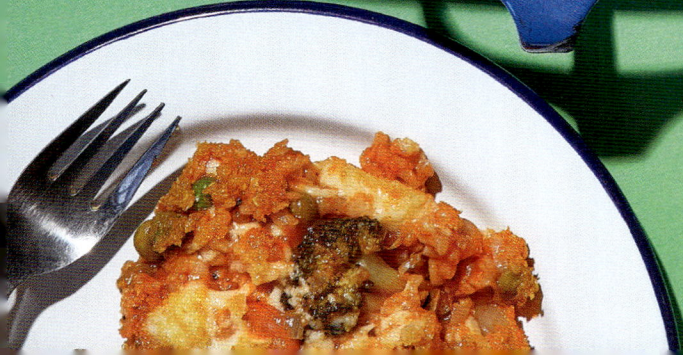

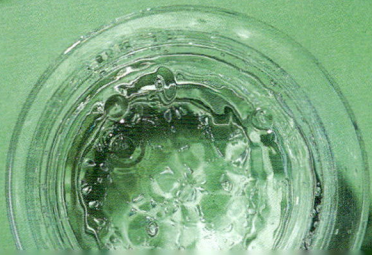

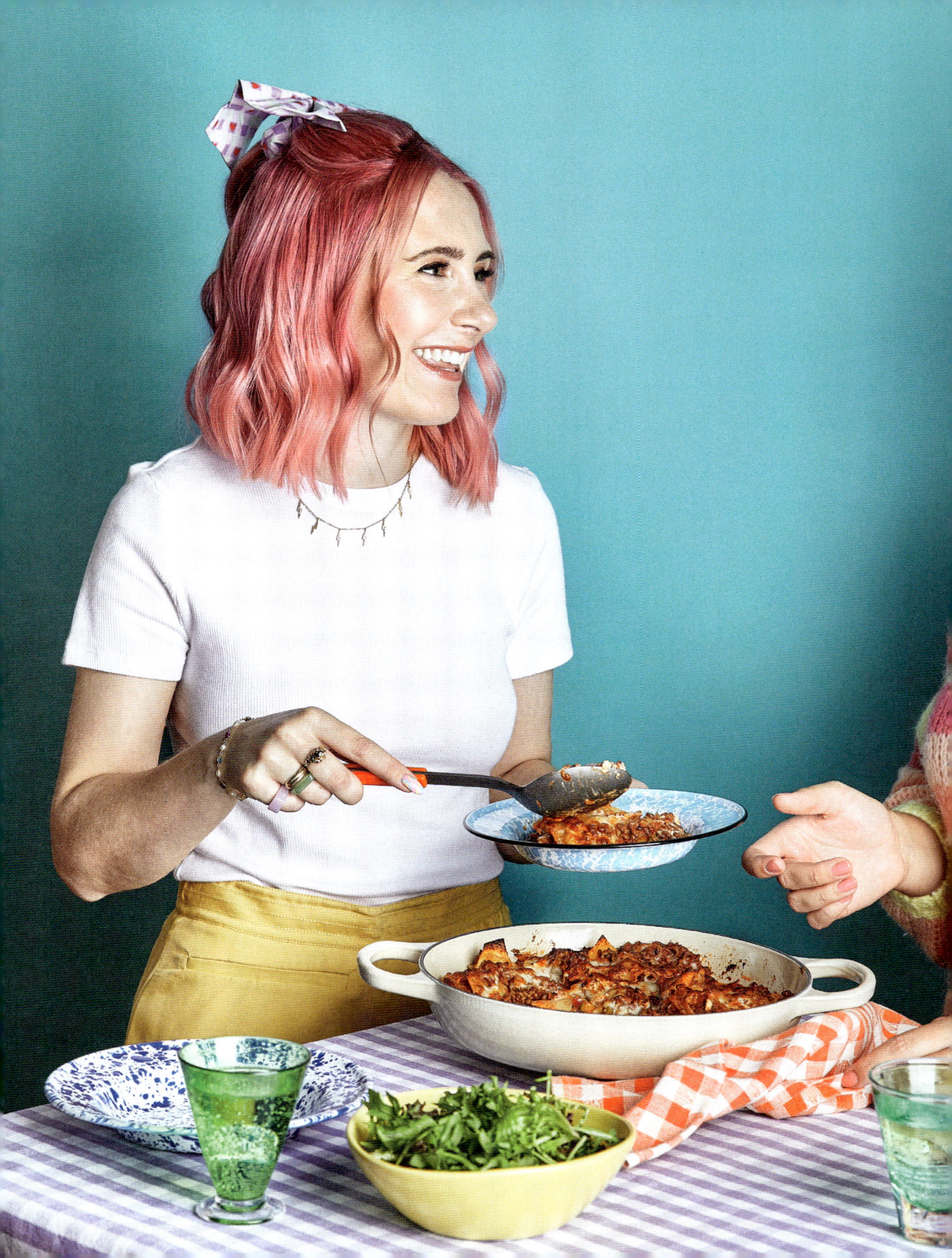

ONE-PAN BEEF OR LENTIL LASAGNE

This recipe has been proudly sitting on the blog for a couple of years and has more than stood the test of time as a reader favourite – and I can see why! Normally, you'd need to make a separate beef ragu and white sauce in two pans, then transfer to a roasting dish, layer up and bake for an hour. However, with this recipe, not only is everything fast tracked, it's all done in one pot! Best of all, it's all made from humble, affordable ingredients and you can optionally make it veggie and infinitely more budget-friendly using canned lentils, if you fancy. Serve with a rocket (arugula) salad.

Serves 2–4

Prep 5 mins

Hob + Grill (Broiler) 30 mins

DF Use dairy-free cream cheese and dairy-free cheese instead of mozzarella and Cheddar.

LL Use lactose-free cream cheese.

V Use lentils instead of beef and veggie/vegan-friendly stock.

VE Combine the dairy-free and veggie advice.

❄ See freezing and defrosting guidance for pasta dishes on page 28.

- Vegetable oil spray
- 100g (3½oz) frozen chopped onion **or** ½ medium leek, finely chopped
- 1 medium courgette (zucchini), finely diced
- 500g (1lb 2oz) minced (ground) beef **or** 2 x 400g (14oz) cans of lentils, drained
- 1 x 400g (14oz) can of chopped tomatoes
- 2 tbsp tomato purée (paste)
- 150ml (⅝ cup) gluten-free beef stock
- 1 tbsp dried mixed herbs
- Pinch each of salt and ground black pepper
- 6–8 gluten-free dried lasagne sheets
- 3 tbsp cream cheese
- 2 handfuls each of grated mozzarella and mature Cheddar

Spray the base of a large ovenproof pot that has a lid with oil and place over a medium heat. Once hot, add the onion or leek and fry until softened. Add the courgette and fry until it is also a little softened.

If using beef, add it to the pot and fry until browned, breaking it up as it cooks. Add the chopped tomatoes, purée, stock, mixed herbs, salt and pepper and mix until all combined. If using lentils, add them now.

Break each lasagne sheet into 2–4 pieces and push them down into the sauce. Space them apart equally so that they're not sitting on top of each other. Allow to simmer until the pasta is al dente – as it becomes more flexible you can move the pieces about a little (I like to have some bits more visible and some beneath the sauce).

Dollop in the cream cheese, then swirl it around in the sauce a little – you don't need to fully mix it in. Sprinkle the grated cheeses over the top of the dish then pop under a hot grill (broiler) on a medium heat for 5 minutes, or until the cheese is golden brown.

PERI-PERI HALLOUMI PASTA

Serves 4

Prep 5 mins

Oven + Hob 40 mins or
Air Fryer + Hob 25 mins

LL **V**

DF
Either omit the halloumi completely or replace it with 400g (14oz) skinless, boneless chicken thighs (chopped into 1cm/½in strips) and follow the cooking instructions as though it were halloumi.

❄ See freezing and defrosting guidance for pasta dishes on page 28.

This recipe combines my love of many things, namely traybakes, all-in-one pasta dishes, crispy halloumi and my homemade mild peri-peri seasoning (which, if you've been savvy shopping using my tips on page 12, will work out cheaper than buying a pre-made blend).

- 400g (14oz) frozen sliced red, green and yellow (bell) peppers
- 500g (1lb 2oz) frozen sweet potato or butternut squash cubes
- 1 tsp salt
- 450g (1lb) halloumi, cut into 5mm (¼in) slices

For the peri-peri seasoning
- 3½ tsp chilli powder

- 3½ tsp smoked paprika
- 3½ tsp dried mixed herbs
- 3½ tbsp vegetable oil
- 3 tbsp red wine vinegar
- Grated zest of 1 lemon
- 2 tbsp vegetable oil

For the pasta and sauce
- Vegetable oil spray
- 100g (3½oz) frozen chopped onion **or** ½ medium leek, finely chopped

- 2 x 400g (14oz) cans of chopped tomatoes
- 1 tbsp tomato purée (paste)
- 800ml (3⅓ cups) gluten-free vegetable stock
- 400g (14oz) gluten-free dried pasta
- 400g (14oz) frozen or canned sweetcorn (drained weight)

In a small bowl, combine the peri-peri seasoning ingredients, reserving a quarter of the lemon zest for serving.

Add the peppers and frozen sweet potato or butternut squash to a large bowl, followed by half the peri-per seasoning and the salt. Mix well.

To prepare the veg and halloumi in the oven, preheat the oven to 190°C fan/210°C (410°F). Spread the coated veg out on 2 baking trays and bake in the oven for 10 minutes.

Meanwhile, add the halloumi to the now empty bowl, followed by half of the remaining peri-peri seasoning (leaving you a quarter of the original quantity). Mix well, then add to the baking trays, placing it in the gaps between the veg, and bake for a further 40 minutes, or until the halloumi is nicely browned on both sides.

To prepare the veg and halloumi in the air fryer, heat the air fryer to 180°C (350°F). Add the coated veg to the air fryer, spread out in an even layer (use both drawers if your air fryer has two), and air fry for 10 minutes, turning it

halfway. Meanwhile, mix the halloumi with half of the remaining peri-peri seasoning (leaving you a quarter of the original quantity), then add it to the air fryer in the gaps between the veg. Air fry for a further 12–15 minutes, turning everything halfway, or until the halloumi is browned on both sides.

Meanwhile, for the pasta and sauce, spray the base of a large pot that has a lid with oil and place over a medium heat. Once hot, add the onion or leek and fry until the onion is browned or the leek has softened. Add the remaining peri-peri seasoning and fry until fragrant. Stir in the chopped tomatoes, purée and stock. Add the pasta and ensure it is submerged under the liquid. Place the lid on, turn the heat to low and simmer for 10–15 minutes until the pasta is al dente and the sauce is a little thickened, then stir through the sweetcorn. Simmer with the lid removed for 5 more minutes.

Stir the roasted veg and halloumi through the pasta and sauce, then serve topped with the reserved lemon zest.

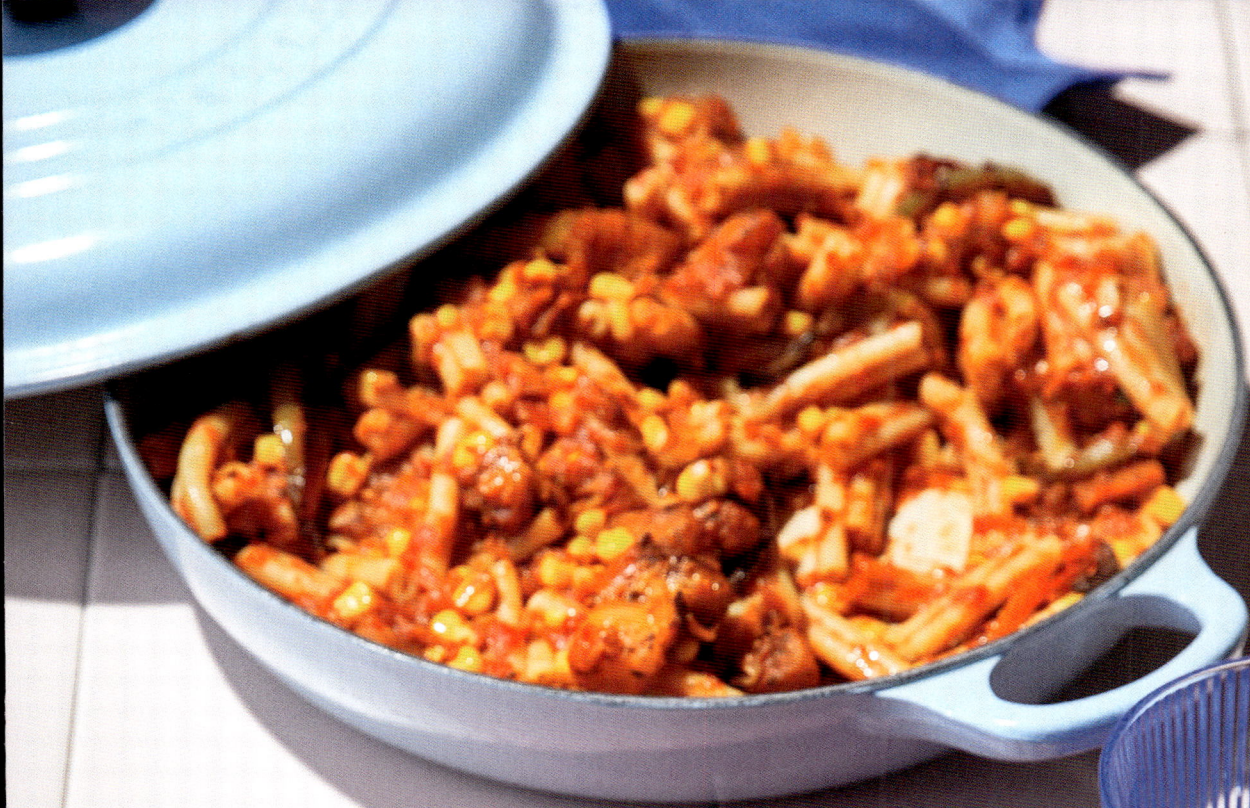

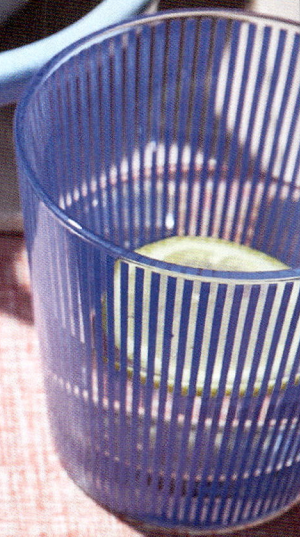

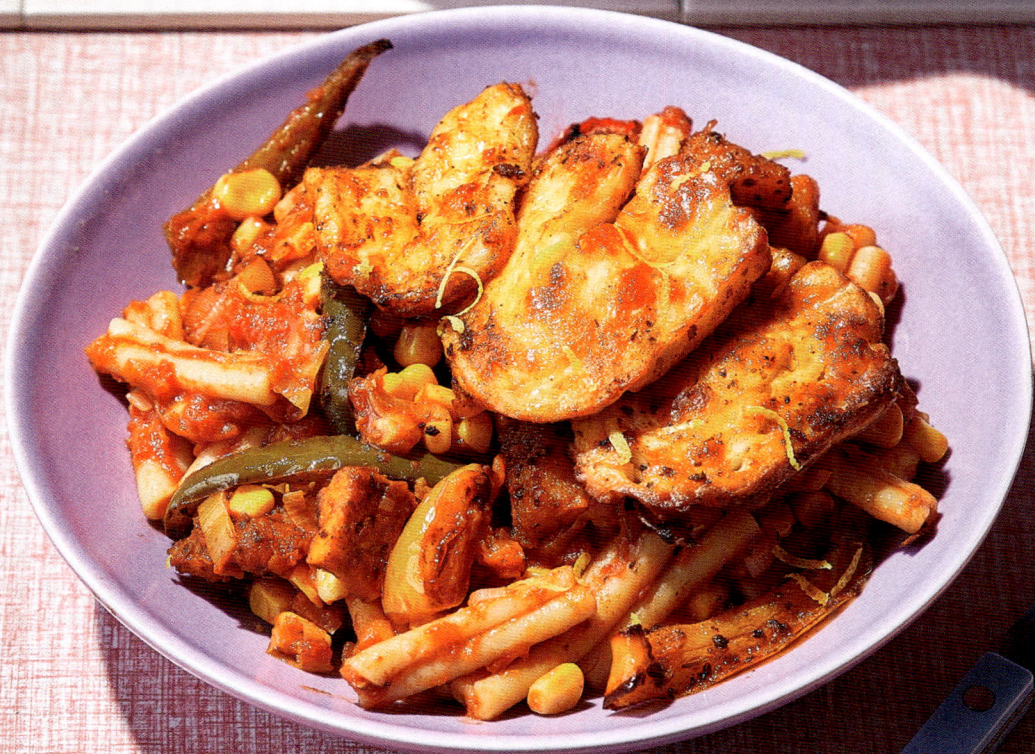

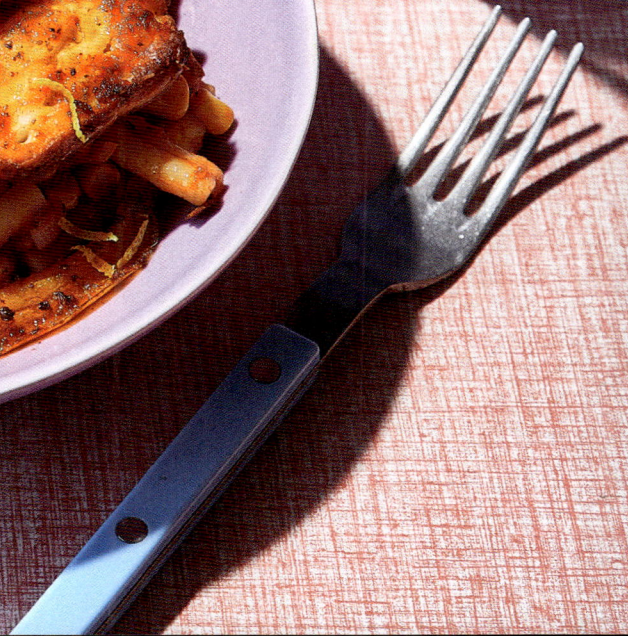

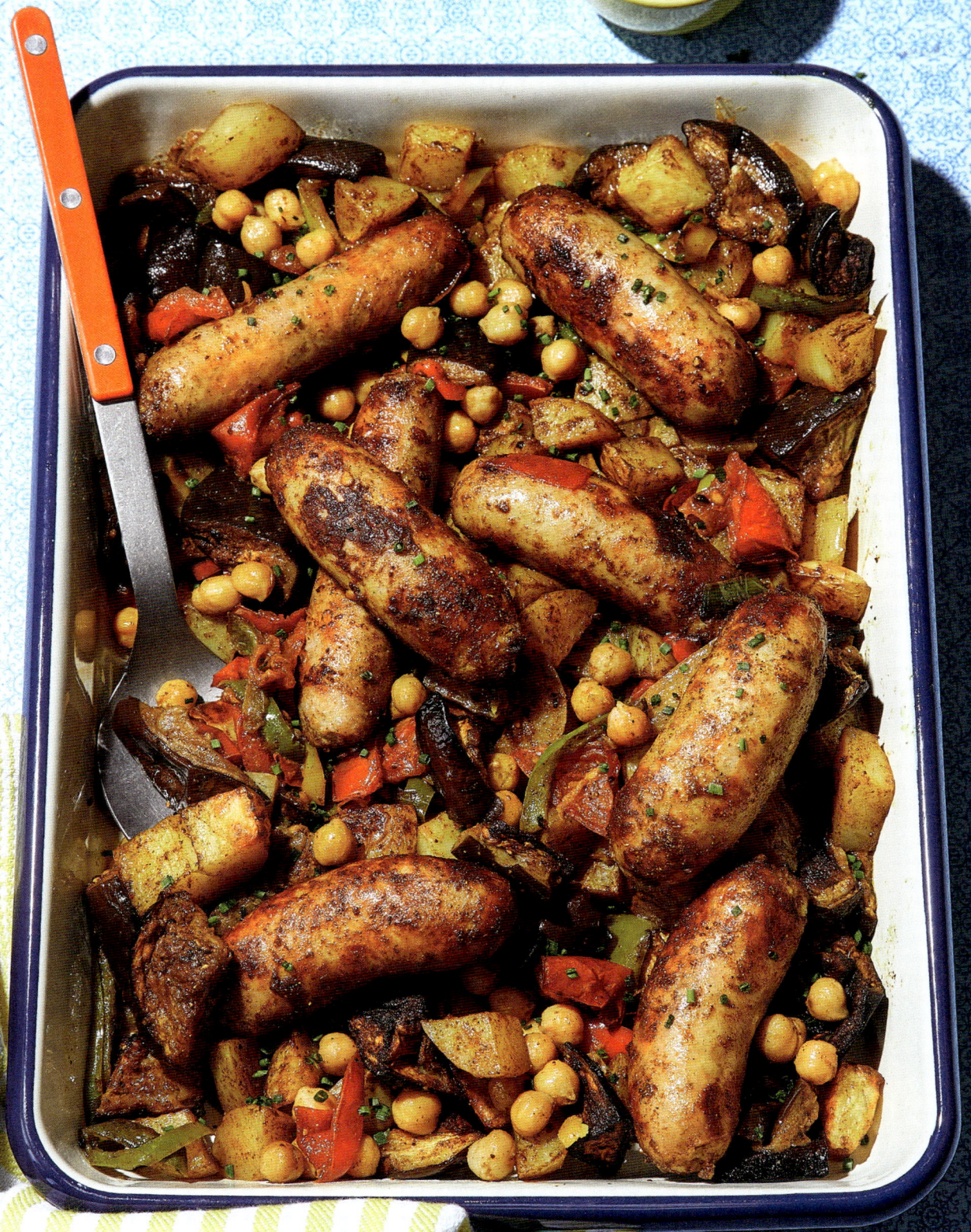

MOROCCAN-STYLE SAUSAGE TRAYBAKE

Serves 4 (oven) or 2 (air fryer)
Prep 10 mins
Oven 50–60 mins or
Air Fryer 30 mins

One of the best things about any traybake recipe is its hands-off nature (you wouldn't believe how productive I am about the house when the oven timer is counting down!). My homemade Moroccan-style spice blend here is a little cost saver and wonderfully ties together every ingredient in this super-easy, all-in-one supper.

DF **LF**

V Use gluten-free veggie-friendly sausages.

VE Use gluten-free vegan-friendly sausages.

❄ Once cooled, store in airtight containers in the freezer for 2–3 months. Allow to defrost completely in the fridge, then reheat in the air fryer for 10 minutes at 200°C (400°F). Check the internal temperature of the sausages with a digital food thermometer against those given on page 255.

- 2 medium aubergines (eggplants), cut into 3cm (1¼in) chunks
- 5 small potatoes (peeled or unpeeled), cut into 1.5cm (⅔in) chunks
- 4 tomatoes, cut into 2.5cm (1in) chunks
- 400g (14oz) frozen sliced red, green and yellow (bell) peppers, or frozen sweet potato cubes

- 8 gluten-free sausages
- Grated zest of 1 lemon
- 1 x 400g (14oz) can of chickpeas, drained
- Large handful of chives, finely chopped, to serve (optional)

For the spice blend
- 5 tbsp vegetable oil
- 2 tsp mild curry powder
- 1 tsp ground cinnamon
- 1 tsp ground allspice
- 1 tsp salt
- 1 tsp ground black pepper

TIP

If using an air fryer for this recipe, before starting you should know that this is quite a large quantity of food to cook in an air fryer! Though the quantity of veg might fit into deep air fryer drawers, piling it up will massively increase the cooking time and the veg will also cook very unevenly. So, for that reason, I'd recommend you halve the quantities for the recipe or air fry the given quantities in 2 batches. The air fryer method opposite assumes you have halved the recipe to serve 2 people.

To cook in an oven, preheat the oven to 220°C fan/240°C (460°F). In a small dish, combine all the ingredients for the spice blend.

Divide the aubergines, potatoes, tomatoes, frozen peppers or sweet potato and sausages between 2 bowls (because it'll probably be way too much to fit into just one and therefore much easier to mix in 2 bowls). Add half the spice blend and lemon zest to each, then stir both until everything is well coated.

Spread the contents of each bowl onto 2 baking trays and spread out into a flat, even layer. Bake in the oven for 50–60 minutes or until the veg and sausages are golden brown, turning everything over halfway and scattering over the chickpeas after you do so.

To cook in an air fryer (see TIP before starting!), in a large bowl, combine the spice blend, lemon zest and prepared veg and sausages and mix well to coat, then remove the sausages to a plate and set aside. Heat the air fryer to 180°C (350°F). Add the veg and spread it out into an even layer (use both drawers if your machine has 2) and air fry for 15 minutes, turning everything over halfway.

Add the chickpeas and turn the veg over once more, then add the sausages on top and air fry for 15 minutes, turning everything over halfway, or until the sausages are nicely browned on both sides and all the vegetables are fork-tender.

Sprinkle with chopped chives, if using, and serve.

ONE-POT LEBANESE-STYLE CHICKEN + RICE

Serves 4–6

Prep 10 mins + 15 mins marinating

Hob 45 mins

LL

DF Use a dairy-free alternative to feta, if using.

F Omit the garlic paste or use 1 tbsp garlic-infused oil, and use leek (green parts only) instead of onion. Use no more than 225g (8oz) green (bell) peppers instead of mixed colours, and use low FODMAP stock.

❄ See freezing and defrosting guidance for risotto and rice dishes on page 28.

TIP

Once simmered (and if you used an ovenproof lidded pot) you can optionally place the finished dish in an 180°C fan/200°C (400°F) oven for 25 minutes for a crispy, baked-rice-style finish.

If only all cooking from scratch was this simple! I'm a huge fan of one-pot rice dishes for that exact reason – not only does it usually mean a lot of hands-off cooking time, but because the rice, chicken and veg is cooked all in the same pot, there's so much less washing up. With gyros-style chicken on the bone (even if you prefer boneless, simply strip the chicken from the bone before serving – it's a super cost-effective ingredient!) and chicken-infused rice with creamy feta-style cheese (again, it's far cheaper than proper feta and still really, really nice), this meal is a winner in so many different ways.

- 5–6 skin-on, bone-in chicken thighs
- 2 tbsp smoked paprika
- ½ tbsp ground cumin or mild curry powder
- ½ tbsp ground coriander or mild curry powder
- 2 tbsp dried mixed herbs
- Grated zest of 1 small lemon
- 1 tsp garlic paste (optional)

- 1 tsp salt
- 1 tsp ground black pepper
- Vegetable oil spray
- 100g (3½oz) frozen chopped onion **or** ½ medium leek, finely chopped
- 400g (14oz) frozen sliced red, green and yellow (bell) peppers

- 300g (1⅔ cups) long-grain rice
- 600ml (2½ cups) gluten-free chicken stock (see page 163 for homemade)
- 200g (7oz) feta-style salad cheese, crumbled or cubed (optional)
- Small handful of coriander (cilantro) leaves, roughly chopped, to serve (optional)

To a large bowl, add the chicken, smoked paprika, cumin or curry powder, ground coriander or curry powder, mixed herbs, lemon zest, garlic paste, if using, salt and pepper. Stir to combine, cover and place in the fridge to marinate for anywhere from 15 minutes to 12 hours.

Spray the base of a large pot that has a lid with oil and place over a medium heat. Add the marinated chicken and fry for 4–5 minutes on each side, until golden brown.

Remove the chicken to a plate. Add the onion or leek and the frozen peppers to the pot and fry until softened, then stir in the rice. Fry for a few minutes until the rice has absorbed any moisture then add the chicken back to the pan. Add the stock and bring to the boil, then turn down the heat to low, pop the lid on and simmer for 30 minutes, turning over any visible rice on top after 20 minutes. Remove the lid and simmer for 5–10 minutes or until the rice is cooked.

Optionally scatter over the feta-style cheese and coriander, then serve.

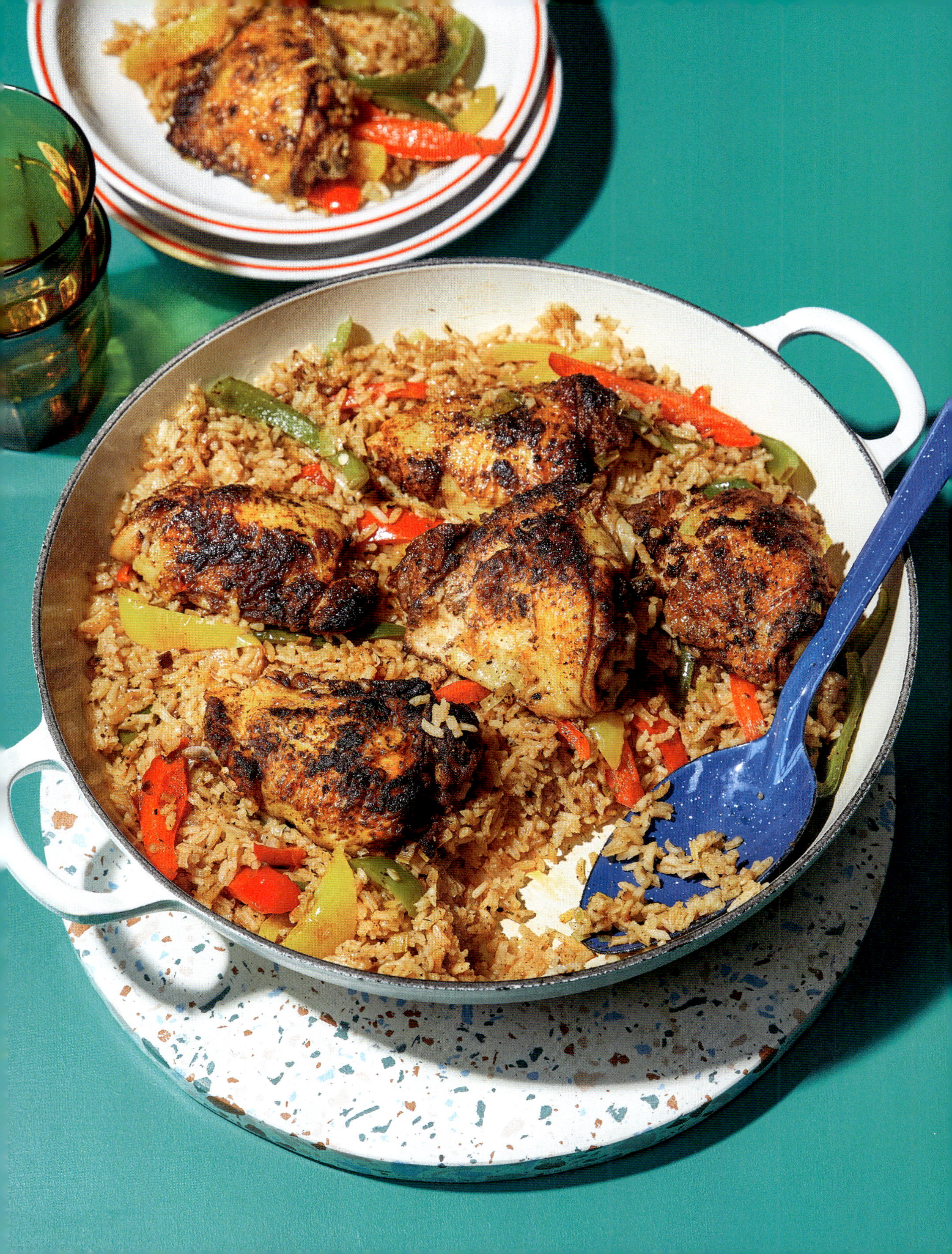

OUMA'S TANGY BEEF BABOTIE

First of all, if you have no idea what this is, then you already have a reason to make it and find out! It's a classic South African beef casserole adopted by the Cape Malay community that my Ouma (my South African grandma) used to absolutely love. Think of a curried cottage pie filling with a fruity tang thanks to the chutney, topped off with a custardy egg layer. If you like steak and eggs, then you will probably love this! It's traditionally made with a slice of white bread soaked in milk to help thicken the filling, but I've opted for naturally gluten-free starch, as bread isn't as cheap for us as it is for others! Serve with rice and a little extra chutney on the side.

Serves 5–6

Prep 10 mins

Hob + Oven 1 hour

DF Use dairy-free milk.

LF Use lactose-free milk.

V Swap the beef for 500g (1lb 2oz) gluten-free vegetarian mince (ground meat) alternative and a 400g (14oz) can of drained lentils.

TIPS

You have the option here of either using all minced (ground) beef or a mix of beef and lentils. The reason I give you this choice is because substituting part of the beef with lentils is an easy and convenient way to make this recipe even more cost-effective with almost no difference to the taste or texture of the finished dish. Whether you opt to do that though is entirely up to you!

Due to the egg layer not turning out particularly well after freezing and reheating, I haven't provided freezing advice here. However, you can still keep leftover portions in the fridge for 3–4 days in airtight containers. To reheat, simply microwave on full power (loosely covered) until piping hot in the middle.

- Vegetable oil spray
- 100g (3½oz) frozen chopped onion **or** ½ medium leek, finely chopped
- 750g (1lb 10oz) minced (ground) beef **or** 500g (1lb 2oz) minced beef and 1 x 400g (14oz) can of lentils, drained
- 300g (10½oz) frozen peas
- 2 tbsp mild curry powder
- 4 tbsp cornflour (cornstarch) or potato starch
- 1 tsp salt
- ½ tsp ground black pepper
- 3 tbsp lemon juice
- 4 tbsp fruit-based chutney (I like Mrs H.S. Ball's), plus extra to serve
- 90g (3¼oz) raisins or finely chopped dried apricot
- 4 large eggs
- 200ml (generous ¾ cup) milk
- 5–6 small dried bay leaves

Preheat the oven to 160°C fan/ 180°C (350°F).

Spray the base of a large ovenproof pot that has a lid with oil and place over a medium heat. Once hot, add the onion or leek and fry until the onion is browned or the leek has softened.

Add the beef and, once it releases a little moisture, scrape anything stuck to the bottom of the pan until it's deglazed. Once the beef has browned, add the lentils, if using, the frozen peas, curry powder, cornflour or potato starch, salt and black pepper. Stir well and fry until fragrant and until there's no liquid left in the pan. Add the lemon juice, chutney and raisins or apricots, stir in and fry for 2–3 minutes. Meanwhile, add the eggs and milk to a jug (pitcher) and beat well with a fork.

Pour the egg and milk mixture over the beef mixture, scatter the bay leaves on top and bake in the oven for 45–50 minutes. Remove the bay leaves before serving.

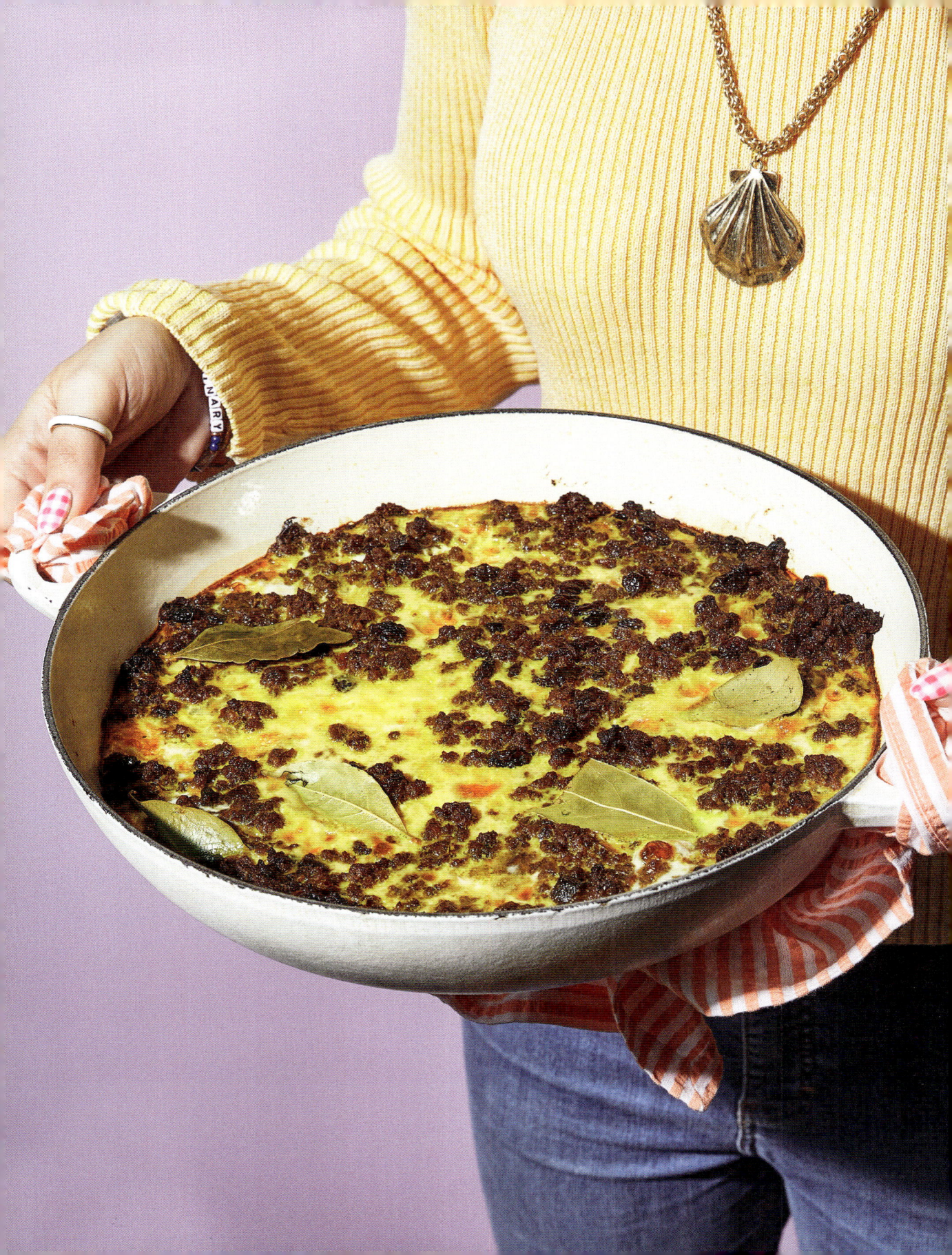

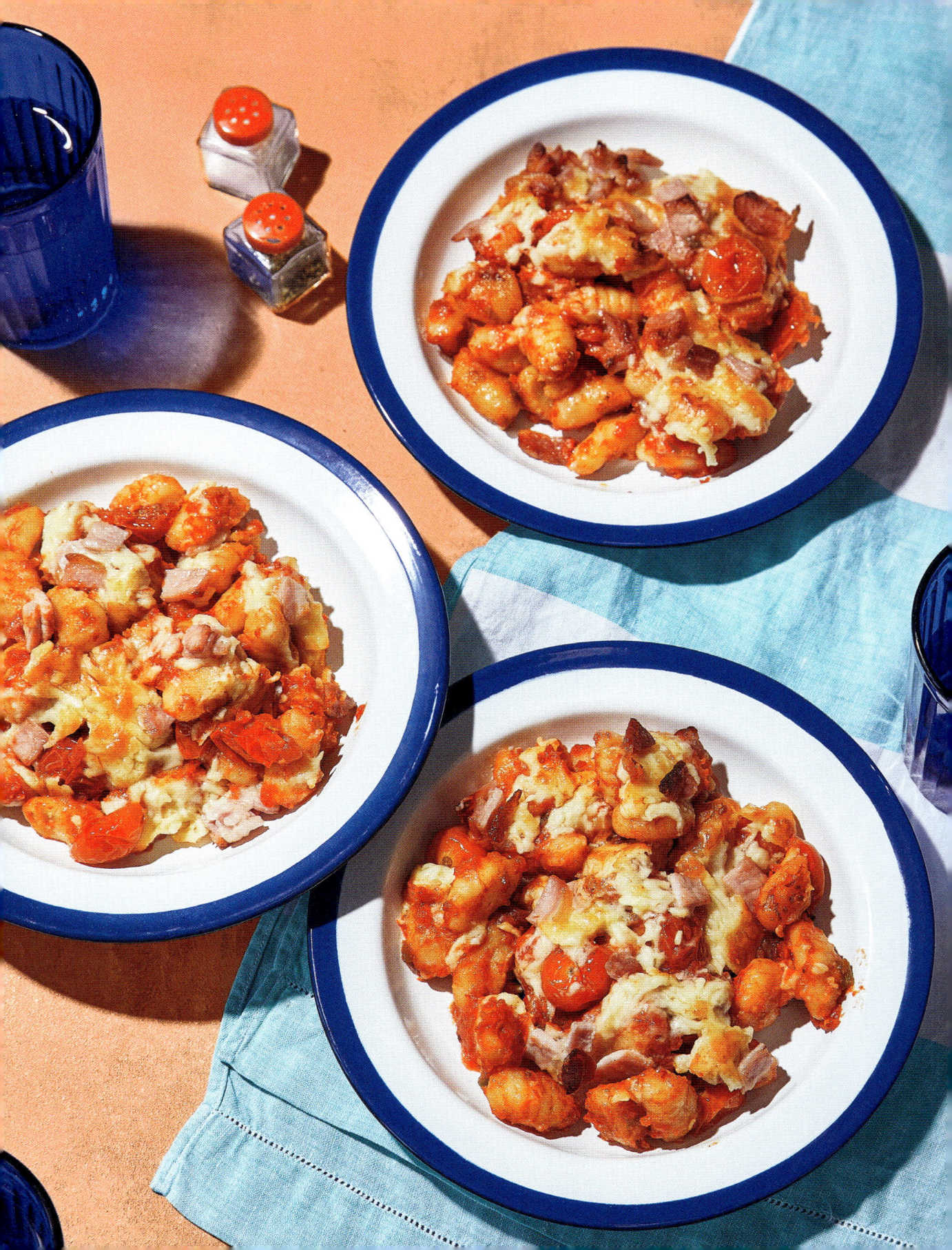

SMOKY BACON + CHEDDAR GNOCCHI AL FORNO

Serves 5–6

Prep 5 mins

Hob + Air Fryer 30 mins or
Hob + Oven 45 mins

LL

DF Use dairy-free cheese.

V Use leftover or stale gluten-free bread, crumbled and sprayed well with vegetable oil instead of bacon.

VE Combine dairy-free and veggie advice.

F Swap the cherry tomatoes for 300g (10½oz) courgette (zucchini), sliced into 1cm (½in) cubes (no need to squish them!).

❄ See freezing and defrosting guidance for pasta dishes on page 28. Once defrosted, cook in the oven at 180°C fan/200°C (400°F) for 15 minutes or the air fryer at 200°C (400°F) for 8–10 minutes once more to crisp up the top.

TIP

Struggling to find gluten-free gnocchi at reasonable prices? You can always turn this into a pasta bake by boiling 350–400g (12½–14oz) gluten-free dried pasta or orzo, then skip the first step of frying the gnocchi and proceed as directed.

Believe it or not, it's possible to find 'accidentally' gluten-free fresh gnocchi in supermarkets, which means that not only is it back on the menu, but at 'normal people' prices! So celebrate that fact by using great-value gnocchi in this comforting Italian-style dish, inspired by one of my favourite dishes: gnocchi all'amatriciana. My version is a little more economized in all the right places, yet still retains everything I love about the original. Serve with rocket (arugula).

- Vegetable oil spray
- 2 x 500g (1lb 2oz) packets of fresh gluten-free gnocchi
- 250g (9oz) cherry tomatoes, halved
- 1 x 400g (14oz) can of chopped tomatoes
- 15g (½oz) jarred jalapeños, finely chopped
- 1 tsp salt
- 100g (3½oz) mature Cheddar, grated
- 6 rashers of smoked back bacon, finely diced

To prepare the gnocchi on the hob, spray the base of a large ovenproof pot that has a lid with oil and place over a medium heat. Once hot, add the gnocchi and spray all over with oil once more. Fry until the gnocchi is golden brown in places, then transfer to a dinner plate and set aside.

To prepare the gnocchi in the air fryer, heat the air fryer to 200°C (400°F). Lightly spray the base of the air fryer basket or crisping tray with oil. Add the gnocchi in an even layer, generously spray with oil and air fry for 8 minutes until a little golden, turning it halfway.

For the sauce, spray the base of a large ovenproof pot that has a lid with oil (no need to clean the pot first if you just used it to prepare the gnocchi) and place over a medium heat. Add the cherry tomatoes cut-side down and place the lid on top. Allow to cook for 3–4 minutes or until you can easily squish them with a wooden spoon.

Add the chopped tomatoes, jalapeños and salt, then reduce the heat to low–medium and allow to gently bubble for 5–10 minutes. Stir in the prepared gnocchi and remove the pan from the heat.

To cook the gnocchi bake in the oven, preheat the oven to 180°C fan/ 200°C (400°F). Pat the gnocchi and sauce flat with the back of a wooden spoon, then top with the cheese and scatter the bacon all over the top. Bake in the oven for 25 minutes or until the bacon is crisp and golden brown.

To cook the gnocchi bake in the air fryer, heat the air fryer to 200°C (400°F), with the crisping tray or basket removed. Transfer the gnocchi and sauce to the air fryer (if you have 2 drawers in your air fryer, it'd be best to use both drawers or you won't get much crispy top at all!) then top with cheese and scatter the bacon all over the top. Air fry for 6–8 minutes or until the bacon is crisp and golden brown.

CHEDDAR + HERB GARDENER'S PIE

Serves 4–6

Prep 10 mins

Hob + Oven 1 hour

With a creamy, cheesy, mustard and spinach mash with a crispy top concealing a herby sauce with a chunky veg and butter bean filling, any gardener would be lucky to come back from the shed and sit down to a plate of this! It's my idea of veggie comfort food at its finest: a dish that provides a welcome reminder that not every single meal must contain meat to be deeply satisfying and nutritious!

V

DF Use dairy-free milk, a dairy-free 'buttery' margarine and a dairy-free cheese.

LL Use lactose-free milk and lactose-free 'buttery' margarine.

F See low lactose advice and use leek (green parts only) instead of onion. Use 140g (5oz) of butter beans (drained weight) and 3 carrots instead of 2.

VE See dairy-free advice.

❄ See freezing and defrosting guidance for soups, stews and curries on page 28 (ensure you store leftovers with the mashed potato layer facing up). Once defrosted, cook in the oven at 180°C fan/200°C (400°F) for 15 minutes or the air fryer at 200°C (400°F) for 8–10 minutes once more to crisp up the top.

TIP

If you didn't make the filling in an ovenproof pot, you can instead transfer the filling to a large, deep roasting dish (around 33 x 25cm/ 13 x 10in) before topping with mash and baking as directed.

For the mash top
- 1kg (2lb 3oz) potatoes, peeled and cut into 2.5cm (1in) chunks
- 125g (4½oz) frozen spinach
- 2 tbsp milk
- 2 tbsp 'buttery' margarine
- 1 tsp Dijon mustard
- 1 tsp salt
- ½ tsp ground black pepper

For the creamy bean and chunky veg filling
- Vegetable oil spray
- 100g (3½oz) frozen chopped onion **or** ½ medium leek, finely chopped
- 2 medium carrots, sliced into 5mm (¼in) rounds
- 1 medium courgette (zucchini), sliced into 5mm (¼in) rounds

- 2 tbsp cornflour (cornstarch) or potato starch
- 2 tsp dried mixed herbs
- 1 tsp salt
- ½ tsp ground black pepper
- 500ml (generous 2 cups) milk
- 1 x 400g (14oz) can butter (lima) beans, drained
- ½ tsp Dijon mustard
- 125g (4½oz) mature Cheddar, grated

Place the potatoes in a large saucepan of boiling water. Bring to the boil again, then simmer for 15–20 minutes until you can poke a fork through them without much force. Around 5 minutes before they're done, add the spinach. Drain and set aside.

Meanwhile, for the filling, preheat the oven to 180°C fan/200°C (400°F). Spray the base of a large ovenproof pot that has a lid with oil and place over a medium heat. Once hot, add the onion or leek and fry until a little softened. Add the carrots and courgette, then fry for 2–3 minutes, pop the lid on and cook for 7–8 minutes until softened; lift the lid and stir halfway.

Stir in the cornflour or potato starch, mixed herbs, salt and pepper. Add the milk, bring to the boil, then reduce the heat to low–medium and simmer until it thickens a little. Add the butter beans and mustard and stir in half the

cheese. Simmer for 4–5 minutes or until nicely thickened.

Return the cooked, drained potatoes and spinach to their large saucepan and add the milk, margarine, mustard, salt and pepper and remaining grated cheese. Use a potato masher to mash until super smooth – it should be a little looser than you'd usually serve mash so it's easier to spread on top of the pie. If yours is a little thick and stodgy, gradually add a little more milk and mix in until easily spreadable.

Use a large serving spoon to dollop the mash on top of the filling, then use the back of a spoon to spread out into a flat, even layer. Use a fork to create wavy lines all over the top and bake in the oven for 30 minutes, or until the top is golden and crisp.

Serve with a dollop of your favourite chutney and a side salad.

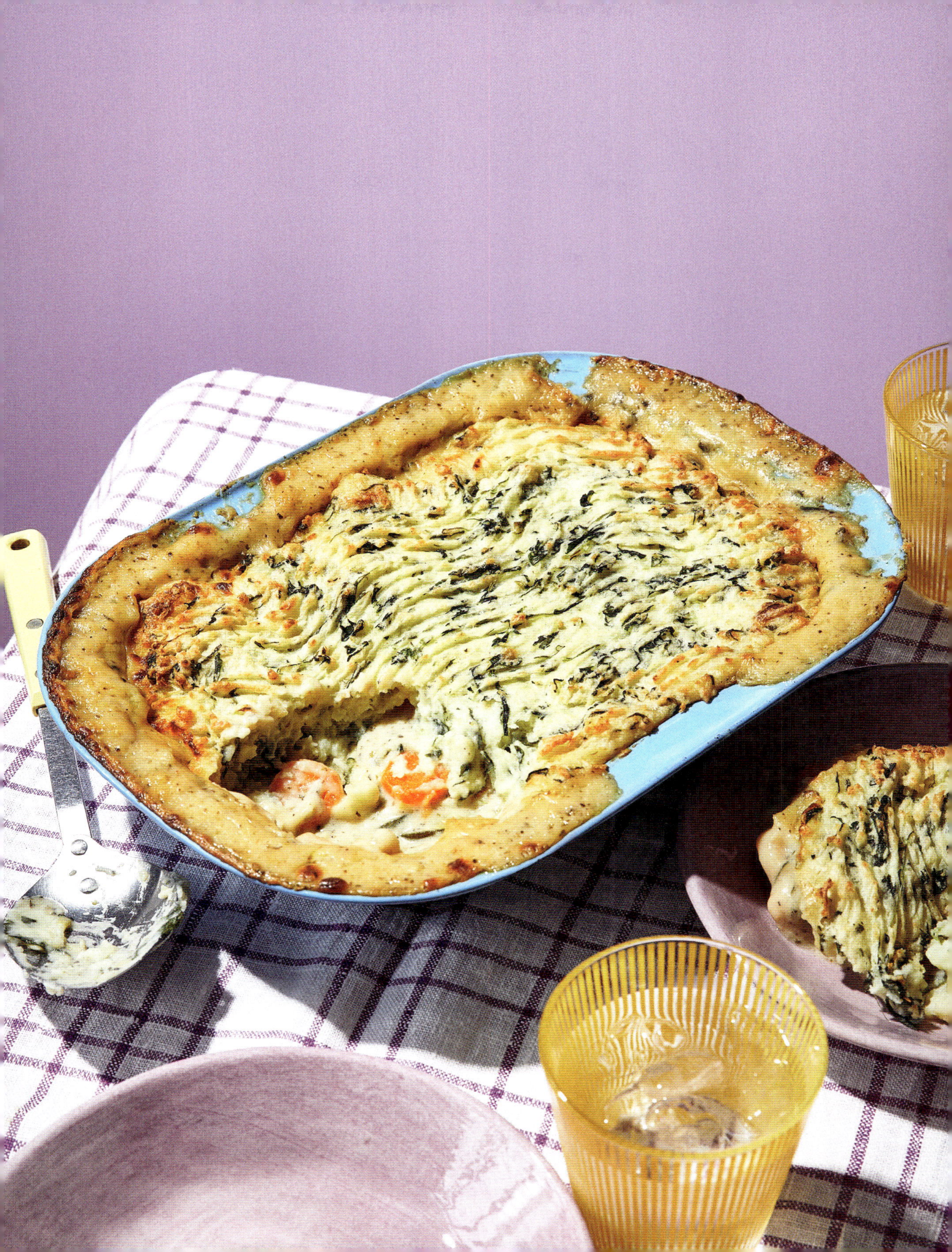

SAUSAGE BALLS IN PEPPERCORN SAUCE

Serves 3

Prep 10 mins

Hob + Oven 35 mins or
Hob + Air Fryer 35 mins

This easy-to-throw-together dish uses ever-affordable pork mince fashioned into crispy meatballs, enveloped in a creamy peppercorn sauce with mixed peppers and peas. It's exactly the type of comfort food I crave after a busy, long day and, fortunately for me, requires *just* the right level of effort I can muster when I'm in that state. Simply serve with pasta, rice or mashed potato and get back to the sofa!

DF Use a dairy-free 'buttery' margarine and dairy-free cream cheese.

LF Use a lactose-free 'buttery' margarine and lactose-free cream cheese.

F See lactose-free advice and use low FODMAP stock. Use leek (green parts only) instead of onion, no more than 225g (8oz) of green (bell) pepper instead of mixed colours, and 150g (5½oz) of canned peas (drained weight) instead of frozen peas. Add 2 medium carrots (sliced into 5mm/¼in rounds) when frying the peppers.

❄ See freezing and defrosting guidance for soups, stews and curries on page 28.

- 2 tbsp 'buttery' margarine
- 100g (3½oz) frozen chopped onion **or** ½ medium leek, finely chopped
- 500g (1lb 2oz) frozen sliced red, green and yellow (bell) peppers
- 500g (1lb 2oz) minced (ground) pork

- ½ tsp salt
- ¼ tsp ground black pepper
- 4 tbsp cornflour (cornstarch) or potato starch
- Vegetable oil spray

For the sauce

- 2 tbsp cornflour (cornstarch) or potato starch

- 1½ tsp coarsely ground black pepper
- 700ml (scant 3 cups) gluten-free ham or vegetable stock
- 150g (⅔ cup) cream cheese
- 200g (7oz) frozen peas

Add the margarine to a large pot that has a lid and place over a medium-high heat. Once melted, add the onion or leek and fry until the onion is browned or the leek has softened. Transfer to a large bowl. Add the frozen peppers to the pot and fry until softened.

Add the pork, salt, pepper and cornflour or potato starch to the onion/leek bowl, and mix well until everything is evenly dispersed and the mince looks smooth. Roll into ping-pong-sized balls (about 35g/1¼oz each).

To cook the meatballs in the oven, preheat the oven to 200°C fan/220°C (425°F). Spray a large baking sheet with oil. Place the meatballs on the prepared baking sheet and spray well with oil, then bake in the oven for 20 minutes or until golden brown.

To cook the meatballs in the air fryer, heat the air fryer to 190°C (375°F). Generously spray the base of the air fryer basket or crisping tray with oil. If you have an air fryer with 2 drawers, use both. Place as many meatballs as will fit in the air fryer basket(s) without touching and generously spray with oil. Air fry for 12–15 minutes until crisp and golden brown, turning over halfway.

Meanwhile, add the cornflour or potato starch for the sauce to the pot with the peppers, followed by the coarsely ground pepper, and stir in. Add the stock and simmer over a low heat for 20 minutes until thickened. Stir in the cream cheese and frozen peas, then simmer for a further 5–10 minutes.

Add the cooked meatballs to the sauce and serve, with mashed potato, pasta or rice.

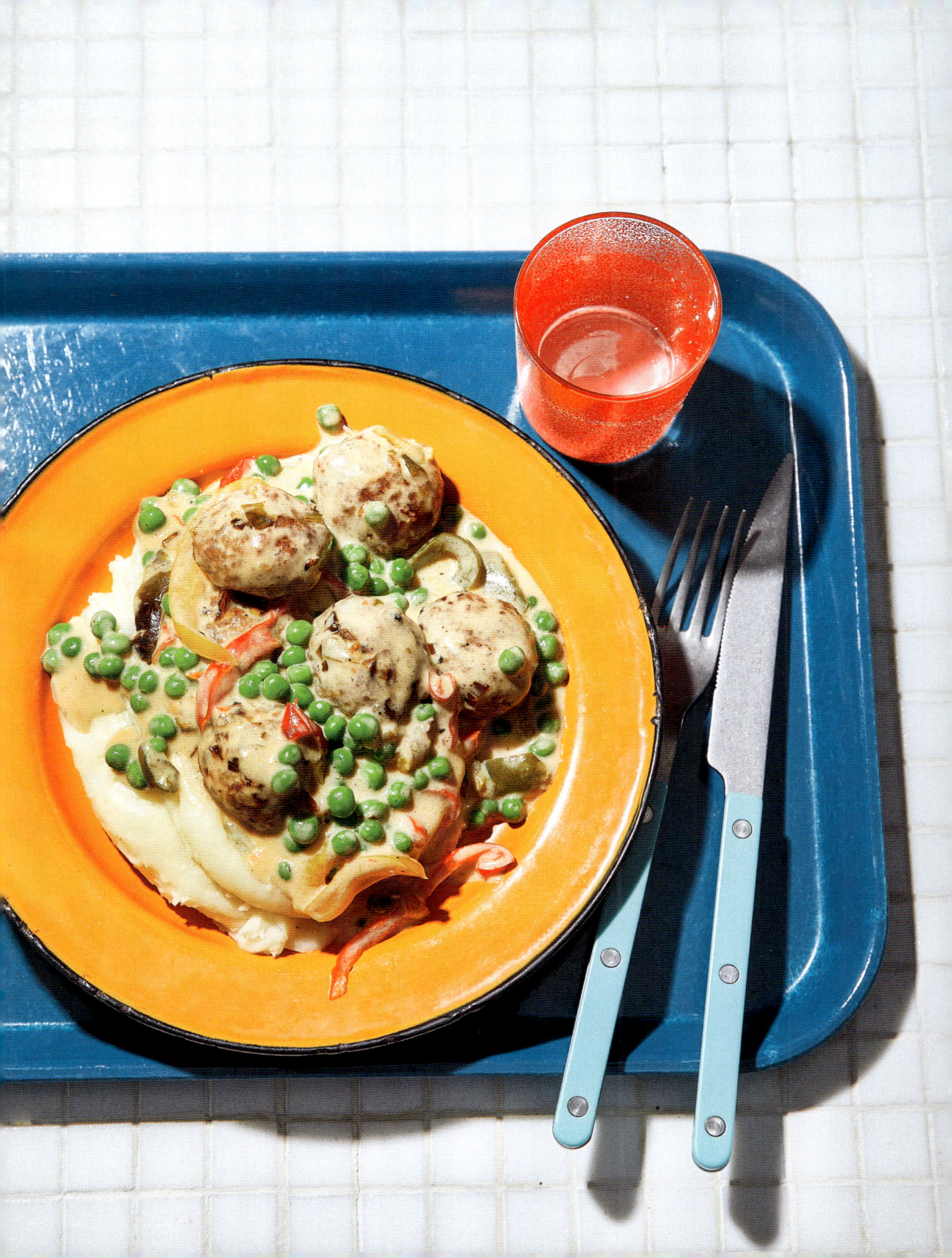

MARK'S MUM'S FIVE SPICE STICKY CHICKEN TRAYBAKE

Serves 4

Prep 5 mins + 15 mins marinating

Oven 35 mins or
Air Fryer 25 mins

DF **LF**

F Use the green part of the leek only. Use light brown sugar instead of honey and use crushed, salted, roasted peanuts (ensure gluten-free) instead of cashews.

❄ Once the chicken has cooled, store in airtight containers in the freezer for up to 2–3 months. Allow to defrost completely in the fridge, then reheat in the air fryer for 8–9 minutes at 200°C (400°F). Check the internal temp with a digital food thermometer against those given on page 255.

TIP

If you'd prefer not to use bone-in chicken (it's amazing value!) then around 750g (1lb 10oz) skinless, boneless chicken thighs would work well here too.

This marinade is one that Mark's mum has been using to coat chicken (be it bone-in chicken here or when frying chopped chicken breast for a quick meal) for decades. She has always simply called it 'black chicken' due to the dark colour achieved using dark soy sauce, but with gluten-free dark soy sauce not being readily available in shops, you can always opt to use black treacle or dark brown sugar instead of honey in the marinade to achieve the same effect. Mark and I use the marinade to make it into a full-on traybake that's perfect served with rice or noodles, which is exactly what you'll find here. Time efficient, cost effective and downright delicious!

- 4 skin-on, bone-in chicken thighs and 4 drumsticks
- Vegetable oil spray
- 3 medium carrots, halved lengthways then sliced into 1cm (½in) half-moons
- ½ medium leek, sliced into 5mm (¼in) rounds

- 75g (2½oz) cashew nuts, crushed a little with the end of a rolling pin
- Small handful of spring onion (scallion) greens, thinly sliced on the diagonal

For the marinade
- 1 tbsp vegetable oil

- 3 tbsp honey, black treacle or light/dark brown sugar
- 1 tbsp Chinese five spice
- 3 tbsp gluten-free soy sauce
- 2 tsp ginger paste
- ½ tsp ground black pepper
- 1 tsp fish sauce (optional)

In a large bowl, combine all the marinade ingredients until smooth. Add the chicken pieces, mix until well coated, cover and place in the fridge to marinate for anywhere from 15 minutes to 12 hours.

To cook in an oven, preheat the oven to 180°C fan/200°C (400°F). Spray a large baking tray with oil. Place the marinated chicken pieces on the baking tray, then place the carrots in any gaps, then the leek in the smaller leftover gaps or on top of the carrots a little if space is lacking. Bake in the oven for 30–35 minutes, turning over the chicken and carrots halfway, until the chicken is nicely browned and fully cooked.

To cook in an air fryer, heat the air fryer to 200°C (400°F). Generously spray the base of the air fryer basket or crisping tray with oil. If you have an air fryer with 2 drawers, you'll likely need to employ both, so grease both if necessary. Place as many chicken pieces as will fit into the air fryer basket without touching, then place the carrots in any gaps, then the leek in the smaller leftover gaps or on top of the carrots a little if space is lacking. Generously spray with oil and air fry for 22–25 minutes, turning them over halfway.

To serve, scatter over the cashews and spring onion greens, and serve with rice or rice noodles.

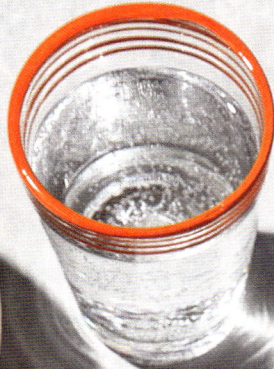

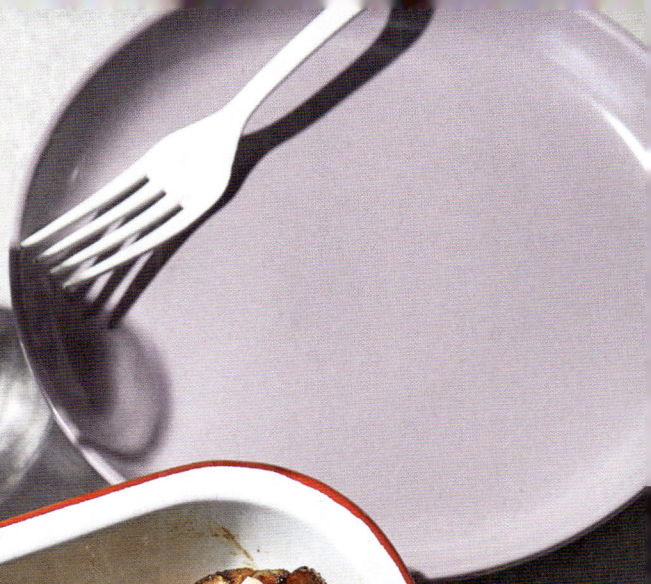

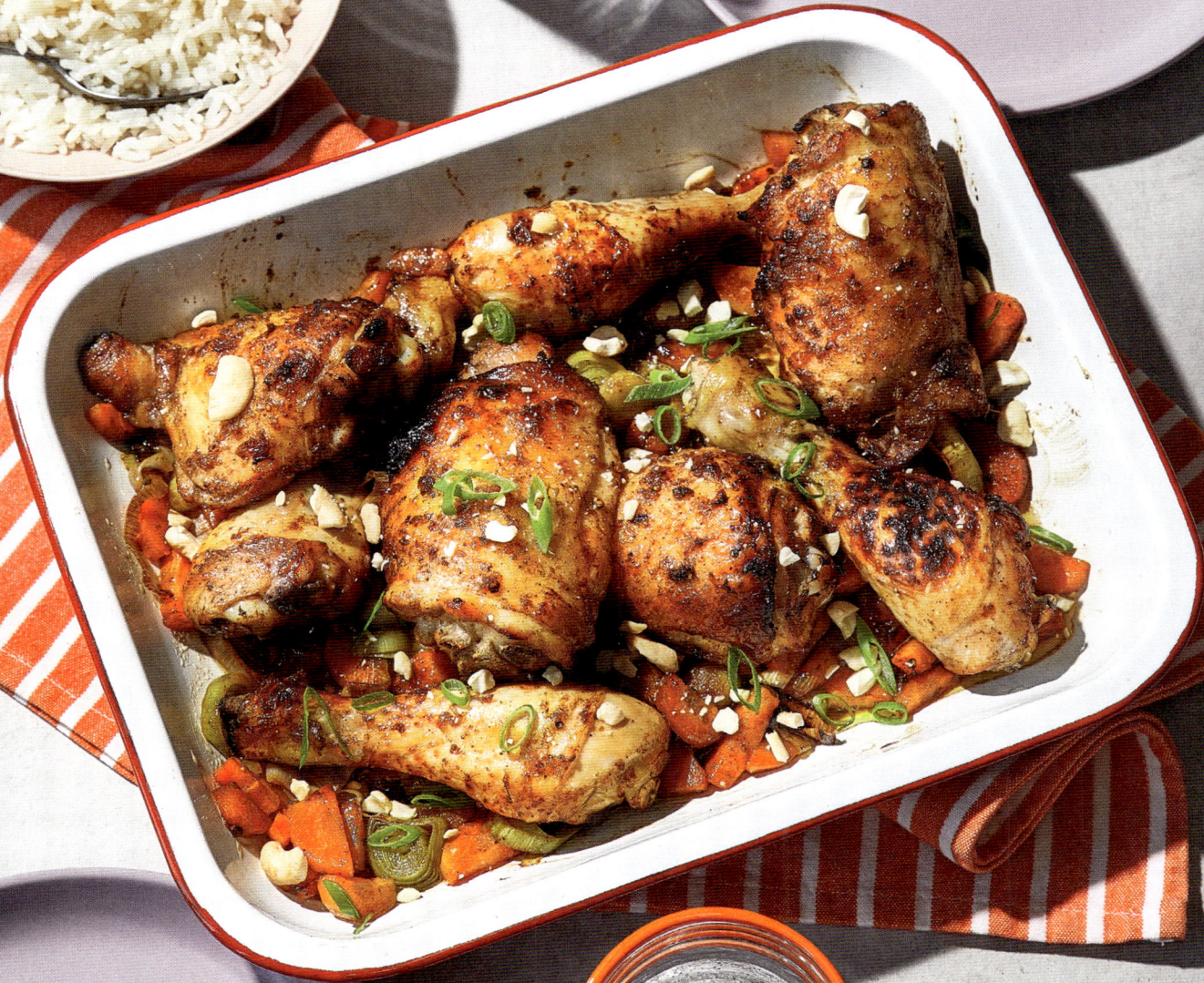

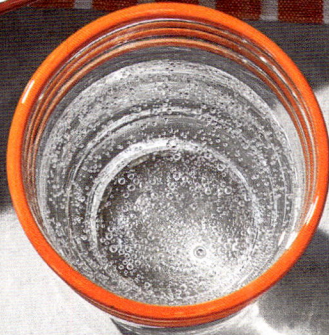

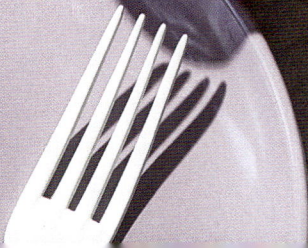

ONE CHICKEN, THREE DINNERS

This little mini subchapter completes the Comfort Food chapter of this book with a simple concept: roasting or air frying one whole chicken at the start of the week and using the cooked meat to make three delicious meals. Why? Firstly, value: it's just way more cost effective than buying smaller, separate packs of chicken. In fact, a 1.9kg (4lb) whole chicken yields around 900g (2lb) cooked chicken, making buying a whole chicken around 35–45% cheaper than buying 900g raw chicken breasts, which would also weigh even less (closer to 600g/1lb 5oz) once cooked. Plus, let's not forget that for every chicken you roast, you can also optionally use the drippings for a nice portion of gluten-free gravy, and use the carcass to make chicken stock at extremely little extra cost using the recipe opposite.

Secondly, not only will doing this save you money, it also brings back something we all crave with dinner: convenience! How? Well, with a main part of your meal already cooked, you'll massively reduce prep and cooking time. And last but not least... who wouldn't want tender chunks of juicy roast chicken in their dinner?!

So give this mini crash course to my 'one chicken, three dinners' concept a go, alongside the three mouthwatering recipes that follow it: Mark's Curry Mee, 'Marry Me' Chicken Pasta and Chicken Special Fried Rice. Of course, you can use the stripped, cooked chicken in any of the other recipes throughout this book too – just bear in mind it only needs to be heated up briefly as it's already cooked!

SALT + PEPPER ROAST CHICKEN
WITH GRAVY + STOCK

Serves 4–6

Prep 2 mins

Air Fryer 55 mins or
Oven 1 hour 20 mins

DF **LF** **F**

F Use the green parts of the leek only and use an extra carrot instead of the celery stalk.

❄ Once the chicken meat has cooled and been stripped from the carcass, store in airtight containers in the fridge for up to 3–4 days or in the freezer for up to 2–3 months. Allow to completely defrost in the fridge before using.

TIPS

Flipping a hot whole chicken in a very hot, very confined air fryer drawer can be a little tricky! I usually just use a large meat fork (the kind you'd use to help carve a turkey) to impale the entire chicken beneath the breast and lift it out, then flip.

Throughout this book you'll find I use fresh lemons for juice and zest fairly often. When you're left with used lemon halves, please always remember that this recipe exists; after all, they can be put to good use here! Regardless of if they've been grated or squeezed already, they'll still add great flavour to the chicken and help to steam it a little from the inside during cooking. So don't throw away your used lemons if you intend to make this!

- 4 tbsp vegetable oil
- 1 tsp salt
- ½ tsp ground black pepper
- 1 x 1.6kg (3½lb) whole chicken (for air fryer) **or** 1.9kg (4lb) whole chicken (for oven)
- 4–5 leftover lemon halves (optional)

For the gravy (optional)
- Chicken juices/drippings from the roasting tin
- 2 tbsp cornflour (cornstarch)
- 500ml (generous 2 cups) gluten-free chicken stock (see below for homemade)

For the stock (optional)
- Leftover chicken carcass and bones, stripped of all the meat
- ½ leek, roughly chopped
- 1 celery stalk, roughly chopped
- 2 medium carrots, roughly chopped
- 1 tbsp dried mixed herbs
- 1.5 litres (6¼ cups) boiling water

To roast the chicken

Combine the oil, salt and pepper in a small dish. Brush the chicken all over with the salt and pepper coating. If you have any leftover lemon halves, stuff them inside the cavity of the chicken.

To cook in an air fryer, heat the air fryer to 190°C (375°F). Tie both ends of the chicken legs together with string (this will make getting the chicken in and out of the air fryer a lot easier), then place the chicken, breast-side down, in the air fryer basket and air fry for 30 minutes. Flip it over (see **TIP**), brush with any remaining coating and air fry for a further 25 minutes. Check the inner thigh with a digital cooking thermometer to ensure it's done – it should read 74°C (165°F) or higher.

Remove from the air fryer (allow any juices to drip back into the air fryer), transfer to a board and allow to rest for 5–10 minutes before carving.

To cook in an oven, preheat the oven to 190°C fan/210°C (410°F). Place the chicken in a roasting tray and roast in the oven for 1 hour 20 minutes until the skin is super-crispy. Check the inner thigh with a digital cooking thermometer to ensure it's done – it should read 74°C (165°F) or higher.

Remove the chicken from the roasting tin (allow any juices to drip back into the tin) and transfer to a board. Allow the chicken to rest for 5–10 minutes before carving.

To serve

Strip the chicken as well as you can to remove every scrap of meat, then use in any of the recipes on the following few pages (or use instead of chicken breast in other recipes, bearing in mind it doesn't need to be heated for long), or simply use for lunch in salads and sandwiches.

To make the gravy

Pour the juices and drippings from the roasting tin or air fryer basket into a small pan and mix in the flour until smooth. Place over a low heat and gently heat for 2–3 minutes.

Pour in the stock and simmer for 5–10 minutes until it thickens to your liking. Strain and transfer to a serving jug (pitcher) or, once cooled, store in airtight containers in the fridge for up to 3–4 days or freezer for up to 2–3 months.

To make the stock

Place the carcass and any other bones into a large pot, along with the leek, celery, carrots and dried mixed herbs. Place over a low heat and pour in the boiling water.

Bring to the boil and allow to very gently bubble for 3–4 hours. Strain and allow to cool, then store in airtight containers in the fridge for up to 3–4 days, or freezer for up to 2–3 months.

MARK'S CURRY MEE

(CURRY NOODLES)

Here's Mark's version of his favourite Malaysian-style dish: creamy coconut curried soup noodles, packed with broccoli, leftover roasted chicken – and curried boiled eggs for good measure. It's a bowlful of flavour and variety that only gets better and better with each mouthful. You'll often find minced lemongrass in small jars (or squeezy tubes) alongside all the spices in supermarkets; alternatively, you could also use the equivalent amount of thinly sliced lemongrass stalk. Don't let the cooking time fool you – for most of that, you can be doing something else entirely!

Serves 3
Prep 10 mins
Hob 1 hour 15 mins

DF **LF**

V Use a veggie-friendly alternative to fish sauce, use 200g (7oz) frozen green beans instead of cooked chicken and use veggie-friendly stock.

VE See veggie advice and omit the eggs.

❄ See freezing and defrosting guidance for soups, stews and curries on page 28. Stir very gently and minimally while reheating to avoid breaking the noodles.

- 4 large eggs
- Vegetable oil spray, plus 2 tbsp vegetable oil for the sauce
- 100g (3½oz) frozen chopped onion **or** ½ medium leek, finely chopped
- 2 tsp fish sauce
- 1 tsp garlic paste (optional)
- 1 tsp lemongrass paste

- 20g (¾oz) jarred jalapeños, finely chopped
- 2 tbsp mild curry powder
- ¼ tsp ground black pepper
- 2 tbsp honey
- 1 x 400g (14oz) can of coconut milk
- 1.4–1.5 litres (6–6¼ cups) gluten-free chicken stock (see page 163 for homemade, or made using 2 stock cubes)

- 300g (10½oz) dried ribbon rice noodles
- 250–300g (9–10½oz) leftover cooked chicken, shredded **or** 300g (10½oz) skinless, boneless chicken breast, thinly sliced
- 300g (10½oz) frozen broccoli florets
- 150g (5½oz) beansprouts
- Small handful of coriander (cilantro) leaves, roughly chopped, to serve (optional)

Cook the eggs in a pan of boiling water for 7–8 minutes. (Alternatively heat the air fryer to 150°C/300°F, place the eggs in the air fryer and air fry for 10 minutes). Remove and leave until cool enough to peel, about 10 minutes, then halve them.

Meanwhile, spray the base of a large pot that has a lid with oil and place over a medium heat. Once hot, add the onion or leek and fry until the onion is browned or the leek has softened. Transfer to a jug (pitcher).

Add the fish sauce, garlic paste, if using, lemongrass paste, jalapeños, curry powder, pepper, honey and the 2 tablespoons of oil to the jug. Use a stick blender to blend until smooth, then return to the pan.

Fry the paste until it starts to brown a little, then stir in a third of the coconut milk. Once it starts bubbling, allow to bubble for 1 minute, then add the rest of the coconut milk and the stock. Bring to the boil, then turn the heat down to low and simmer for 45–55 minutes or until reduced and slightly thickened.

Add the dried rice noodles, chicken and broccoli, then simmer for 10–12 minutes or until the noodles are cooked and the chicken is piping hot (and cooked through if using raw). Add the beansprouts and allow to slightly soften for 1–2 minutes.

Serve the noodles in large serving bowls and garnish with the egg halves and coriander, if using.

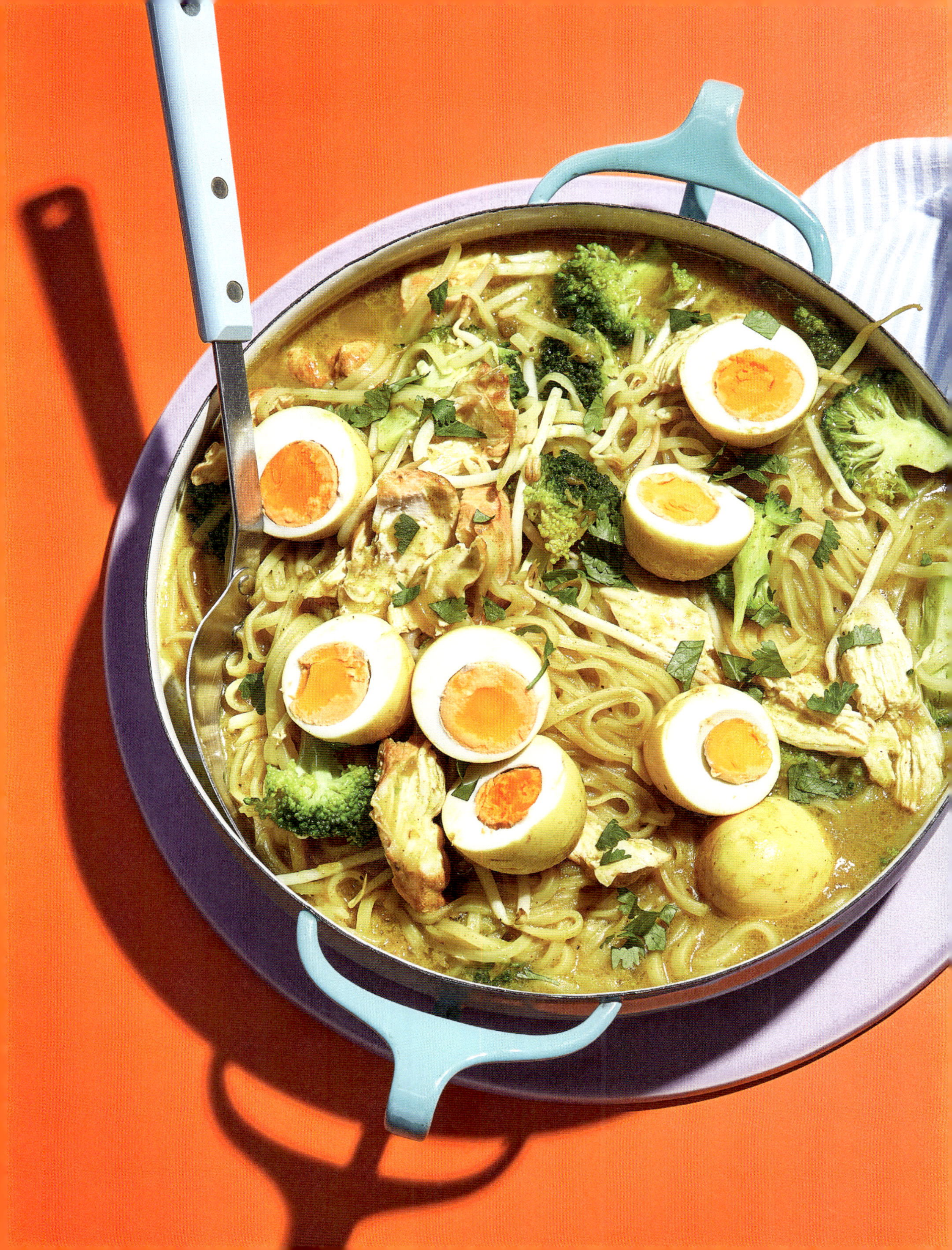

'MARRY ME' CHICKEN PASTA

Get ready to say 'I do' to my budget-friendly, one-pot pasta version of the viral recipe that swept the internet. Though we all prefer the more matrimonial title, it's essentially just Tuscan chicken – a creamy, cheesy, herby sauce and tender chicken, often paired with smoked paprika and sun-dried tomatoes. But as sun-dried tomatoes are currently even more expensive than the chicken required to make this dish, I've opted to make my own 'oven dried' or 'air fryer dried' tomatoes instead at a fraction of the price! Oh, and as I like to avoid the common crisis of 'what on earth shall I serve this dish with?' when I make dinner, I've opted to make this a pasta dish; best of all, I always cook the pasta in the sauce, which saves on washing up.

Serves 3

Prep 5 mins

Hob + Oven 45 mins or
Hob + Air Fryer 35 mins

DF Use dairy-free cheese and dairy-free cream cheese.

LL Use lactose-free cream cheese.

V Swap the chicken for 400g (14oz) firm tofu, prepared and cooked as in the crispy chilli tofu recipe on page 98, and use veggie/vegan-friendly stock.

VE Combine the dairy-free and veggie advice.

❄ See freezing and defrosting guidance for pasta dishes on page 28.

TIP

Don't overcook the pasta once it's added along with the stock, or when you add the remaining ingredients and keep stirring the pot, it can easily break and disintegrate!

- Vegetable oil spray
- 500g (1lb 2oz) cherry tomatoes
- 300g (10½oz) frozen sliced red, green and yellow (bell) peppers
- 1½ tbsp smoked paprika
- 1 tsp salt
- ¼ tsp ground black pepper
- 700ml (scant 3 cups) gluten-free chicken stock (see page 163 for homemade, or made using 1 stock cube)
- 1½ tbsp dried mixed herbs
- 250g (9oz) gluten-free dried penne, fusilli or orzo
- 120g (generous ½ cup) cream cheese
- 250–300g (9–10½oz) leftover cooked chicken, shredded **or** 300g (10½oz) raw skinless, boneless chicken breast, thinly sliced
- 100g (3½oz) frozen spinach
- 50g (1¾oz) mature Cheddar, grated

To make the roasted tomatoes in an oven, preheat the oven to 180°C fan/200°C (400°F). Spray a large baking tray with oil.

Spread the cherry tomatoes out on the baking tray and generously spray with more oil. Roast in the oven for 25 minutes, turning them over halfway. Turn the oven off and leave the tomatoes in the oven with the door ajar for 10–20 minutes.

To make the roasted tomatoes in an air fryer, heat the air fryer to 170°C (340°F). Generously spray the base of the air fryer basket or crisping tray with oil. If you have an air fryer with 2 drawers, use both. Place as many tomatoes as will fit in the air fryer basket(s) without touching and generously spray with oil. Air fry for 12–15 minutes, turning them halfway. Keep warm in the air fryer drawer (closed) for around 10–20 minutes.

Meanwhile, spray the base of a large pot that has a lid with oil and place over a medium heat. Once hot, add the frozen peppers and fry until softened. It's likely that they'll release lots of water as they defrost but just allow it to evaporate off before continuing.

Add the smoked paprika, salt and pepper and fry until fragrant. Add the stock, mixed herbs and pasta, briefly stir and ensure all the pasta is submerged under the stock. Simmer for 6–8 minutes, stirring occasionally, until the pasta is al dente and the stock is nicely reduced and thickened.

Add the cream cheese, chicken and spinach and turn the heat up a little (the cold ingredients will reduce the heat of everything) until gently bubbling again. Simmer for another 5 minutes until the spinach has completely defrosted and dispersed, the sauce is thick and creamy and the chicken is piping hot (and cooked through if using raw).

Add the roasted tomatoes to the pot with the grated cheese, and stir in.

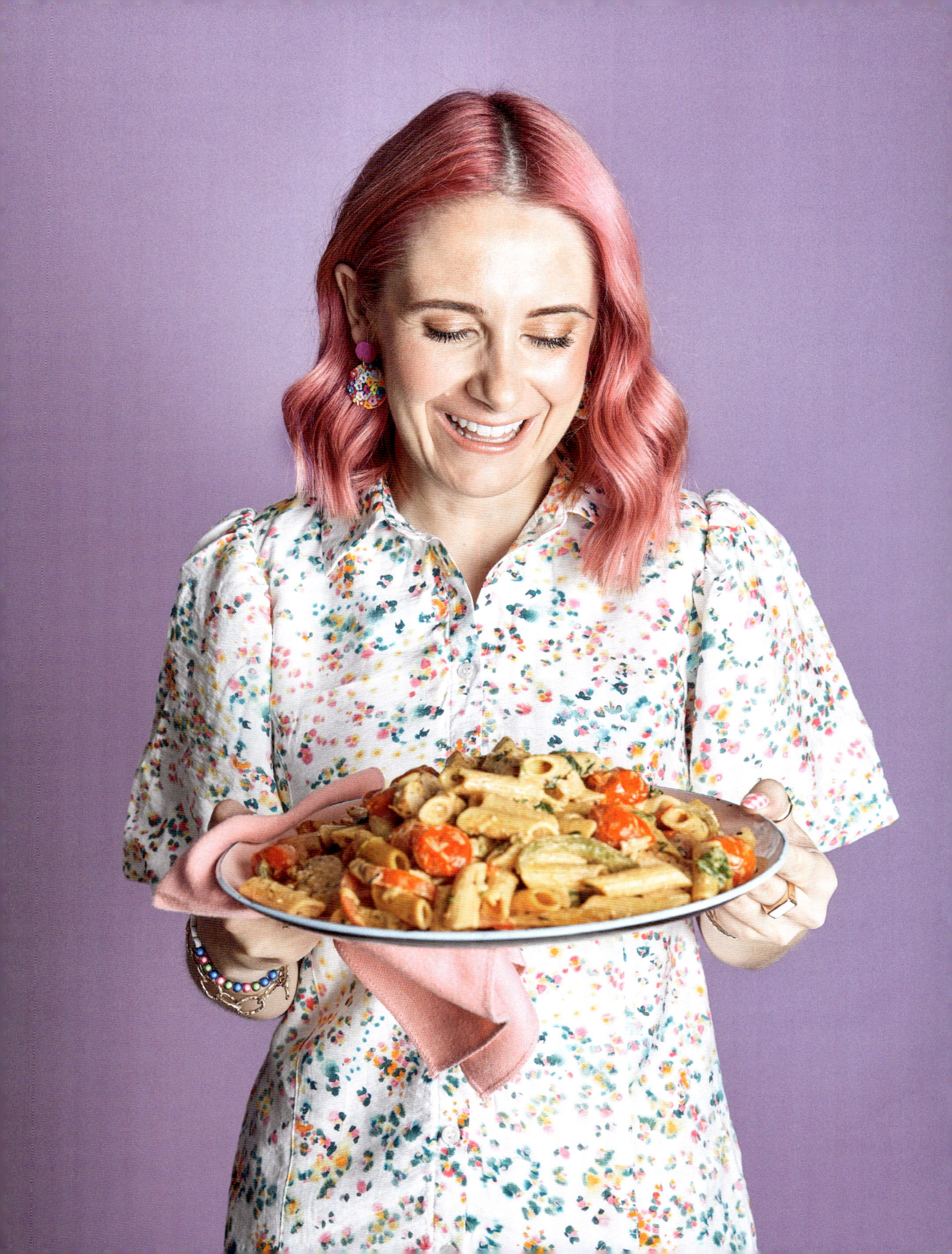

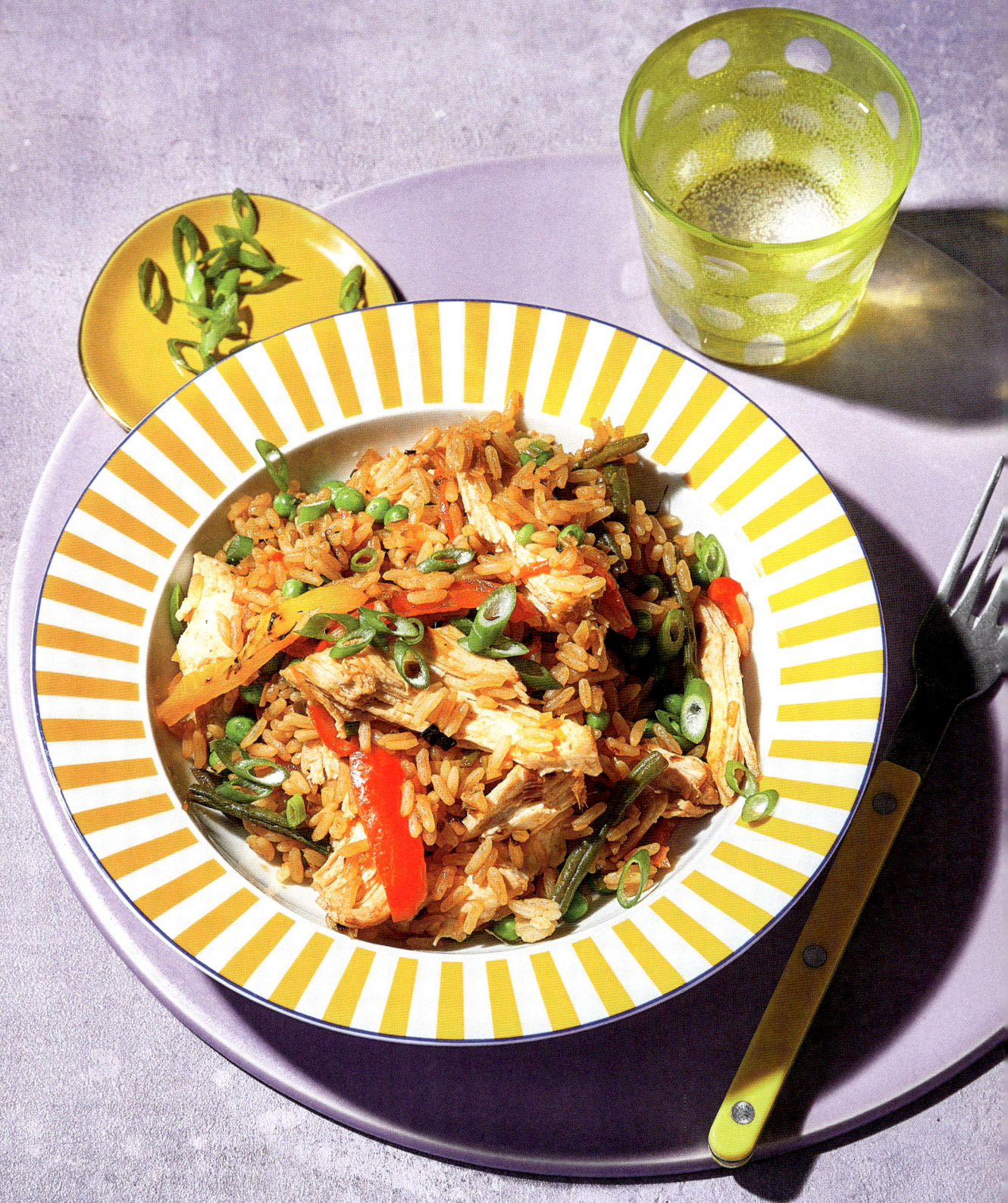

CHICKEN SPECIAL FRIED RICE

As much as I love fried rice as a side alongside all of my fakeaway favourites from past and present books, Mark has made me realize that a good fried rice with lots of variety hidden in between each grain is a glorious thing. Plus, it's an amazing way to use up leftovers, random bits and bobs in the fridge nearing their use-by date, as well as cost-effective frozen ingredients, when there's nothing in the fridge. So please bear in mind that, though this is the version that Mark and I have settled on, this recipe is one you can absolutely make your own – just use the weight of chicken as a rough measurement for how much protein you'll need, and the same goes for the veg. Cook the rice as far ahead of time as possible.

Serves 3
Prep 5 mins
Hob 40 mins

DF **LF**

F Use light brown sugar instead of honey, leek (green parts only) instead of onion, 225g (8oz) green (bell) pepper instead of mixed colours and canned peas instead of frozen peas.

V Swap the chicken for 400g (14oz) firm tofu, prepared and cooked as in the crispy chilli tofu recipe on page 98.

VE See veggie advice and use light brown sugar instead of honey.

❄ See freezing and defrosting guidance for risotto and rice dishes on page 28.

TIP

Frozen ingredients can introduce a lot of excessive moisture, which is the enemy of any good fried rice dish! It can unfortunately make the end product quite claggy. Be sure to evaporate it all off by making sure your wok is nice and hot before continuing to add the next ingredient.

See my microwave sweet and sour chicken on page 128 for guidance on how to cook the rice in the microwave – use the measurements for rice and boiling water given here.

- 600ml (2½ cups) boiling water
- 300g (1⅔ cups) long-grain rice
- 100g (3½oz) frozen chopped onion **or** ½ medium leek, finely chopped
- 250g (9oz) frozen sliced red, green and yellow (bell) peppers
- 150g (5½oz) frozen green beans
- 200g (7oz) frozen peas
- 15g (½oz) jarred jalapeños, finely chopped
- 1 tbsp ginger paste
- 250–300g (9–10½oz) leftover cooked chicken, shredded **or** 300g (10½oz) raw skinless, boneless chicken breast, thinly sliced
- Small handful of spring onion (scallion) greens, thinly sliced on the diagonal, to garnish

For the stir fry sauce
- 4 tbsp gluten-free soy sauce
- 3 tbsp honey
- 2 tbsp vegetable oil, plus extra oil spray for the wok
- 1 tsp tomato purée (paste)
- 1 tbsp pickling juice from the jalapeño jar
- ½ tsp salt

Add the boiling water to a medium saucepan and bring back to a rapid boil, then add the rice, pop the lid on and turn the heat down to low. Allow the rice to cook for 20 minutes, then take off the heat. Remove the lid and allow to cool for as long as you can (ideally allow to cool completely and store covered in the fridge until you need it) for the best texture.

Once the rice has cooled for as long as you can, in a small dish, combine the stir fry sauce ingredients until smooth. Set aside.

Lightly spray the base and sides of a large wok with oil and place over a high heat. (If using raw chicken, add to the hot wok and stir fry until golden and cooked through. Remove to a plate and respray the wok with oil before continuing with the recipe

as normal.) Add the leek or onion to the pan and stir fry until softened, then add the peppers, green beans and peas. Continue to stir fry until any water released has evaporated (the cold ingredients will lower the temperature of the wok so increase the heat until all the liquid is gone). Add the jalapeños and ginger paste, then stir well to coat everything.

Pour in the sauce and allow it to excitedly bubble until reduced a little and starting to look a little sticky. Add the cooled rice and stir fry for 1–2 minutes until the rice is well coated and everything is evenly dispersed.

Stir through the chicken and stir fry for 2–3 minutes (3–5 minutes if it's fridge cold) until the chicken is piping hot.

Garnish with the spring onion greens and serve.

BIG BATCH SLOW COOKING

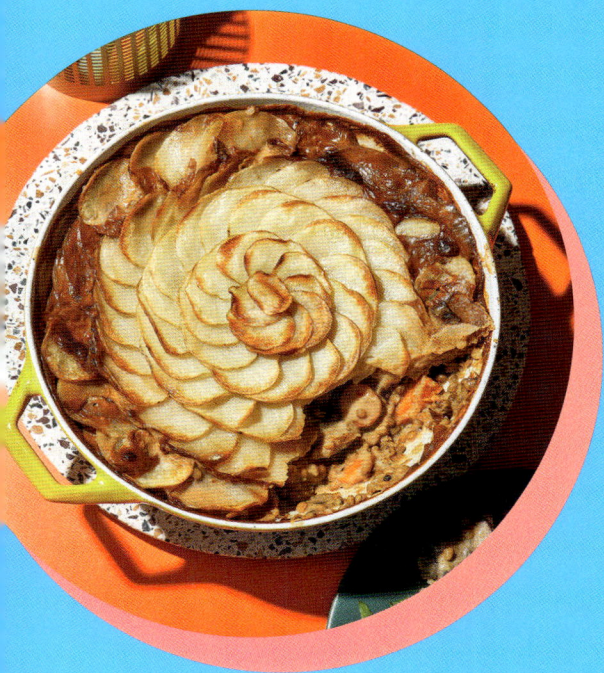

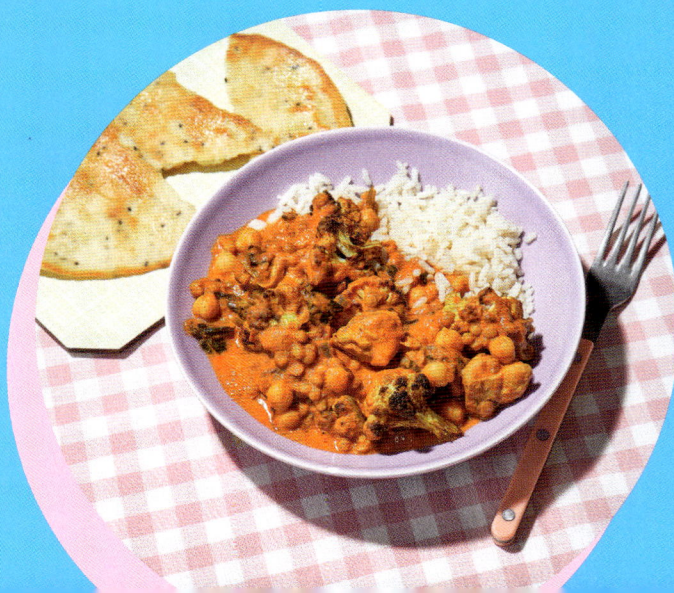

What if I told you that you could save money and time by always cooking too much food? This chapter aims to harness all the benefits of meal prep, bulk cooking and your freezer space. In a nutshell, the entire point of these recipes is to ensure you have leftovers that you can then portion out and freeze as future ready meals. After that, you'll simply need to follow the defrosting guidance on page 28 to reheat them straight from frozen. Since these are larger quantities of food, <u>you'll need either a large lidded pot (if making these recipes on the hob) or at least a 6.5l (7 quart) slow cooker</u> (which is larger than average).

By always ensuring you have plentiful amounts of leftovers that can live in your freezer until you need them, you'll be able to reap the rewards by:

- <u>Cooking less often:</u> Not only will having homemade ready meals in your freezer mean you'll now have days where you won't need to cook at all, but it'll also save on your energy bills on those days too, as there will be less washing up and fewer appliances whirring away!

- <u>Taking advantage of the lower prices that come with buying larger quantities of meat and veg:</u> By cooking extra meals in advance to freeze, you can benefit from the cost savings of buying larger quantities of ingredients without the risk of them going to waste.

- <u>Using lots of repeated ingredients:</u> Although this chapter has lots of different dishes to choose from, it actually uses a very modest pool of spices, seasonings, vegetables and store-cupboard ingredients. That way, you won't need to buy an entire new collection of ingredients to make them!

- <u>Taking advantage of the cost savings that come with bulking out meals with veg, beans, lentils and pulses:</u> Not only are these ingredients incredibly cost effective (and 100% delicious), they're also really good for you! So naturally you'll see them feature regularly throughout these recipes. Though see the answer to the question concerning not liking 'X, Y or Z ingredients' on page 27 if you'd still prefer not to use them!

- <u>Using a slow cooker to save switching on the oven:</u> Slow cookers are incredibly cost effective to run, which is why they became the sole focus of this chapter! However, even though they're one of the most affordable small appliances to purchase, you can also make all of these recipes on the hob using a large pot that has a lid (mine is 5.3 litres/5½ quarts).

The content of this chapter is a reflection of how my cooking habits have shifted over recent years when I've been time-poor but still wanted to enjoy flavourful yet cost-friendly meals. On the days I cook, it simply involves throwing everything into my trusty big lidded pot or slow cooker in the morning, then simply serving/portioning it up in the evening. And when I need a last-minute emergency meal, I simply defrost a portion of a past slow-cooked meal – much cheaper than a takeaway! So I hope you'll come to embrace slow cooking like I have, as the cost and time-saving benefits are exceptionally quick to come around!

SMOKIN' COWBOY BEANS

This smoky and sweet tomato stew takes full advantage of one of the most cost-effective, filling and protein-packed ingredients: canned beans! Packed with peppers, carrots and smoky bacon, this one-pot wonder takes just 10 minutes of effort, so you can do absolutely anything else except watching it cook.

Serves 6–8

Prep 10 mins

Hob 1 hour or
Slow Cooker 6–7 hours

DF **LF**

V Swap the bacon for 250g (9oz) frozen sliced mushrooms.

VE See veggie advice and use caster (superfine) sugar instead of honey.

❄ See freezing and defrosting guidance for soups, stews and curries on page 28.

- Vegetable oil spray
- 10–12 rashers of smoked back bacon, finely chopped
- 2 tbsp smoked paprika
- 1 tbsp mild curry powder
- 400g (14oz) frozen sliced red, green and yellow (bell) peppers
- 3 medium carrots, sliced into 1cm (½in) rounds
- 150g (5½oz) frozen chopped onion **or** ½ large leek, finely chopped
- 25g (1oz) jarred jalapeños, finely chopped, plus 2 tbsp pickling juice from the jar
- 3 tbsp honey
- 2 x 400g (14oz) cans of red kidney beans, drained
- 1 x 400g (14oz) can of cannellini beans, drained
- 2 x 400g (14oz) cans of chopped tomatoes
- 2 tbsp dried mixed herbs
- 100ml (generous ⅓ cup) boiling water
- 2 tsp salt
- ¼ tsp ground black pepper

Optional extras
- 1 tbsp tomato purée (paste)
- 4 tbsp gluten-free BBQ sauce
- Handful of coriander (cilantro) leaves, roughly chopped, to serve

To cook on the hob, spray the base of a large pot that has a lid with oil and place over a medium heat. When hot, add the bacon and fry until starting to crisp.

Add the smoked paprika and curry powder, then stir in and fry until fragrant. You might notice a lot of crispy brown goodness getting stuck to the bottom of the pot. Add the frozen peppers and, as they begin to soften, the moisture they release after around a minute will help to deglaze the pan. Stir everything until the base is deglazed.

Stir in the carrots, onion or leek, jalapeños, plus the juice from the jar, and the honey, then add the kidney beans, cannellini beans and chopped tomatoes. Stir well, then add the dried mixed herbs and pour in the boiling water.

Place the lid on top and turn the heat down to low. Simmer for 1 hour until nicely thickened and the carrots are cooked. Optionally, stir in the tomato purée to thicken the sauce and/or the gluten-free BBQ sauce for an extra punch of flavour, then cook for a further 5–10 minutes with the lid removed. Add the salt and pepper and serve with the coriander sprinkled on top, if using.

To cook in a slow cooker, spray the base of a frying pan with oil and place over a medium heat. When hot, add the bacon and fry until starting to crisp. Add the smoked paprika and curry powder, then stir in and fry until fragrant.

Meanwhile, add the remaining ingredients to the slow cooker and stir well. Once the bacon is crisp, add to the slow cooker and stir in. Pop the lid on and cook on low for 6–7 hours or on high for 3½ hours. Once cooked, optionally add the tomato purée and/or BBQ sauce and slow cook for a further 10–15 minutes with the lid removed. Sprinkle with the coriander, if using.

Serve with long-grain rice, potato wedges or mashed potatoes.

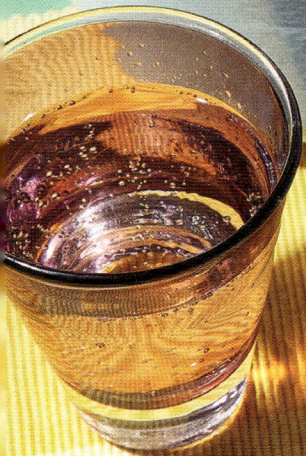

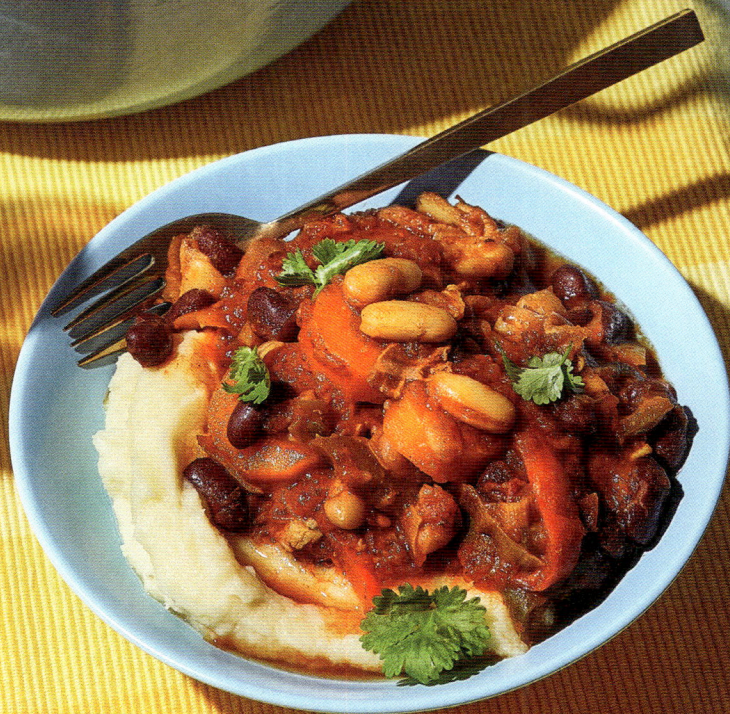

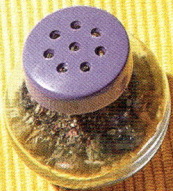

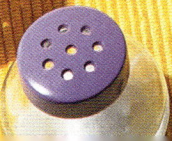

BACON, MUSHROOM + CHEDDAR RISOTTO

Serves 6–8

Prep 10 mins

Hob 35 mins or
Slow Cooker 5–6 hours

LL

DF Use dairy-free cheese.

F Use leek instead of onion (green parts only), oyster mushrooms (roughly chopped) instead of frozen sliced mushrooms, and canned peas instead of frozen. Use 2 low FODMAP stock cubes.

V Swap the bacon for 100g (3½oz) extra onion/leek, and use veggie/vegan-friendly stock.

VE Combine the dairy-free and veggie advice.

❄ See freezing and defrosting guidance for risotto and rice dishes on page 28.

TIP

If making this in a slow cooker, after you've fried the bacon, you can also fry the onion (until browned) or leek (until softened) too. It adds a little extra flavour! Once crisp, simply add the bacon to the slow cooker, then re-use the pan (no need to clean it or add any extra oil) to fry the onion or leek.

This recipe centres around yet another one of my favourite affordable ingredients: smoked bacon. When chopped finely, its bold, smoky flavour will magically spread to every grain of rice and, of course, it pairs perfectly with the mushrooms. The final result is a gloriously cheesy, smoky risotto that's surprisingly filling, meaning a little goes a long way at the dinner table! Cooking it on the hob will give the rice more texture, whereas the slow cooker will make the finished risotto stickier. There's no right or wrong way to do it, so choose whichever method or finish you prefer! Simply serve with rocket (arugula).

- Vegetable oil spray
- 150g (5½oz) frozen chopped onion **or** ½ large leek, finely chopped
- 10–12 rashers of smoked back bacon, finely chopped
- 600g (1lb 5oz) frozen sliced mushrooms
- 500g (2⅔ cups) risotto rice
- About 1.5 litres (6¼ cups) hot gluten-free chicken stock (see page 163 for homemade, or made using 2 stock cubes)
- 2 tbsp dried mixed herbs
- 1 tsp salt
- ½ tsp ground black pepper
- 200g (7oz) mature Cheddar, grated
- 300g (10½oz) frozen peas

To cook on the hob, spray the base of a large pot that has a lid with oil and place over a medium-high heat. Once hot, add the onion or leek and fry until the onion is browned or the leek has softened.

Add the bacon and fry until browned – if lots of liquid comes out of the bacon, the heat of the pan should evaporate it in a few minutes and you'll then be able to crisp it up a little. Add the mushrooms and stir in; they'll introduce a lot of liquid as they defrost. Once the water has released, stir in the rice. Stir occasionally until the rice has absorbed all the liquid, then stir more often for 2–3 minutes. Turn the heat down to medium.

Add about 200ml (generous ¾ cup) of stock to the pot at a time, stirring it in immediately, then stir occasionally until the rice has absorbed almost all of it. Repeat until the rice is essentially translucent and not a brighter white

colour anymore, which means it's cooked – if you're not sure, just try a bit to ensure it's not still hard. You may not need all of the stock, as it can vary a little depending on how much moisture came out of the mushrooms earlier. This entire process should take around 20–25 minutes.

Stir in the mixed herbs, salt and pepper, Cheddar and peas, then allow to simmer for a few minutes to defrost the peas. Serve immediately.

To cook in a slow cooker, spray the base of a frying pan with oil and place over a medium heat. Once hot, add the bacon and fry until crisp and golden.

Add everything except the cheese and peas to the slow cooker and stir well. Stir in the crisp bacon, pop the lid on and cook on low for 5–6 hours or on high for 2½ hours. Around 10–20 minutes before it's done, stir in the cheese and peas, then cover with the lid for the remaining time.

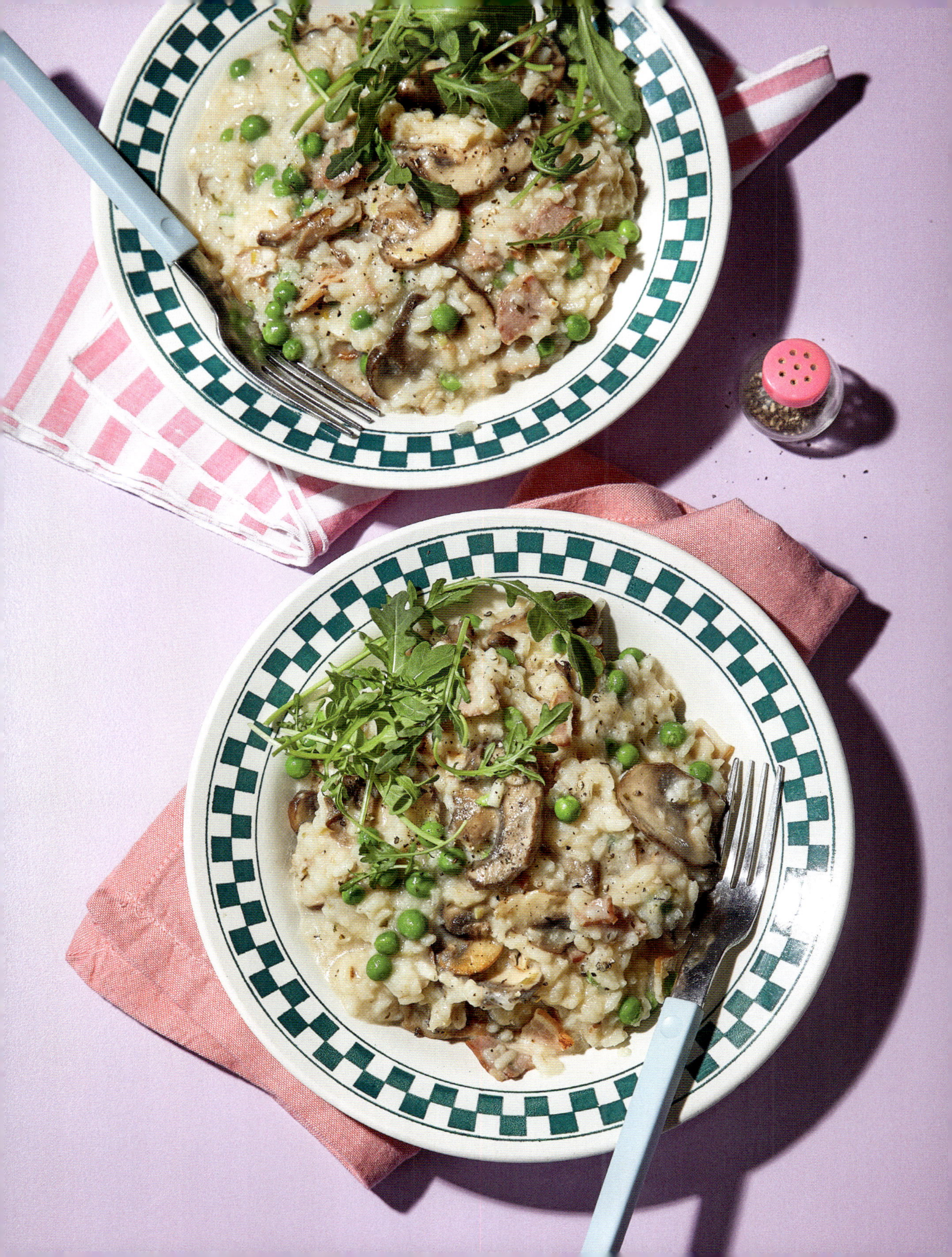

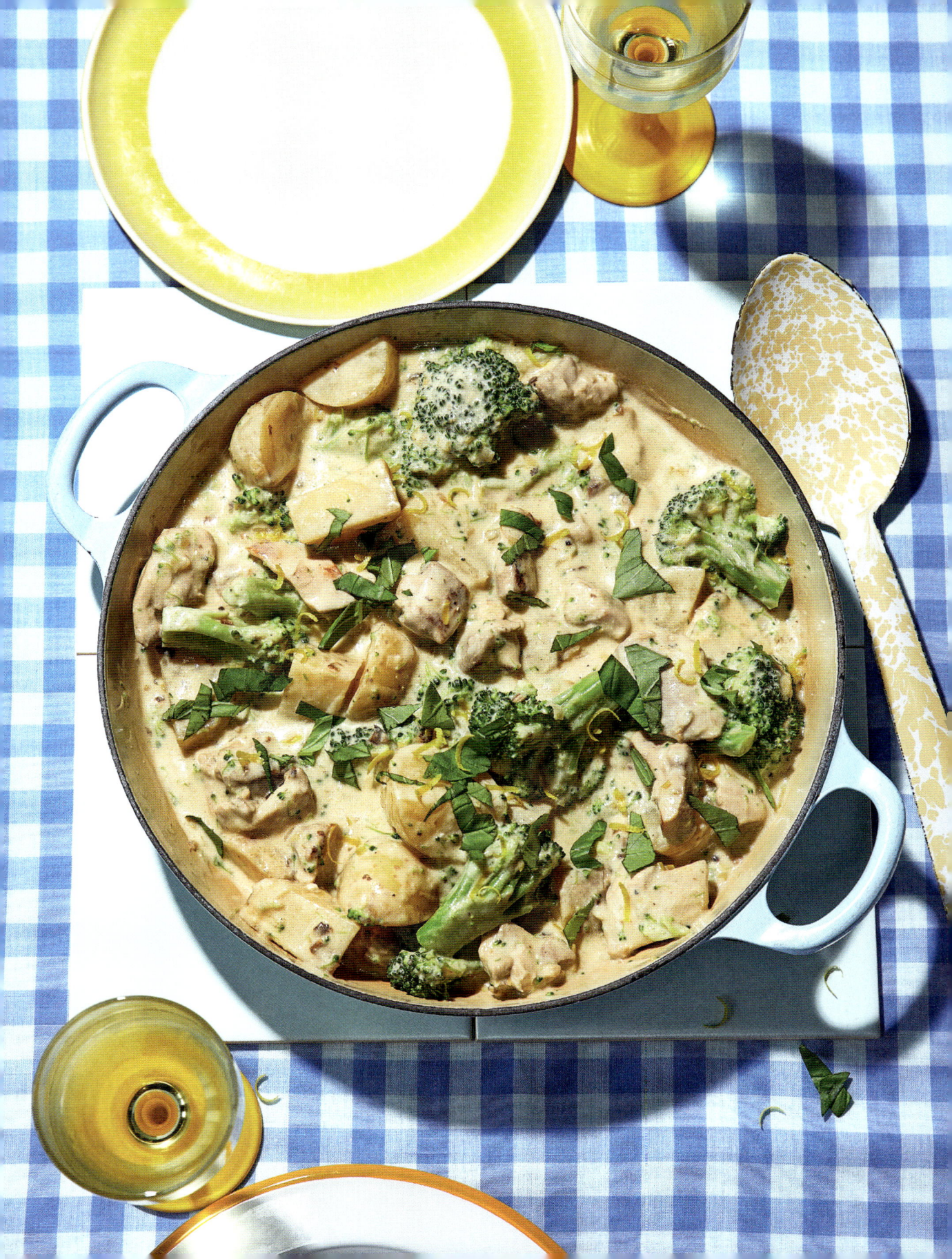

ONE-POT CREAMY LEMON MUSTARD CHICKEN

This easy-peasy stew combines a punch of mustard with zesty lemon in a creamy sauce, brimming with melt-in-the-mouth chicken and broccoli. The addition of the potato is not only because it's an affordable ingredient that makes the meal go further, but it also means you don't have to prepare anything else to serve it with. It reheats especially well from frozen, so you can bet I always have a portion or two in my freezer in case of a dinner emergency!

Serves 4–6

Prep 10 mins

Hob 45 mins or
Slow Cooker 5–6 hours

- Vegetable oil spray
- 150g (5½oz) frozen chopped onion **or** ½ large leek, finely chopped
- 500g (1lb 2oz) skinless, boneless chicken thighs, cut into bite-sized pieces
- ½ tsp ground black pepper
- 3 tbsp Dijon mustard

- 700ml (scant 3 cups) gluten-free chicken stock, for the hob, **or** 550ml (2¼ cups) stock, for the slow cooker (see page 163 for homemade)
- 700–800g (1lb 9oz–1lb 12oz) small to medium potatoes, cut into 2.5cm (1in) chunks
- Grated zest of 1 lemon and juice of ½

- 1 tsp salt
- 500g (1lb 2oz) frozen broccoli florets
- 150g (⅔ cup) cream cheese
- 3 tbsp cornflour (cornstarch) or potato starch, mixed with 6 tbsp water
- Handful of basil leaves, roughly chopped, to serve

DF Use dairy-free cream cheese.

LF Use lactose-free cream cheese.

F Use leek (green parts only) instead of onion, swap the frozen broccoli for 4–5 medium carrots, sliced into 1.5cm (⅔in) rounds, and use lactose-free cream cheese. Use low FODMAP stock.

V Swap the chicken for 2 x 400g (14oz) drained cans of lentils, and use veggie/vegan-friendly stock.

VE Combine dairy-free and veggie advice.

❄ See freezing and defrosting guidance for soups, stews and curries on page 28.

TIP

Don't forget to use the lower measurement of chicken stock if making this in the slow cooker, otherwise the resulting stew can be quite watery. Keep an eye out during this chapter for other recipes where the slow cooker version of a dish requires less stock or water being added.

To cook on the hob, spray the base of a large pot that has a lid with oil and place over a medium heat. Once hot, add the onion or leek and fry until the onion is browned or the leek has softened. Add the chicken and black pepper and continue to fry until sealed.

Stir in the mustard, then add the stock, potatoes, lemon zest (reserve a little for serving), lemon juice and salt. Briefly stir and ensure all the potato is submerged under the stock. Pop the lid on and simmer for 30 minutes or until the potatoes are cooked.

Add the frozen broccoli and cream cheese and turn the heat up a little until everything is gently bubbling again. Simmer for another 5 minutes until the broccoli has completely cooked through, then quickly stir in the starch slurry, which will almost instantly thicken the sauce. Serve sprinkled with the basil and reserved lemon zest.

To cook in a slow cooker, lightly spray the base of the slow cooker with oil, then add everything except the broccoli, cream cheese, starch slurry and basil – don't forget to reserve a little lemon zest to serve at the end – and stir well. Pop the lid on and cook on low for 5–6 hours or on high for 2½ hours. Around 2 hours (low) or 45 minutes (high) before it's done, add the broccoli. Around 20 minutes before it's done, stir in the cream cheese and starch slurry, then cover with the lid for the remaining time. Serve sprinkled with the basil and reserved lemon zest.

CARAMELIZED LEEK, POTATO + FETA SOUP

Serves 6–8

Prep 10 mins

Hob 55 mins or
Slow Cooker 6–7 hours

A big theme of this book involves getting extra flavour out of your ingredients at very little extra cost, and caramelizing your leeks is a perfect example of this. Especially when combined with the honey, it gives the leeks a delicate sweetness and a more complex flavour. So why not?! It works so well with the tang of the feta, and the result is a soup that's bursting with flavour, which absolutely anyone can pull off. Serve alongside a gluten-free cheese toastie or with slices of buttered gluten-free bread.

LL **V**

DF Use a dairy-free 'buttery' margarine instead of butter, and a dairy-free alternative to feta.

VE See dairy-free advice and use maple syrup instead of honey. Ensure stock is vegan-friendly.

❄ See freezing and defrosting guidance for soups, stews and curries on page 28.

- 3 tbsp butter
- 750g (1lb 10oz) leeks (about 4–5 medium leeks), each sliced into thirds then halved lengthways
- 2½ tbsp honey
- 4 medium potatoes, peeled and cut into 5mm (¼in) slices
- 450g (1lb) parsnips, peeled and cut into 1cm (½in) discs
- 2.25 litres (4¾ pints) gluten-free vegetable stock (made using 3 stock cubes)
- 1½ tsp salt
- 1 tsp ground black pepper
- 300g (10½oz) feta-style salad cheese, grated

TIPS

Add a splash of boiling water if the soup is a little too thick or, if it's too thin for your liking, simply simmer the blended soup until thickened.

Once the leeks have been halved lengthways, they can easily fall apart into lots of separate layers. Once cut, try not to handle them or move them around too much to prevent this; or else they will be hard to caramelize.

To cook on the hob, add the butter to a large pot that has a lid, and place over a medium heat. Once the butter has melted and started to turn a little foamy, add the leek sections, cut-side down. Fry until golden brown, then drizzle over the honey and stir until all the leeks are coated. Flip them so the browned side is facing upwards and fry on the other side until golden.

Add the potatoes and parsnips, stir well, then fry for 3–4 minutes. Pour in the stock, add the salt and pepper and turn the heat down to low. Simmer for 35–40 minutes until the potato and parsnips are cooked, then use a stick blender to blend until smooth and thickened.

Stir through the grated feta-style cheese and simmer until it's all melted and disappeared.

To cook in a slow cooker, caramelize the leeks in the butter and honey as instructed opposite, then add to the slow cooker with the potatoes, parsnips, stock, salt and pepper. Pop the lid on and cook on low for 6–7 hours or on high for 3½ hours. Around 30 minutes before it's done, stir in the feta-style cheese and cover with the lid once again for the remaining time. Blend with a stick blender until smooth and thickened.

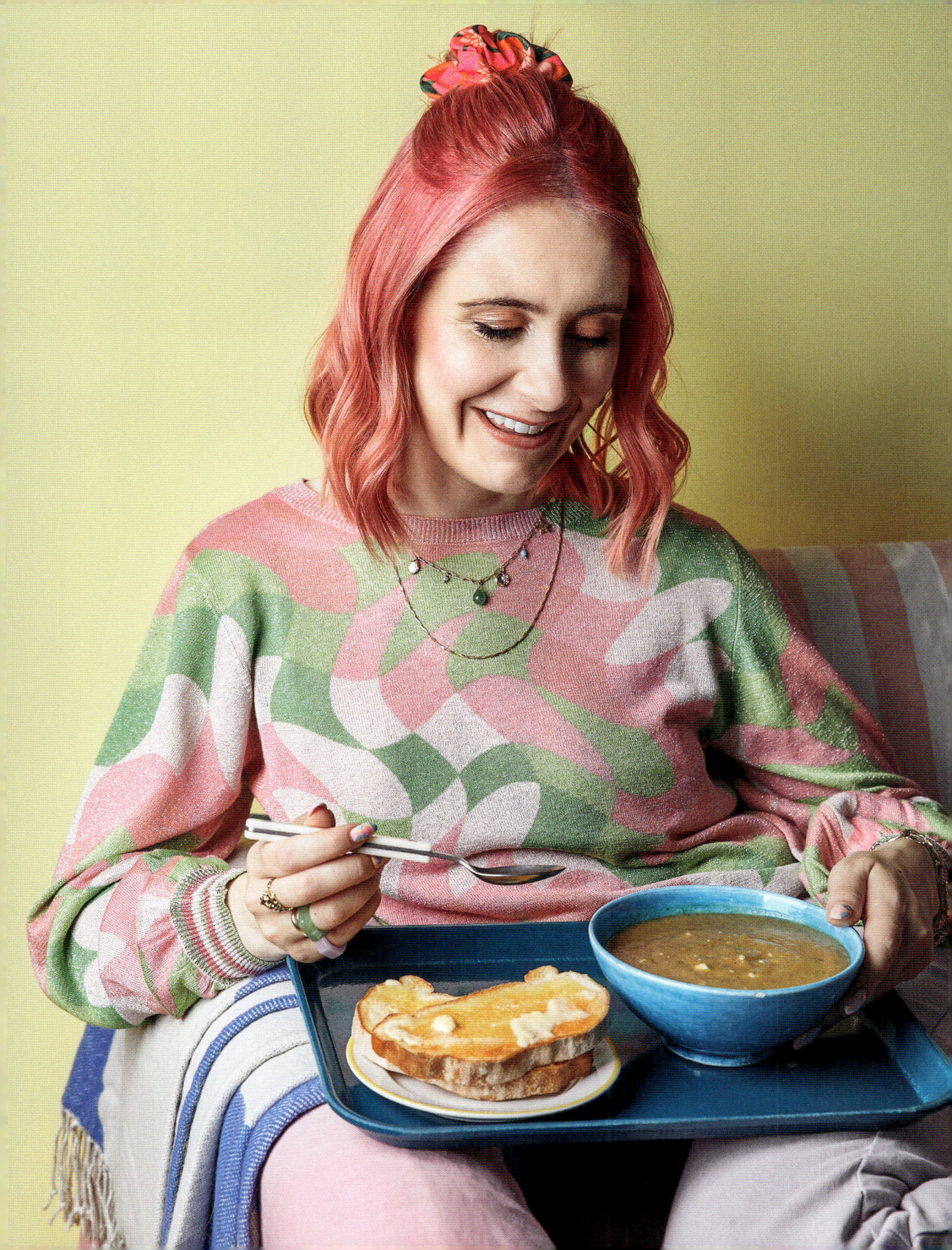

ONE-POT ARROZ CON POLLO

(SPANISH-STYLE CHICKEN RICE)

With a tomato and smoked paprika flavour profile, this Spanish-inspired one-pot rice dish is a bit like paella (yet fortunately doesn't require mega-costly saffron!), with tender chunks of chicken and dried mixed herbs. Expect the same smoke-tinged flavour with rice that's undeniably delicious, having absorbed that wonderful blend of tomato, stock and chicken juices while in the pot. Remember to use less stock if cooking in the slow cooker, as excess liquid will make the rice claggy! Serve with lemon wedges for squeezing, if you like.

Serves 6–8

Prep 10 mins

Hob + Oven 1 hour or
Slow Cooker 5–6 hours

- Vegetable oil spray
- 150g (5½oz) frozen chopped onion **or** ½ large leek, finely chopped
- 400g (14oz) frozen sliced red, green and yellow (bell) peppers
- 3 medium carrots, sliced into 1cm (½in) rounds
- 500g (1lb 2oz) skinless, boneless chicken thighs
- 2 tsp garlic paste (optional)
- 2 tbsp smoked paprika
- ½ tsp salt
- 1 tsp ground black pepper
- 400g (2¼ cups) long-grain white rice
- 2 x 400g (14oz) cans of chopped tomatoes
- 1½ tbsp dried mixed herbs
- 800ml (3⅓ cups) gluten-free chicken stock, for the hob, **or** 650ml (2¾ cups) stock, for the slow cooker (see page 163 for homemade)
- 300g (10½oz) frozen peas
- Handful of chopped parsley, to serve (optional)

DF **LF**

F Use leek instead of onion (green parts only), all green (bell) peppers instead of mixed colours, low FODMAP stock, canned peas instead of frozen, and omit the garlic paste. One eighth of the finished dish is a safe low FODMAP serving size.

V Swap the chicken for two 400g (14oz) cans of drained chickpeas, and use veggie/vegan-friendly stock.

VE See veggie advice.

❄ See freezing and defrosting guidance for risotto and rice dishes on page 28.

To cook using the hob and oven, spray the base of a large pot that has a lid with oil and place over a medium heat. Once hot, add the onion or leek and fry until the onion is browned or the leek has softened. Add the peppers and carrots, then continue to fry until the peppers have softened. Add the chicken, fry until sealed, then add the garlic paste, if using, smoked paprika, salt and pepper and fry until fragrant.

Add the rice and stir for around 30 seconds until it coats everything. Quickly add the tomatoes, mixed herbs and stock, then briefly stir.

Place the lid on, turn the heat down to low and simmer for 20 minutes. Give it a stir to ensure nothing is getting stuck to the bottom, then place the lid back on and simmer for a further 15 minutes. Remove the lid and mix through the peas. Simmer with the lid removed for a further 10 minutes or until the rice is cooked. Top with the parsley, if using, then serve.

To cook in a slow cooker, lightly spray the base of the slow cooker with oil, then add everything except the peas and parsley. Pop the lid on and cook on low for 5–6 hours or on high for 2½ hours, stirring once or twice within the final hour to prevent it sticking. Around 20 minutes before it's done, stir in the peas and then cover with the lid once again for the remaining time. Top with the parsley, if using, then serve.

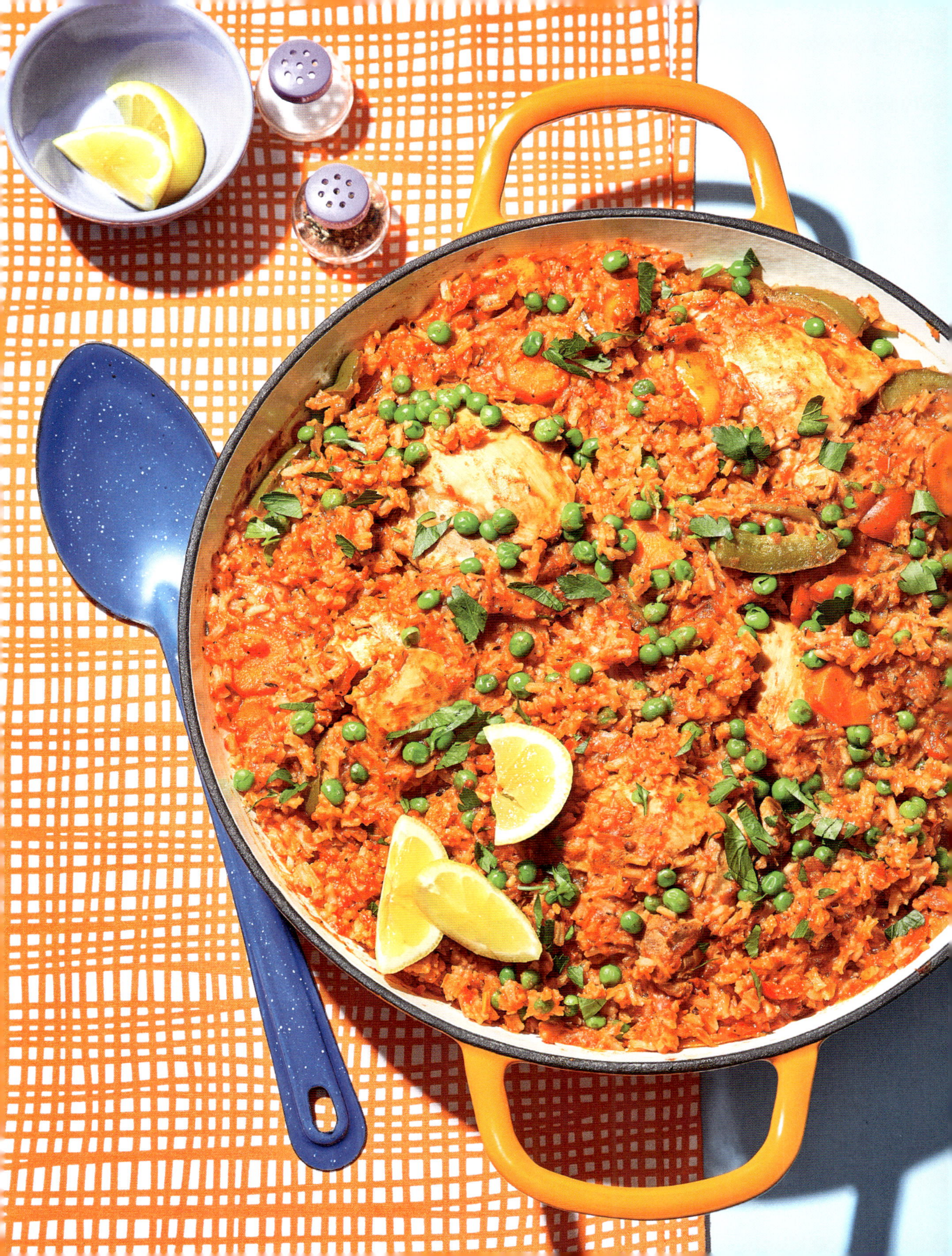

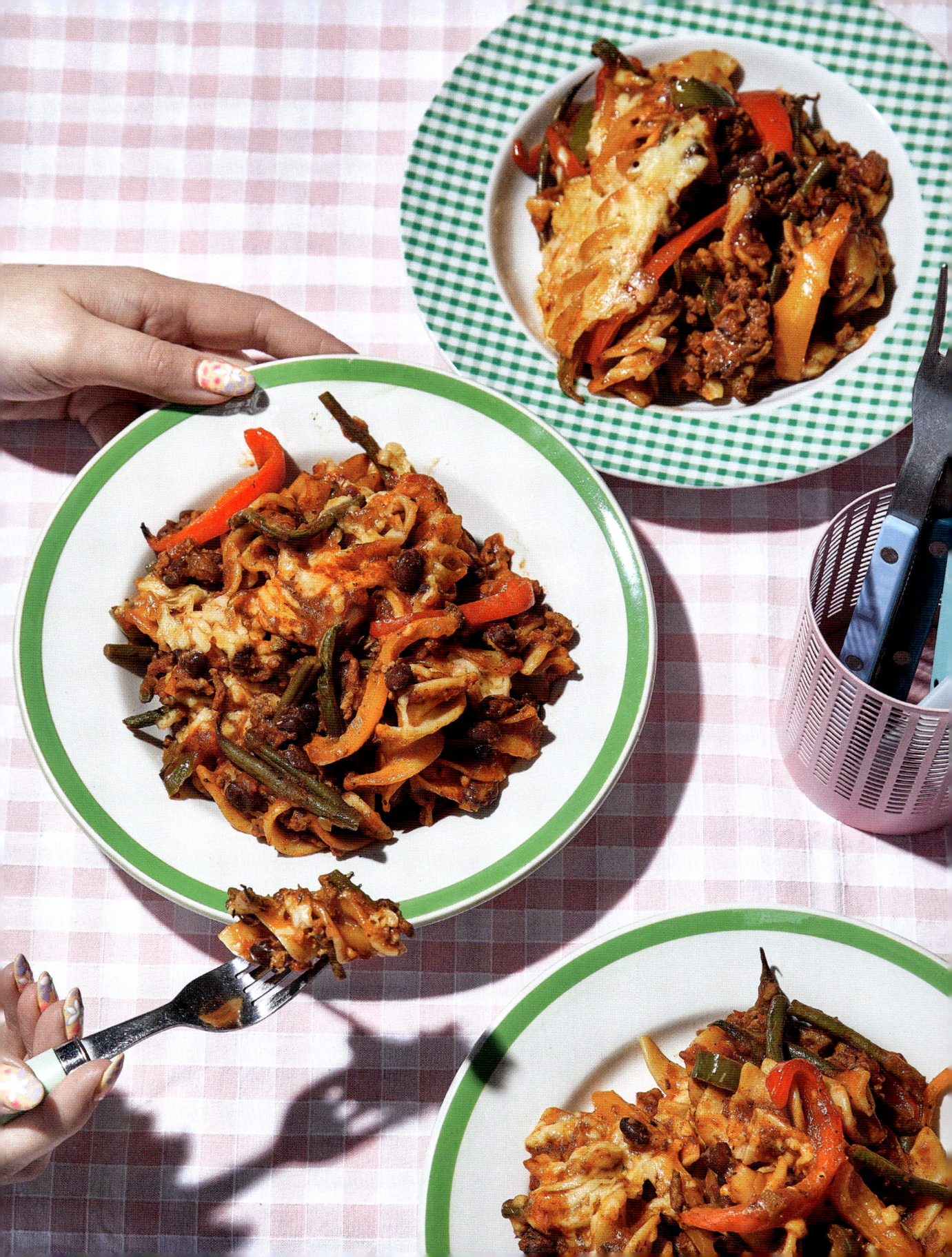

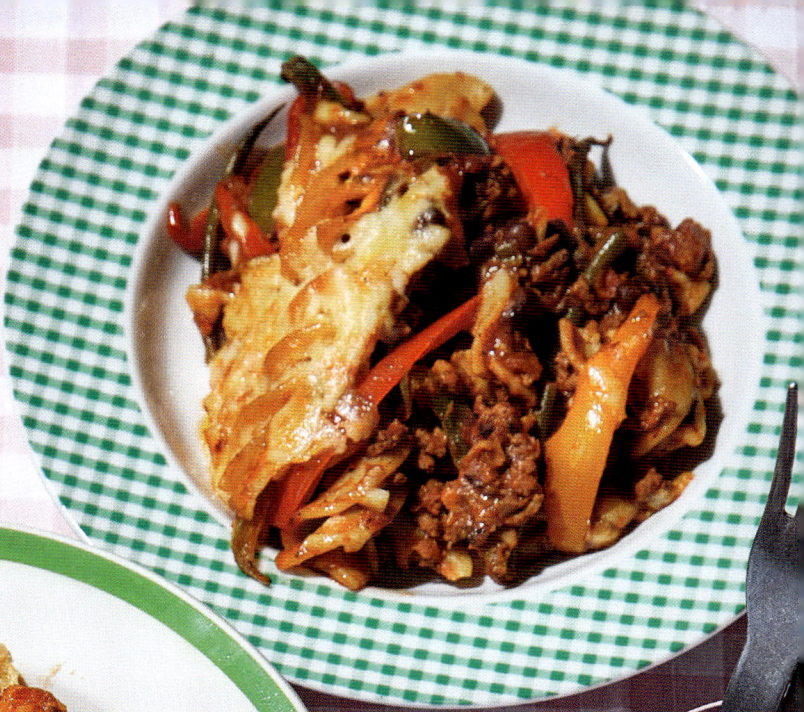

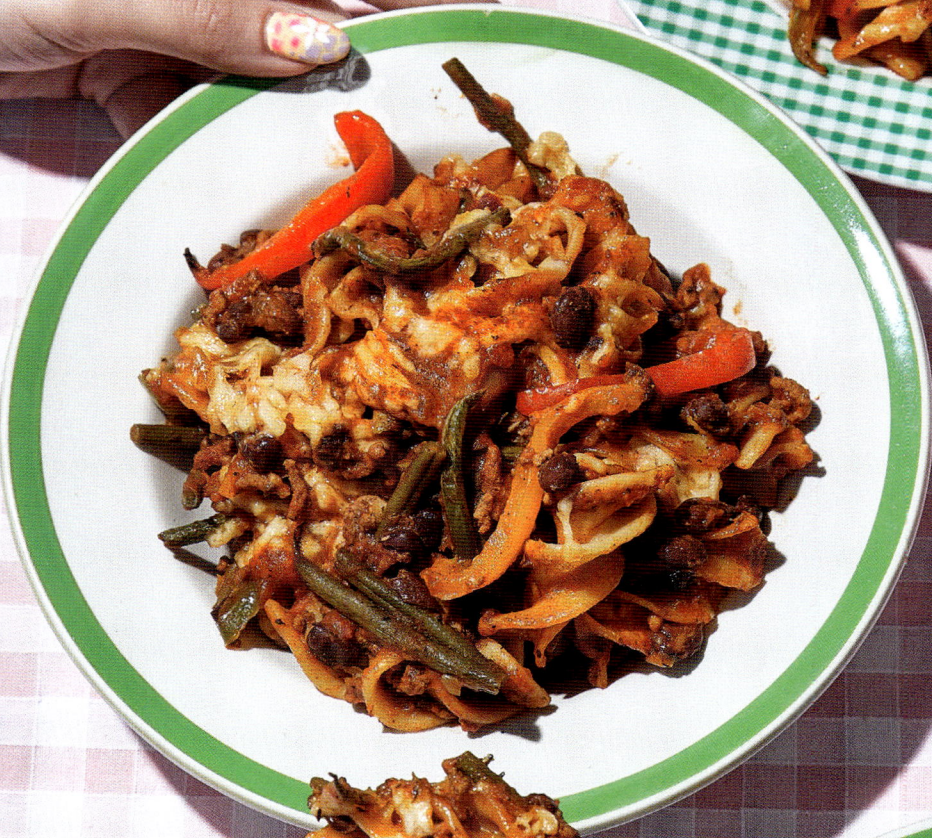

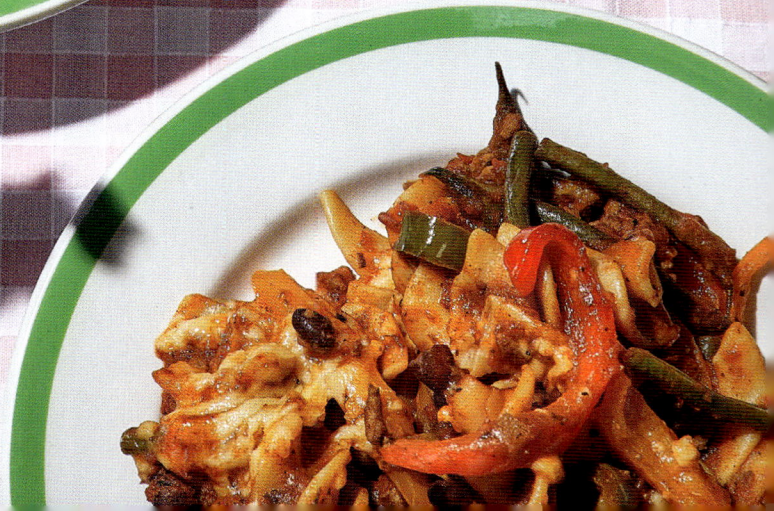

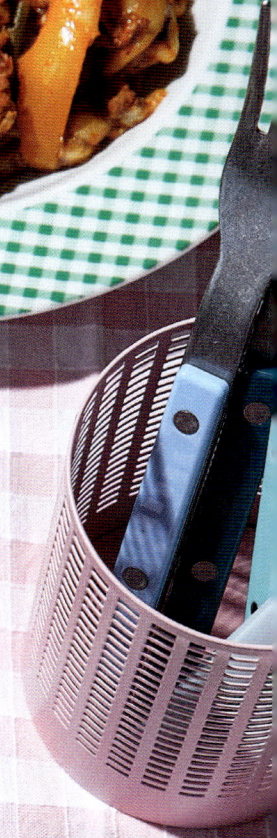

ONE-POT CAJUN BURRITO PASTA

If you're a fan of burritos and the spicy beef, veggies and Cajun-style rice that often features, then this one-pot pasta dish has all of the above and your name written all over it. Of course, the knack with one-pot pasta dishes and using gluten-free pasta simply boils (excuse the pun) down to this: not overcooking the pasta! On the hob, look for an al dente texture, and in the slow cooker keep an eye on it during the final 10 minutes. When it's done, it's done!

Serves 6–8

Prep 10 mins

Hob + Oven 35 mins or
Slow Cooker 6–7 hours

LL

DF Use dairy-free cheese.

V Swap the beef for two 400g (14oz) cans of drained kidney beans, and use veggie/vegan-friendly stock.

VE Combine the dairy-free and veggie advice.

❄ See freezing and defrosting guidance for pasta dishes on page 28.

TIPS

Don't overcook the pasta once it's added to the pot, or when you stir it afterwards, it can easily all break and disintegrate! Take the lid off after 5–8 minutes (hob) or 15 minutes (slow cooker) to check how it's getting on.

This is a reminder that this will be way too much food to cook in a small slow cooker! This recipe is made for a 6.7l (7 quart) slow cooker; if you don't have one, then simply halve the quantity of everything needed to serve 3–4 (and bear this in mind for the other in this chapter).

- Vegetable oil spray
- 150g (5½oz) frozen chopped onion **or** ½ large leek, finely chopped
- 500g (1lb 2oz) minced (ground) beef
- 2 tsp garlic paste (optional)
- 20g (¾oz) jarred jalapeños, finely chopped
- 2 tbsp smoked paprika
- 1 tbsp mild curry powder
- 1½ tbsp dried mixed herbs
- 1 tsp salt
- ½ tsp ground black pepper
- 400g (14oz) frozen sliced red, green and yellow (bell) peppers
- 200g (7oz) frozen green beans
- 1 x 400g (14oz) can of black beans, drained
- 2 x 400g (14oz) cans of chopped tomatoes
- 1 tbsp tomato purée (paste)
- 800ml (3⅓ cups) gluten-free beef or ham stock, for the hob, **or** 600ml (2½ cups) stock, for the slow cooker
- 500g (1lb 2oz) gluten-free dried pasta
- 75g (2½oz) mature Cheddar, grated

To cook using the hob and oven, spray the base of a large ovenproof pot that has a lid with oil and place over a medium heat. Once hot, add the onion or leek and fry until the onion is browned or the leek has softened.

Add the beef and, once it releases a little moisture, scrape anything stuck to the bottom of the pan until it's deglazed. Once the beef has browned, add the garlic paste, if using, jalapeños, smoked paprika, curry powder, mixed herbs, salt and pepper. Stir well and fry until fragrant and until there's no liquid left in the pan. Stir in the peppers, green beans and black beans, and fry for 2–3 minutes.

Add the chopped tomatoes, purée and stock, then stir well once more. Add the pasta and ensure it is all submerged under the stock. Place the lid on, turn the heat down to low and simmer for 10–12 minutes until the pasta is cooked and the sauce is a little thickened.

Preheat the oven to 200°C fan/220°C (425°F).

Remove the lid and briefly stir once or twice (don't stir too much as gluten-free pasta is fragile!) then pat everything down into a flat, even layer and top with the grated cheese. Bake in the oven for 15 minutes, until the cheese is golden brown.

To cook using a slow cooker, spray the base of a large frying pan with oil and place over a medium heat. Once hot, add the onion or leek and fry until the onion is browned or the leek has softened. Add the beef and fry until browned.

Meanwhile, add the remaining ingredients apart from the pasta and cheese to the slow cooker and stir well. Once the beef has browned, add the beef and onion or leek to the slow cooker and stir in. Pop the lid on and cook on low for 6–7 hours or on high for 3½ hours, stirring in the pasta 20–30 minutes before serving. Once the pasta is cooked, sprinkle the grated cheese on top and cover with the lid for 5–10 minutes until melted.

CREAMY MUSHROOM HOTPOT

Serves 6–8

Prep 10 mins

Hob + Oven 1 hour 10 mins or
Slow Cooker + Oven 7–8 hours

A hearty hotpot like this never fails to be a crowd-pleaser, with crispy, golden brown potato slices concealing a mushroom, carrot and lentil filling in a creamy vegetable gravy. It's the ultimate comfort food that nobody will care is gluten-free, with no fancy free-from products required. See the TIPS below for more info on what I use to quickly slice the potato, ensuring they're all the exact same thickness and all cook at the same speed. Serve with a side salad or steamed/boiled veggies.

V

DF Use dairy-free cream cheese.

LF Use lactose-free cream cheese.

VE See dairy-free advice and use vegan-friendly stock.

❄ See freezing and defrosting guidance for soups, stews and curries on page 28 (ensure you store leftovers with the potato slices facing up). Once defrosted, roast in the oven for 20–30 minutes once more to crisp up the potato slices.

- Vegetable oil spray
- 1 small onion **or** 100g (3½oz) leek, finely chopped
- 750g (1lb 10oz) frozen sliced mushrooms
- 4 medium carrots, cut into 1cm (½in) dice
- 1 tsp garlic paste (optional)
- 2 x 400g (14oz) cans of lentils, drained
- 1 tbsp tomato purée (paste)
- 1 tsp salt
- 1½ tsp ground black pepper
- 1 litre (generous 4 cups) gluten-free vegetable stock, for the hob, **or** 800ml (3⅓ cups) stock, for the slow cooker (made with 2 stock cubes)
- 200g (scant 1 cup) cream cheese
- 3 tbsp cornflour (cornstarch) or potato starch, mixed with 6 tbsp water
- 6 medium potatoes, sliced 3mm (⅛in) thick
- 10g (¼oz) parsley leaves, finely chopped, to serve (optional)

TIPS

If making this in a slow cooker, don't slice the potatoes too early! Instead, prepare the potatoes after adding the cream cheese and starch slurry.

A mandoline is a kitchen gadget that you can easily buy in supermarkets or online. Essentially, it's created to make slicing vegetables super-quick and easy and, best of all, it helps to create slices that are all the same thickness – perfect for ensuring your potatoes all cook evenly and at the same time! Use with care, though: the blade is very sharp so be especially wary when slicing small chunks of veg that are hard to grip. If your mandoline comes with a guard and/or protective gloves, do use them!

To cook using the hob and oven, preheat the oven to 180°C fan/200°C (400°F).

Spray the base of a large ovenproof pot with oil and place over a medium heat. Once hot, add the onion or leek and fry until the onion is browned or the leek has softened. Add the mushrooms, carrots and garlic paste, if using, and fry until the mushrooms are defrosted and have released liquid into the pan. Add the lentils, tomato purée, salt, pepper and stock, then stir well.

Stir in the cream cheese, then add the starch slurry and quickly mix it in. Simmer for 10–15 minutes or until the sauce has nicely thickened.

Top with the potato slices, overlapping slightly, then spray generously with vegetable oil and bake in the oven for 40–45 minutes or until the potato slices are crisp at the edges. Top with the chopped parsley, if using, and serve.

To cook using a slow cooker and oven, lightly grease the base of the slow cooker by spraying it with oil. Add all the ingredients except the cream cheese, starch slurry, potatoes and parsley, then stir well.

Pop the lid on and cook on low for 6–7 hours or on high for 3½ hours. Around 20 minutes before it's done, stir in the cream cheese and starch slurry, then cover with the lid once again for the remaining time.

Preheat the oven to 180°C fan/200°C (400°F). Transfer everything to a large ovenproof pot or suitably-sized roasting dish. Top with the potato slices, overlapping slightly, then spray generously with vegetable oil and bake in the oven for 40–45 minutes or until the potato slices are crisp at the edges. Sprinkle over the chopped parsley, if using, and serve.

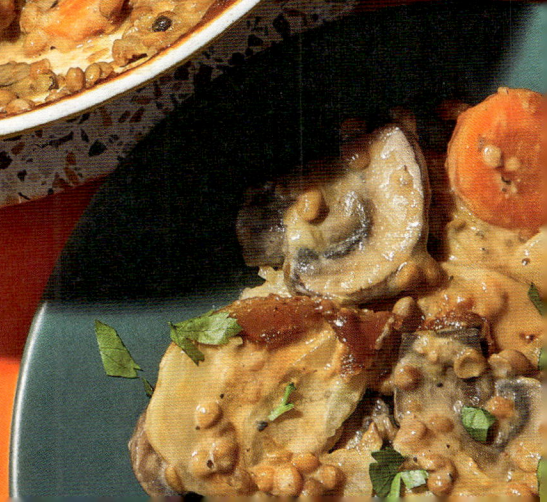

ONE-POT CHICKEN NOODLE SOUP

Sometimes it's the simplest things that you miss eating when you're gluten-free, that most 'normal people' probably don't even look twice at! In this case, I simply missed cracking open a can of chicken noodle soup, and in all my years on a gluten-free diet, I don't think I've ever even seen a dedicated gluten-free version in supermarkets. So I decided to make my own, which is far better value than what I used to buy anyway!

Serves 6

Prep 10 mins

Hob + Oven 40 mins or
Slow Cooker 6–7 hours

- Vegetable oil spray, for the hob and oven
- 150g (5½oz) frozen chopped onion **or** ½ large leek, finely chopped
- 300g (10½oz) celery, roughly chopped
- 4 medium carrots, sliced into 1cm (½in) rounds
- 500g (1lb 2oz) skinless, boneless chicken thighs, cut into 5mm (¼in) strips

- 1 tsp salt
- ½ tsp ground black pepper
- 2.2 litres (4¾ pints) gluten-free chicken stock, for the hob, **or** 2 litres (4¼ pints), for the slow cooker (see page 163 for homemade, or made using 3 stock cubes)

- 1½ tbsp dried mixed herbs
- 300g (2 cups) drained canned or frozen sweetcorn
- 200g (7oz) frozen spinach
- 500g (1lb 2oz) gluten-free dried spaghetti

DF **LF**

V Swap the chicken for 500g (1lb 2oz) frozen sliced mushrooms, and use veggie/vegan-friendly stock.

VE See veggie advice.

F Use leek (green parts only) instead of onion, no more than 60g (2oz) celery (stalks only), and 3 low FODMAP stock cubes.

❄ See freezing and defrosting guidance for pasta dishes on page 28. The soup will thicken a lot once cooled, so add a little extra boiling water when reheating until you reach a thickness you're happy with.

TIPS

Don't overcook the pasta once it's added to the pot, or when you stir it afterwards, it can easily all break and disintegrate! Take the lid off after 5–8 minutes (hob) or 15 minutes (slow cooker) to check how it's getting on.

This recipe also works really well with other shapes or gluten-free pasta like penne, fusilli or orzo.

To cook using the hob and oven, spray the base of a large pot that has a lid with oil and place over a medium heat. Once hot, add the onion or leek and fry until the onion has browned or the leek has softened. Add the celery and carrots and fry for a further 1–2 minutes, then add the chicken, salt and pepper and fry until the chicken is sealed.

Add the stock and mixed herbs, turn the heat down to low and simmer for 20 minutes, then add the sweetcorn, spinach and spaghetti, gently pushing the spaghetti below the surface of the soup as the lower half begins to soften. Simmer for a further 10 minutes or until the spaghetti is cooked and the soup is thickened to your liking.

To cook in a slow cooker, add everything to the slow cooker except the sweetcorn, spinach and spaghetti. Pop the lid on and cook on low for 6–7 hours or on high for 3½ hours. Around 20–30 minutes before it's done, stir in the sweetcorn and spinach, then add the spaghetti and cover with the lid once again for the remaining time.

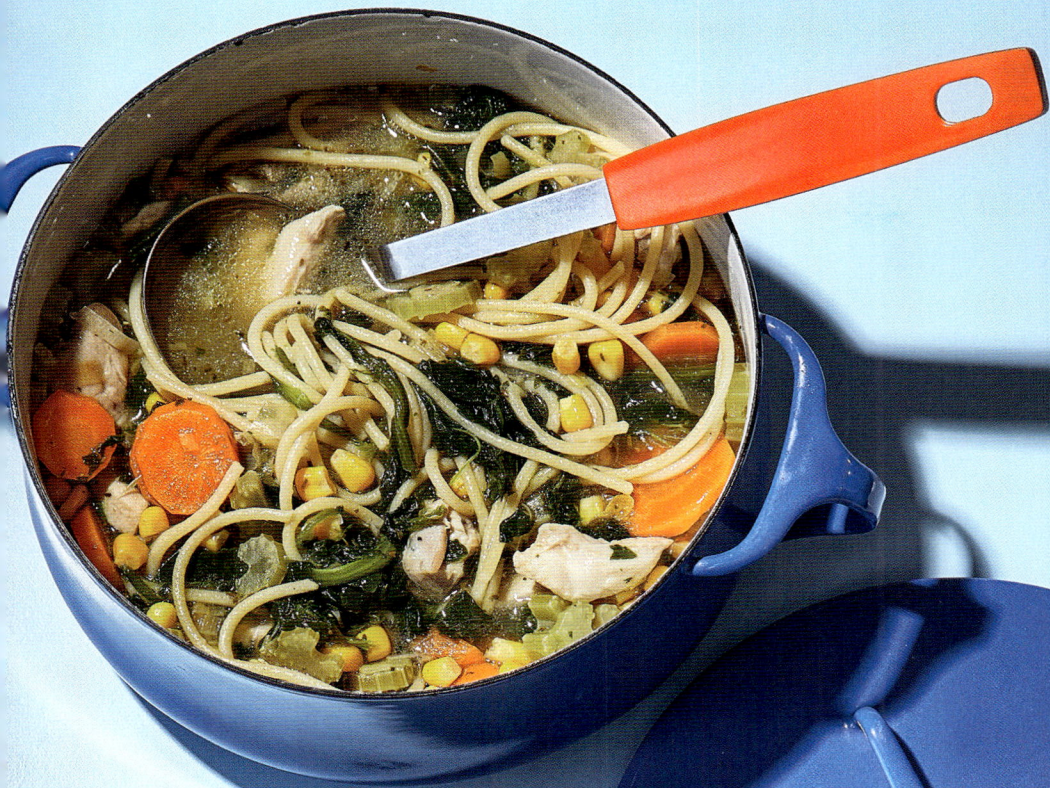

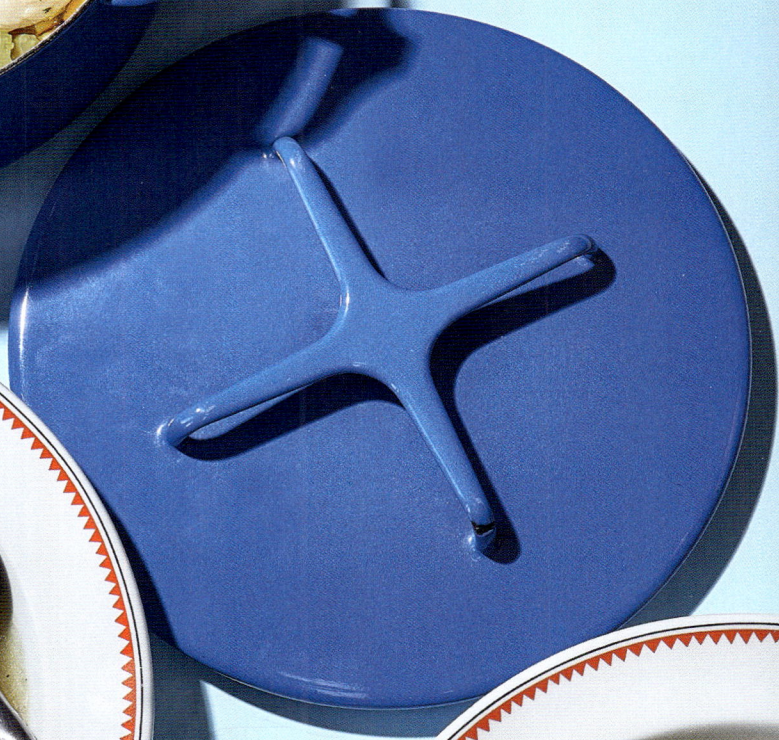

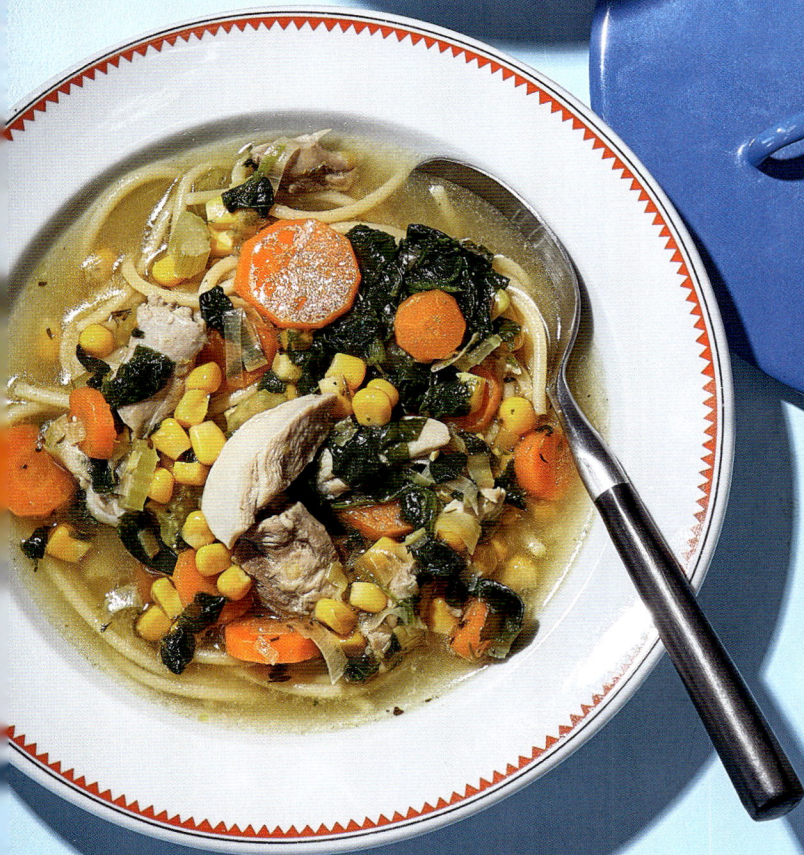

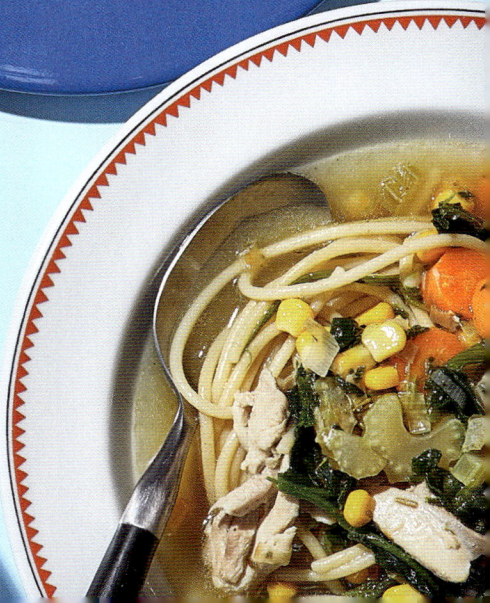

BRAZILIAN-STYLE GAMMON STEW
+ CHEDDAR DUMPLINGS

Serves 6–8

Prep 25 mins

Hob + Oven 5 hours 45 mins or
Slow Cooker 7–8 hours

Say hello to a Brazilian-style remix of one of my childhood favourites: stew and dumplings. This gammon stew is mildly spicy with an exceptionally satisfying smoky flavour (even more so if you use a smoked gammon joint) with cannellini beans, and cheesy, fluffy dumplings on top (and a crispy finish if you cook them in the oven). It is slow cooking at its finest!

LL

DF Use dairy-free cheese and a (hard) dairy-free alternative to butter (ideally chill it in the freezer first).

F Use leek (green parts only) instead of onion, all green (bell) peppers instead of mixed colours, only 450g (1lb) cannellini beans (drained weight), a low FODMAP stock cube, and omit the garlic paste.

❄ See freezing and defrosting guidance for soups, stews and curries on page 28.

TIP

Some gammon joints can be particularly salty, which is why I haven't added any extra salt to this recipe! However, when cooking gammon in the slow cooker for several hours, it can still make the stew taste too salty. So, if you are going to be cooking this in a slow cooker, I'd recommend first soaking the gammon in a bowl of water in the fridge (so that the water is covering the entire gammon) for 12–48 hours (change the water every 12 hours if soaking it longer) to remove any excess salt. I haven't found this to be necessary when cooking this on the hob – just the slow cooker!

- Vegetable oil spray
- 150g (5½oz) frozen chopped onion **or** ½ large leek, finely chopped
- 400g (14oz) frozen sliced red, green and yellow (bell) peppers
- 2 medium parsnips, sliced into 5mm (¼in) rounds
- 3 medium carrots, sliced into 5mm (¼in) rounds
- 2 tbsp garlic paste (optional)
- 25g (1oz) jarred jalapeños, finely chopped
- 2 tbsp smoked paprika
- 1 tbsp mild curry powder
- 1½ tbsp dried mixed herbs
- ½ tsp ground black pepper
- 3 tbsp cornflour (cornstarch) or potato starch
- 2 x 400g (14oz) cans of cannellini beans, drained
- 750g (1lb 10oz) boneless smoked or unsmoked gammon joint
- 1.2 litres (2½ pints) gluten-free ham stock, for the hob, **or** 1 litre (generous 4 cups) stock, for the slow cooker (made using 1 stock cube)
- Handful of parsley leaves, roughly chopped, to garnish (optional)

For the dumplings

- 315g (generous 2¼ cups) gluten-free self-raising flour
- 150g (⅔ cup) cold butter, grated
- 175g (6¼oz) mature Cheddar, grated
- 2 tbsp dried mixed herbs
- 1 tsp salt
- ½ tsp ground black pepper
- 200ml (generous ¾ cup) water

To cook using the hob and oven, spray the base of a large pot that has a lid with oil and place over a medium heat. Once hot, add the onion or leek and fry until the onion is browned or the leek has softened. Stir in the peppers, parsnips and carrots and fry for 2–3 minutes.

Add the garlic paste, if using, jalapeños, smoked paprika, curry powder, mixed herbs and black pepper. Stir well and fry until fragrant and there's no liquid left in the pan, then stir through the cornflour or potato starch.

Stir in the cannellini beans and place the whole gammon joint in the middle of the pan. Pour in the stock, which should just cover the gammon joint. Place the lid on, turn the heat down to low and simmer for 4½–5 hours until the gammon easily falls apart (test by scraping it with a fork) then remove it to a board. Use 2 forks to shred the gammon then stir it back into the pot.

continued overleaf

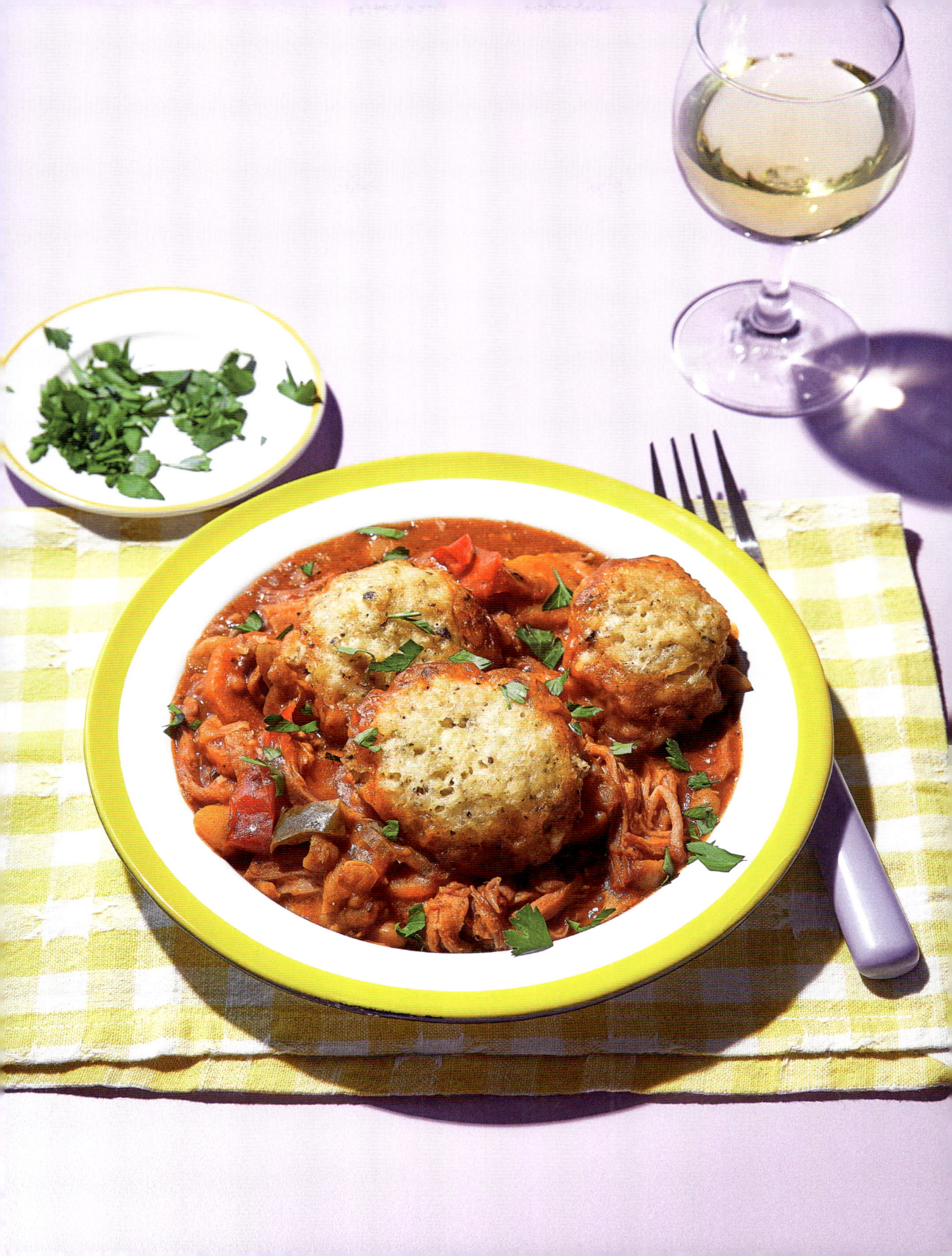

Meanwhile, preheat the oven to 200°C fan/220°C (425°F) and prepare the dumplings.

Add all the dumpling ingredients except the water to a large bowl and mix well. Add a third of the water at a time, stirring after each addition, until it forms a thick, sticky dough, then bring it together into a ball. Far too sticky? Add a little more flour. Too dry to form a ball? Add a little extra water.

Divide the dough into 16 equal golf-ball-sized balls (50g/1¾oz each), then place them back in the bowl and cover until you have shredded the gammon. Push the dumplings into the stew so that just the tops are visible. Pop the lid on and bake in the oven for 15 minutes, then remove the lid and continue to cook for 15–20 minutes until the dumpling tops are golden brown. Serve the stew sprinkled with chopped parsley, if using.

To cook in a slow cooker, lightly spray the base of the slow cooker with oil, then add everything except the parsley and the dumpling ingredients. Pop the lid on and cook on low for 6–7 hours or on high for 3½ hours. Remove the gammon to a board, use 2 forks to shred the meat, then stir it back into the slow cooker.

Around 20 minutes before shredding the gammon, prepare the dumplings as outlined on the left, adding them to the pot with the shredded gammon and submerging them in the stew so that just the tops are visible. Place a clean tea towel (dish cloth) over the slow cooker before putting the lid back on – this helps the dumplings puff up – and continue to slow cook for 60 minutes on low or 45 minutes on high, until soft and puffy. Serve the stew sprinkled with chopped parsley, if using.

TIP

Digital weighing scales can make portioning out the dumpling dough incredibly easy, ensuring that each dumpling is exactly the same size and that they all cook in the same time frame. Simply put the bowl containing the dumpling dough on the scale and press the 'zero' button to set the weight to zero. Once you remove the dough, the scale will now show you how much you've removed, so you can continue to take it out until the scale reads -50g. For each dumpling, simply press the 'zero' button again and portion out once more. Try using this technique when you need to weigh out portions for other recipes and thank me later!

MARK'S RENDANG-STYLE BEEF + BROCCOLI CURRY

Serves 6-8

Prep 10 mins

Hob + Oven 1 hour 55 mins or
Slow Cooker + Air Fryer
6-7 hours

Here's a recipe that Mark and I make regularly, especially after our recent trip to Malaysia. This curry is like no other in this book, with a totally different flavour profile thanks to the combo of tamarind, honey, five spice, curry powder and coconut milk. The beef is melt-in-your-mouth tender and the broccoli (my addition!) works so well alongside it. Serve with sticky jasmine rice.

DF **LF**

V Swap the beef for 2 x 400g (14oz) cans of drained chickpeas, and use veggie/vegan-friendly stock.

VE See veggie advice and use light brown sugar instead of honey.

❄ See freezing and defrosting guidance for soups, stews and curries on page 28.

- Vegetable oil spray
- 150g (5½oz) frozen chopped onion **or** ½ large leek, finely chopped
- 600g (1lb 5oz) beef stewing steak, cut into 2.5cm (1in) chunks
- 25g (1oz) jarred jalapeños, finely chopped
- 1½ tbsp ginger paste
- 2 tsp garlic paste (optional)
- 2 tsp Chinese five spice

- 2 tbsp mild curry powder
- 3 tsp tamarind paste
- 1½ tsp salt
- 3 tbsp honey
- 400g (14oz) frozen sliced red, green and yellow (bell) peppers
- 4 medium carrots, sliced into 1cm (½in) rounds
- 2 x 400g (14oz) cans of coconut milk
- 500ml (generous 2 cups) gluten-free beef stock

- 500g (1lb 2oz) frozen broccoli florets
- 3 tbsp cornflour (cornstarch) or potato starch, mixed with 6 tbsp water

To serve (optional)
- 2 small handfuls of coriander (cilantro) leaves, roughly chopped
- 2 small red chillies, thinly sliced

TIPS

If you're not sure where to find tamarind paste, see the tip over on page 110.

Fancy making this recipe even lazier? Instead of roasting or air frying the broccoli, you can just add it to the curry for the final 45 minutes (or for the final 2 hours, if cooking on low in a slow cooker) of cooking time. Of course, you won't get that more-ish roasted broccoli finish, but I just wanted to give you the option for both ease and simplicity!

To cook using the hob and oven, lightly spray the base of a large pot that has a lid with oil and place over a medium heat. Once hot, add the onion or leek and fry until the onion is browned or the leek has softened. Add the beef and fry until almost sealed, then add the jalapeños, ginger paste, garlic paste, if using, five spice, curry powder, tamarind, salt and honey. Stir well to coat everything and allow to excitedly bubble for 1–2 minutes.

Add the peppers and carrots, then continue to stir fry until the peppers have softened. Stir in a third of the coconut milk and allow to bubble for 1–2 minutes before adding the rest of the coconut milk and the stock. Pop the lid on, turn the heat down to low and simmer for 50–60 minutes. Give it a stir, place the lid back on and simmer for a further 45 minutes.

About 30 minutes before the curry is done, preheat the oven to 200°C fan/220°C (425°F).

Lightly grease a medium baking sheet by spraying it with a little oil. Place the broccoli on top and spray all over with oil once more. Roast in the oven for 25 minutes, turning over halfway, until crisp, lightly browned in places and fork-tender.

Once the curry has finished simmering, stir in the starch slurry and simmer for a few more minutes until the sauce is nicely thickened. Stir in the roasted broccoli just before serving, garnished with the coriander and chilli if using.

continued overleaf

To cook using a slow cooker and air fryer, spray the base of a large frying pan with oil and place over a medium heat. Once hot, add the onion or leek and fry until the onion is browned or the leek has softened. Add the beef and fry until browned.

Add to the slow cooker with the remaining ingredients, apart from the broccoli and starch slurry, and stir well. Pop the lid on and cook on low for 6–7 hours or on high for 3½ hours.

Around 15–20 minutes before it's done, prepare the broccoli. Heat the air fryer to 200°C (400°F), then add the broccoli florets, making sure they're touching as little as possible, and spray generously with oil. Air fry for 10–15 minutes until browned at the edges and fork-tender, shaking them halfway (or 3–4 times if particularly piled up).

Once the curry has finished cooking, stir in the starch slurry and cook for a few more minutes until the sauce is nicely thickened.

Once the curry is ready, turn off the heat and optionally allow to cool for 10 minutes – it will thicken more as it cools. Stir in the air fried broccoli just before serving, garnished with the coriander and chilli, if using.

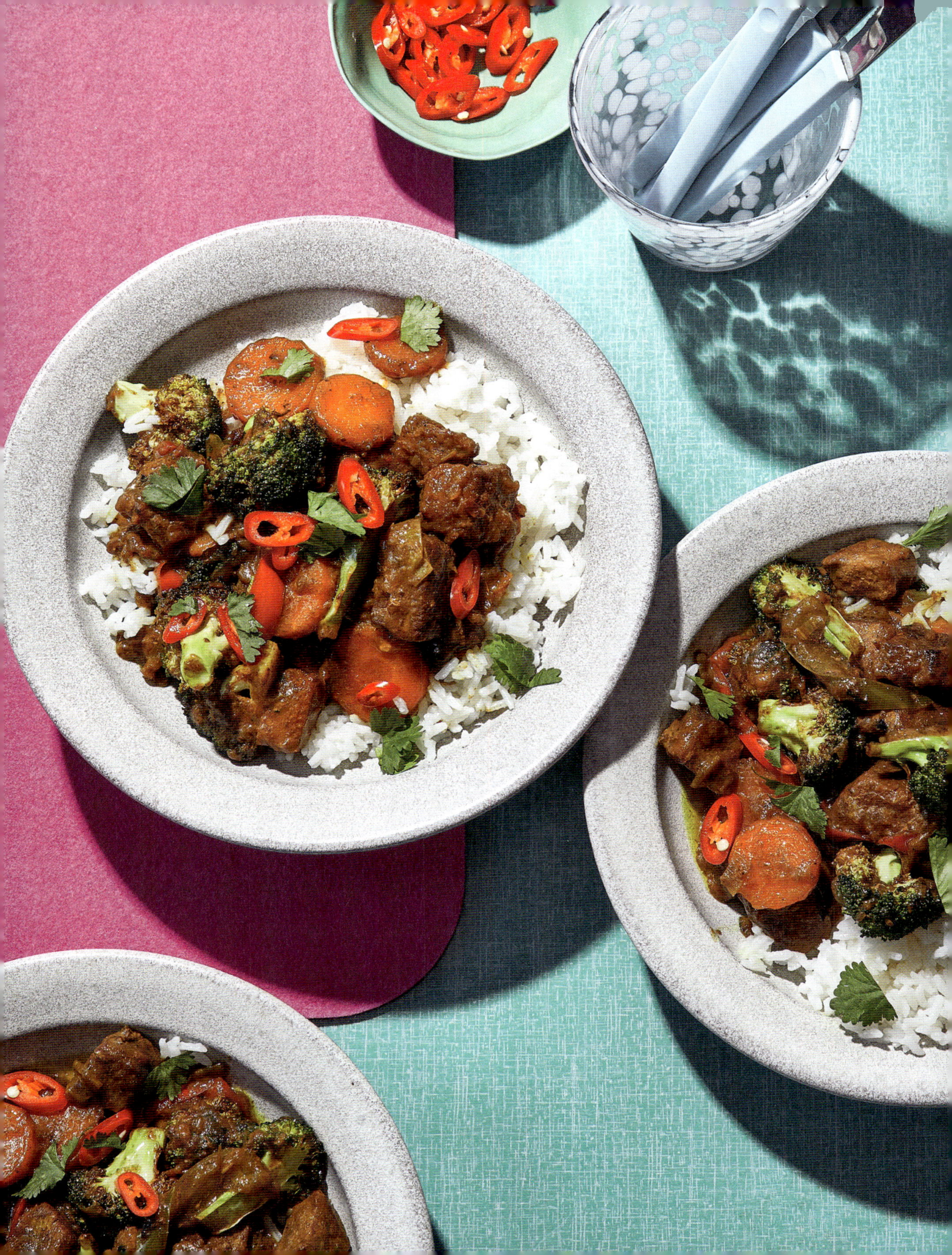

ROASTED SWEET POTATO + CHICKPEA COCONUT CURRY

Serves 6–8

Prep 10 mins

Hob + Oven 1 hour or
Slow Cooker + Air Fryer
6–7 hours

DF **LF** **V** **VE**

❄ See freezing and defrosting guidance for soups, stews and curries on page 28.

TIP

If using fresh spinach instead of frozen, be sure to add it right at the end of the recipe and then stir it in to wilt it down.

This meat-free meal uses lots of affordable, accessible ingredients, with jalapeños added for a little extra kick. In fact, it has one of the lowest costs per portion in this entire book. Treat this recipe as a crash course in how simple budget-friendly cooking from scratch can be! Serve with long-grain rice and/or naan bread (see page 44 for homemade).

- Vegetable oil spray
- 150g (5½oz) frozen chopped onion **or** ½ large leek, finely chopped
- 3 medium carrots, sliced into 1cm (½in) rounds
- 25g (1oz) jarred jalapeños, finely chopped
- 3 tbsp mild curry powder
- 2 tsp salt, plus 2 pinches for the sweet potato
- 1 x 400g (14oz) can of coconut milk
- 2 x 400g (14oz) cans of chopped tomatoes
- 2 x 400g (14oz) cans of chickpeas, drained
- 2 tbsp tomato purée (paste)
- 100ml (generous ⅓ cup) boiling water
- 200g (7oz) frozen spinach
- 1kg (2lb 3oz) sweet potatoes, peeled and cut into 1.5cm (⅔in) cubes
- 1 tsp coarsely ground black pepper

To cook using the hob and oven, preheat the oven to 200°C fan/220°C/425°F. Spray 2 large baking trays with vegetable oil.

Spray the base of a large pot with oil and place over a medium heat. Once hot, add the onion or leek and fry until the onion is browned or the leek has softened. Add the carrots, jalapeños, curry powder and salt, then fry until fragrant.

Add half the coconut milk and bring to the boil. Allow it to bubble for 4–5 minutes before adding the rest of the coconut milk, the chopped tomatoes, chickpeas, tomato purée and boiling water. Stir well and bring to the boil, then reduce to a low heat and simmer, uncovered, for 50–60 minutes. About 20–30 minutes before it's done, add the spinach.

Meanwhile, spread the sweet potato out on the baking trays and spray well with oil before seasoning all over with the 2 pinches of salt and the black pepper. Roast in the oven for 30–35 minutes or until lightly browned all over, turning them over halfway.

Once the curry has reduced and thickened, remove from the heat and allow to cool for 10 minutes (it will thicken more as it cools). Stir in the sweet potato just before serving.

To cook using a slow cooker and air fryer, lightly spray the base of the slow cooker with oil, then add everything except the spinach, sweet potato and black pepper and stir well. Pop the lid on and cook on low for 6–7 hours or on high for 3½ hours. Around 20–30 minutes before it's done, add the spinach and cover with the lid once again for the remaining time.

Place the sweet potato in a large bowl, spray well with oil and season with the 2 pinches of salt and the black pepper. Stir until evenly coated. Heat the air fryer to 200°C (400°F). Add the sweet potato cubes, making sure they're touching as little as possible, and air fry for 20 minutes until browned at the edges, shaking them halfway (or 3–4 times if particularly piled up). Stir the sweet potato into the curry just before serving.

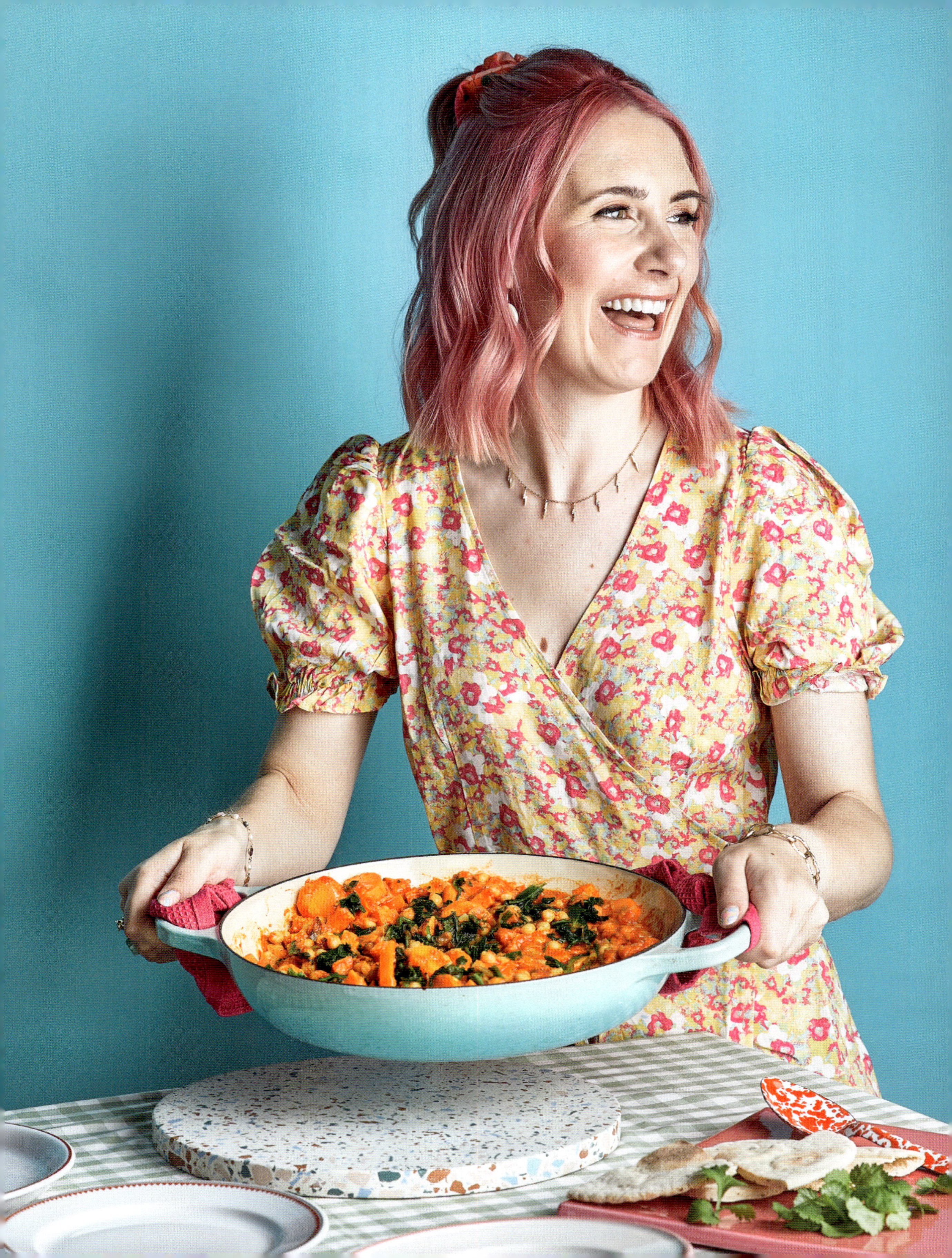

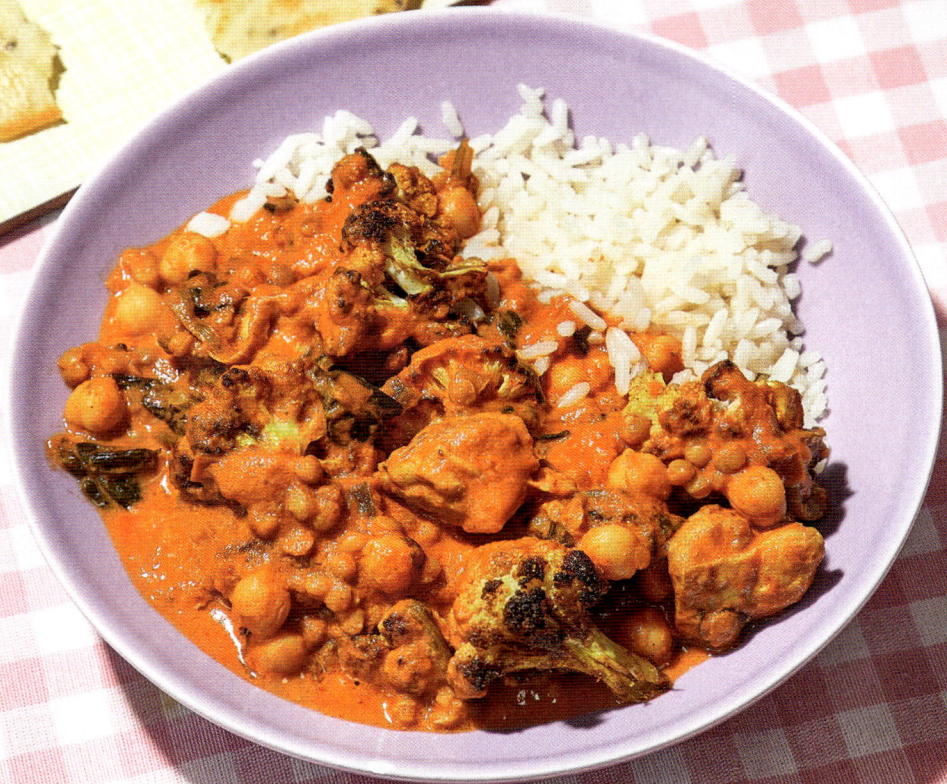

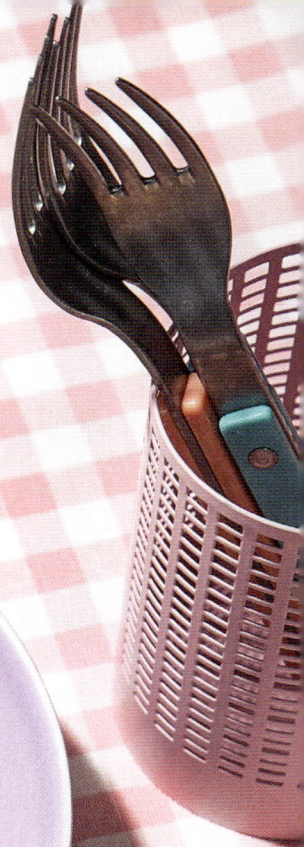

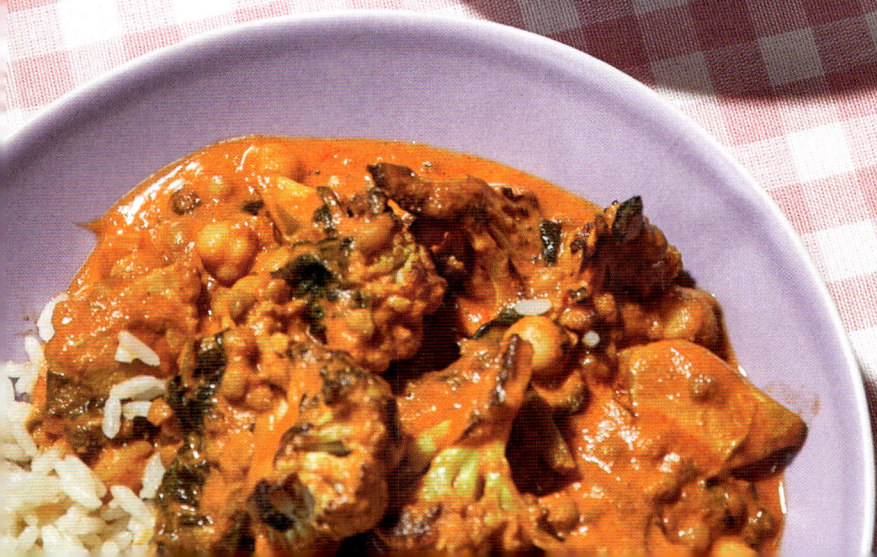

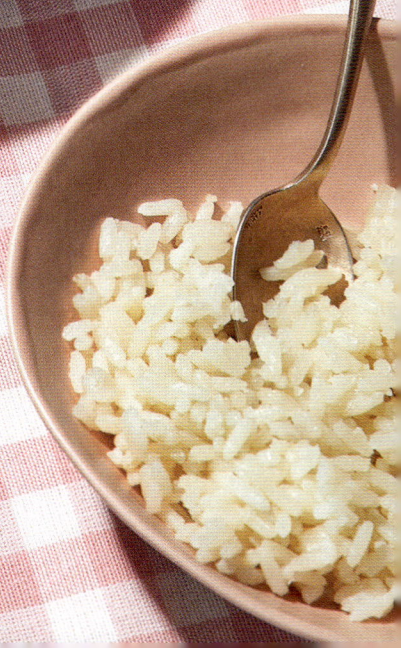

'CURRY VAN' TIKKA MASALA

Inspired by all the curry vans that I wish would pull up directly outside of my house, this curry never fails. Unlike the tikka masala you might find in Indian restaurants here in the UK (which is usually large chunks of chicken in a sauce and absolutely nothing else) my 'curry van' version contains a mix of chicken, lentils, chickpeas and cauliflower. Serve with long-grain rice and/or naan bread (see page 44 for homemade).

Serves 6–8

Prep 10 mins

Hob + Oven 1 hour or
Slow Cooker + Air Fryer 6–7 hours

DF Use a thick dairy-free yoghurt.

LF Use lactose-free Greek yoghurt.

V Swap the chicken for an additional 400g (14oz) can of drained chickpeas, and use veggie/vegan-friendly stock.

VE Combine the dairy-free and veggie advice and use caster (superfine) sugar instead of honey.

❄ See freezing and defrosting guidance for soups, stews and curries on page 28.

TIP

When roasting cauliflower, the aim is for it to be fork-tender after being roasted or air fried. Simply poke it with a fork – if it goes through without much resistance, it's perfect! The same goes for cooking broccoli.

- Vegetable oil spray
- 150g (5½oz) frozen chopped onion **or** ½ large leek, finely chopped
- 500g (1lb 2oz) skinless, boneless chicken thighs, cut into bite-sized chunks
- 2 tsp garlic paste (optional)
- 2 tbsp ginger paste
- 20g (¾oz) jarred jalapeños, finely chopped
- 2½ tbsp mild curry powder, plus 1 tbsp for the cauliflower
- 2 tbsp smoked paprika
- 1½ tsp salt
- 2 x 500g (1lb 2oz) cartons of passata (sieved tomatoes)
- 400ml (1⅔ cups) gluten-free chicken stock, for the hob, **or** 250ml (1 cup), for the slow cooker (see page 163 for homemade)
- 1 x 400g (14oz) can of lentils, drained
- 1 x 400g (14oz) can of chickpeas, drained
- 2 tbsp tomato purée (paste)
- 600g (1lb 5oz) frozen cauliflower florets
- 200g (7oz) frozen spinach
- 2 tbsp honey or caster (superfine) sugar
- 250g (generous 1 cup) natural or Greek yoghurt **or** 150ml (⅝ cup) double (heavy) cream

To cook using the hob and oven, preheat the oven to 200°C fan/220°C (425°F). Spray a large baking tray with oil.

Spray the base of a large pot that has a lid with oil and place over a medium heat. Add the onion or leek and fry until the onion is browned or the leek has softened. Add the chicken and continue to fry until sealed. Stir in the garlic paste, if using, ginger paste, jalapeños, curry powder, smoked paprika and salt. Fry until fragrant then stir in the passata, stock, lentils, chickpeas and tomato purée. Place the lid on, reduce the heat to low and simmer for 30 minutes.

Meanwhile, add the frozen cauliflower to the oiled tray, sprinkle over the 1 tablespoon of curry powder and spray all over with oil. Turn until coated, then roast for 30–35 minutes, turning it over halfway.

Once the curry has simmered for 30 minutes, add the spinach, honey or sugar and yoghurt or cream. Simmer, uncovered, for another 15–20 minutes, then stir in the roasted cauliflower.

To cook using a slow cooker and air fryer, lightly spray the base of the slow cooker with oil, then add everything except the spinach, honey or sugar, yoghurt or cream, and cauliflower to the slow cooker and stir well. Pop the lid on and cook on low for 6–7 hours or on high for 3½ hours.

Around 20–30 minutes before it's done, add the spinach, honey or sugar and the yoghurt or cream and cook, uncovered, for the remaining time.

Meanwhile, heat the air fryer to 200°C (400°F). Place the cauliflower in a large bowl, spray well with oil, then mix with the 1 tablespoon of curry powder. Add the cauliflower to the air fryer, ensuring the florets are touching as little as possible, and spray generously with oil, then air fry for 20 minutes until browned at the edges, shaking them halfway (or 3–4 times if particularly piled up).

Once the curry is ready, allow to cool for 10 minutes – it will thicken more as it cools. Stir in the cauliflower just before serving.

KEEMA CURRY

Serves 6–8

Prep 10 mins

Hob 1 hour 10 mins or
Slow Cooker 6–7 hours

Here's my version of aloo keema, a traditional Pakistani and north Indian dish, that I absolutely adore for it's cost effectiveness and batch-cooking efficiency. Whether you cook it in a pot on the hob or in the slow cooker, you can expect the same mildly spicy, bold curried tomato sauce, potatoes that soak up all that flavour, and a mix of beef and lentils. The frozen peas and lentils essentially bulk out the beef, making it seem like far more than it is at a fraction of the price! However, if you're not partial to lentils and don't mind the extra cost of doing so, you could always use an extra 250g (9oz) of minced (ground) beef instead of lentils. Serve with long-grain rice and/or naan bread (see page 44 for homemade).

DF **LF**

V Swap the beef for 2 x 400g (14oz) cans of drained chickpeas, and use veggie/vegan-friendly stock.

VE See veggie advice.

❄ See freezing and defrosting guidance for soups, stews and curries on page 28.

- Vegetable oil spray
- 150g (5½oz) frozen chopped onion **or** ½ large leek, finely chopped
- 500g (1lb 2oz) minced (ground) beef
- 2 tsp garlic paste (optional)
- 2 tbsp ginger paste
- 20g (¾oz) jarred jalapeños, finely chopped
- 3 tbsp mild curry powder
- 2 tsp salt
- 4 medium potatoes, peeled and cut into 1.5cm (⅔in) cubes
- 2 x 400g (14oz) cans of chopped tomatoes
- 1 x 400g (14oz) can of lentils, drained
- 2 tbsp tomato purée (paste)
- 150ml (⅝ cup) gluten-free beef stock
- 200g (7oz) frozen peas

To cook on the hob, spray the base of a large pot that has a lid with oil and place over a medium heat. Once hot, add the onion or leek and fry until the onion is browned or the leek has softened.

Add the beef and, once it releases a little moisture, scrape anything stuck to the bottom of the pan until it's deglazed. Once the beef has browned, add the garlic paste, if using, ginger paste, jalapeños, curry powder and salt. Stir well and fry until fragrant and there is no liquid left in the pan. Stir in the potatoes and fry for 2–3 minutes.

Add the tomatoes, lentils, tomato purée and stock, then stir well once more. Turn the heat down to low, cover and simmer for 45–50 minutes until nicely thickened. Stir in the peas and simmer, uncovered, for 5 minutes or until the peas are done.

To cook in a slow cooker, spray the base of a large frying pan with oil and place over a medium heat. Once hot, add the onion or leek and fry until the onion is browned or the leek has softened. Add the beef and fry until browned.

Meanwhile, add the remaining ingredients apart from the peas to the slow cooker and stir well. Once the beef has browned, add it along with the onion or leek to the slow cooker and stir in. Pop the lid on and cook on low for 6–7 hours or on high for 3½ hours, stirring in the peas 10 minutes before serving.

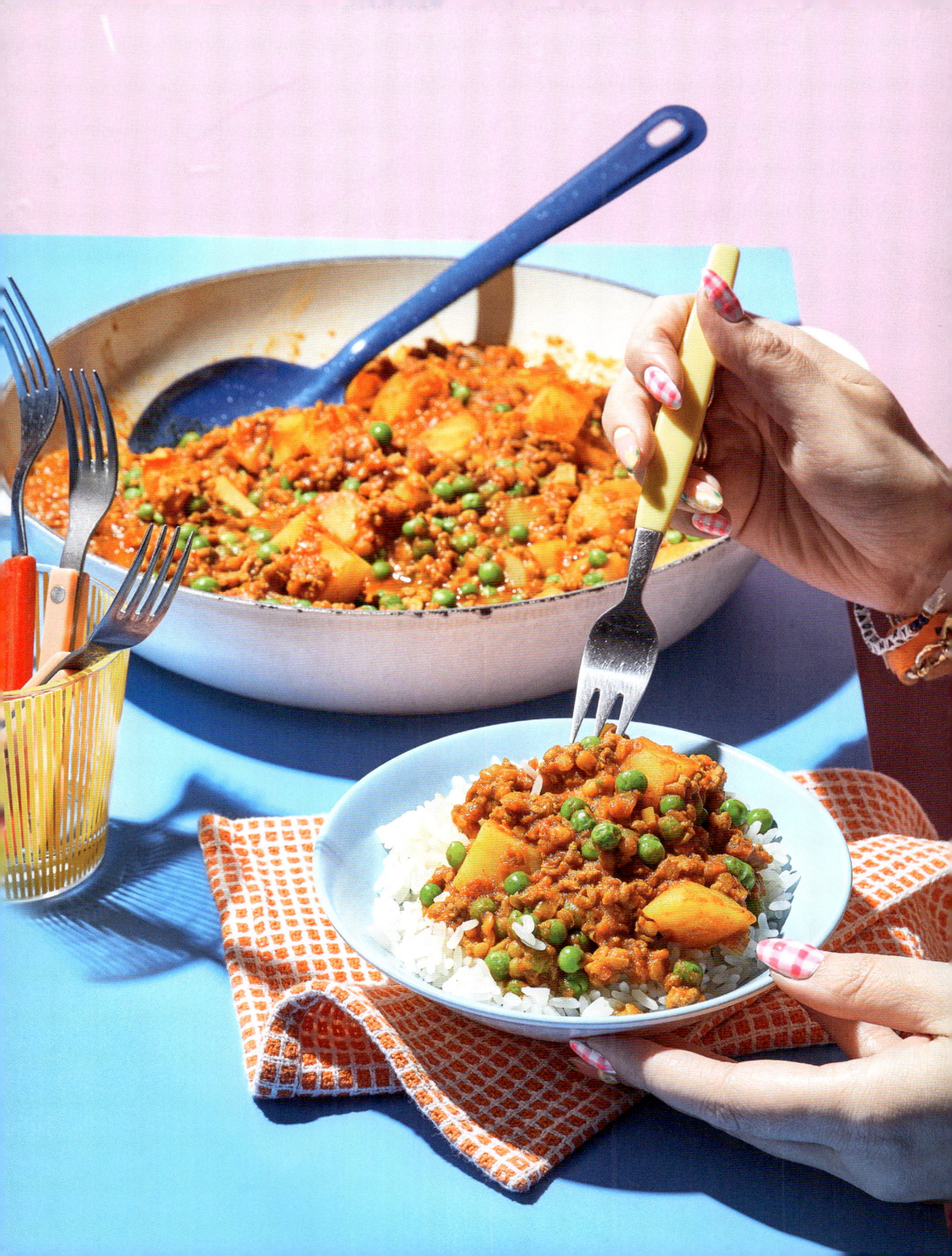

AUBERGINE + COCONUT DHAL

Serves 6–8

Prep 10 mins

Hob 55 mins or
Slow Cooker 7–8 hours

DF **LF** **V** **VE**

❄ See freezing and defrosting guidance for soups, stews and curries on page 28.

A good dhal recipe is worth its weight in gold, and this one is no exception. Yep, it's another one-pot recipe that needs no accompaniment (although a good gluten-free naan goes a long way!) that's hearty, filling, with a velvety coconut, ginger and tomato base packed with tender veg and vibrant red lentils, all tinged with warming spices. Just ensure you always check the ingredients list when buying packets of dried lentils as some have 'may contain' warnings for gluten. And don't try this one with canned lentils or you'll be left with lentil soup!

- Vegetable oil spray
- 150g (5½oz) frozen chopped onion **or** ½ large leek, finely chopped
- 2 medium aubergines (eggplants), sliced into 1cm (½in) rounds
- 3 medium carrots, sliced into 1cm (½in) rounds
- 2 tsp garlic paste (optional)

- 1 tbsp ginger paste
- 25g (1oz) jarred jalapeños, finely chopped
- 3 tbsp mild curry powder
- 1 tsp salt
- ½ tsp ground black pepper
- 450g (1lb) dried red lentils (ensure gluten-free)
- 2 x 400g (14oz) cans of chopped tomatoes

- 1 tbsp tomato purée (paste)
- 1 x 400g (14oz) can of coconut milk
- 1 litre (generous 4 cups) gluten-free vegetable stock
- Handful of coriander (cilantro) leaves, roughly chopped (optional)

To cook on the hob, spray the base of a large pot that has a lid with oil and place over a medium heat. Once hot, add the onion or leek and fry until the onion is browned or the leek has softened. Add the aubergines and continue to fry until lightly browned.

Add the carrots, garlic paste, if using, ginger paste, jalapeños, curry powder, salt and pepper. Stir well and fry until fragrant then add the dried red lentils and continue to fry for a further 2–3 minutes.

Stir in the chopped tomatoes, tomato purée, coconut milk and stock, and bring to the boil. Place the lid on, turn the heat down to low and simmer for 40–45 minutes or until the lentils are cooked and the sauce has thickened. Serve with chopped coriander, if using.

To cook in a slow cooker, spray the base of the slow cooker with oil, then add everything else and stir well. Pop the lid on and cook on low for 7–8 hours or on high for 3½ hours. Serve with chopped coriander, if using.

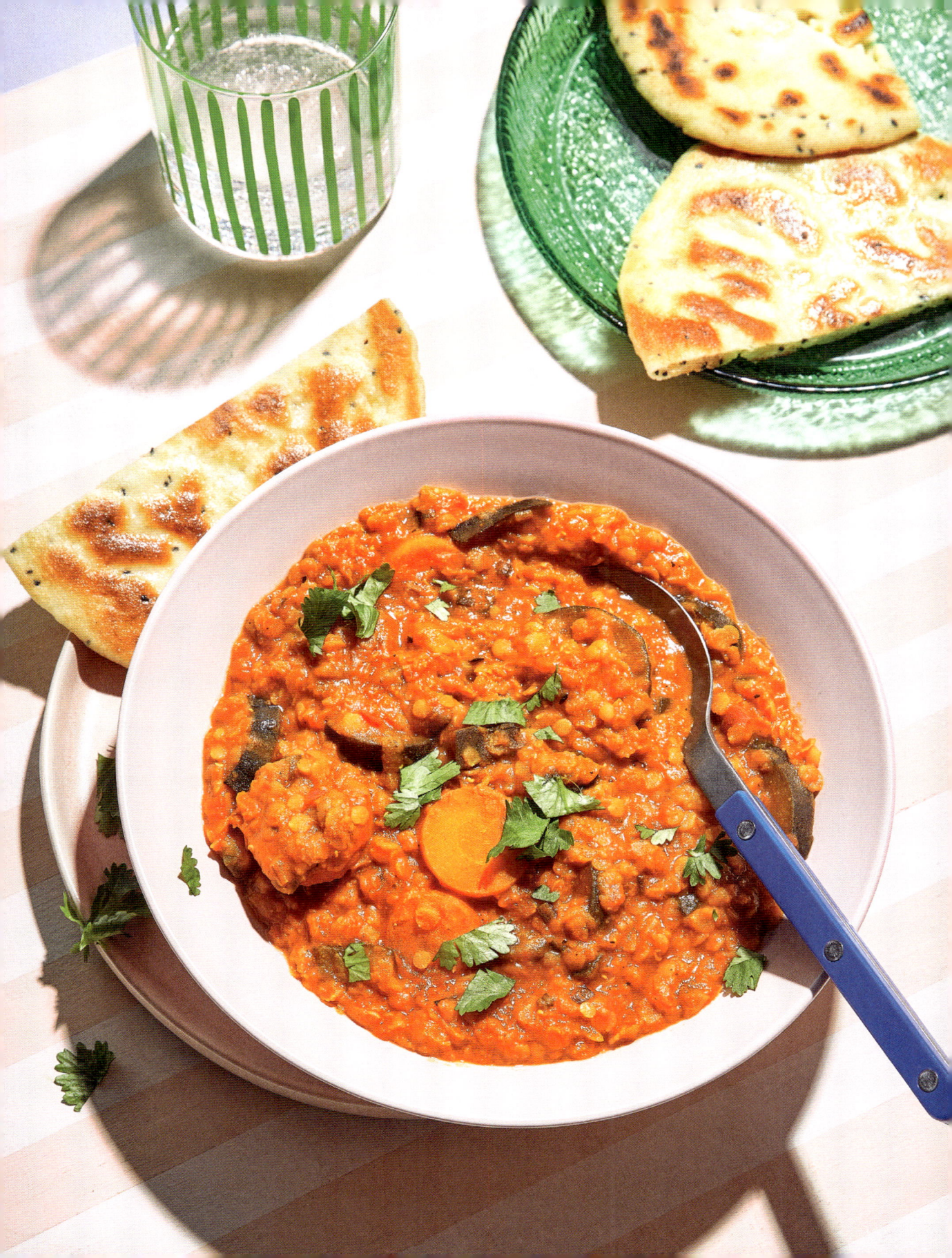

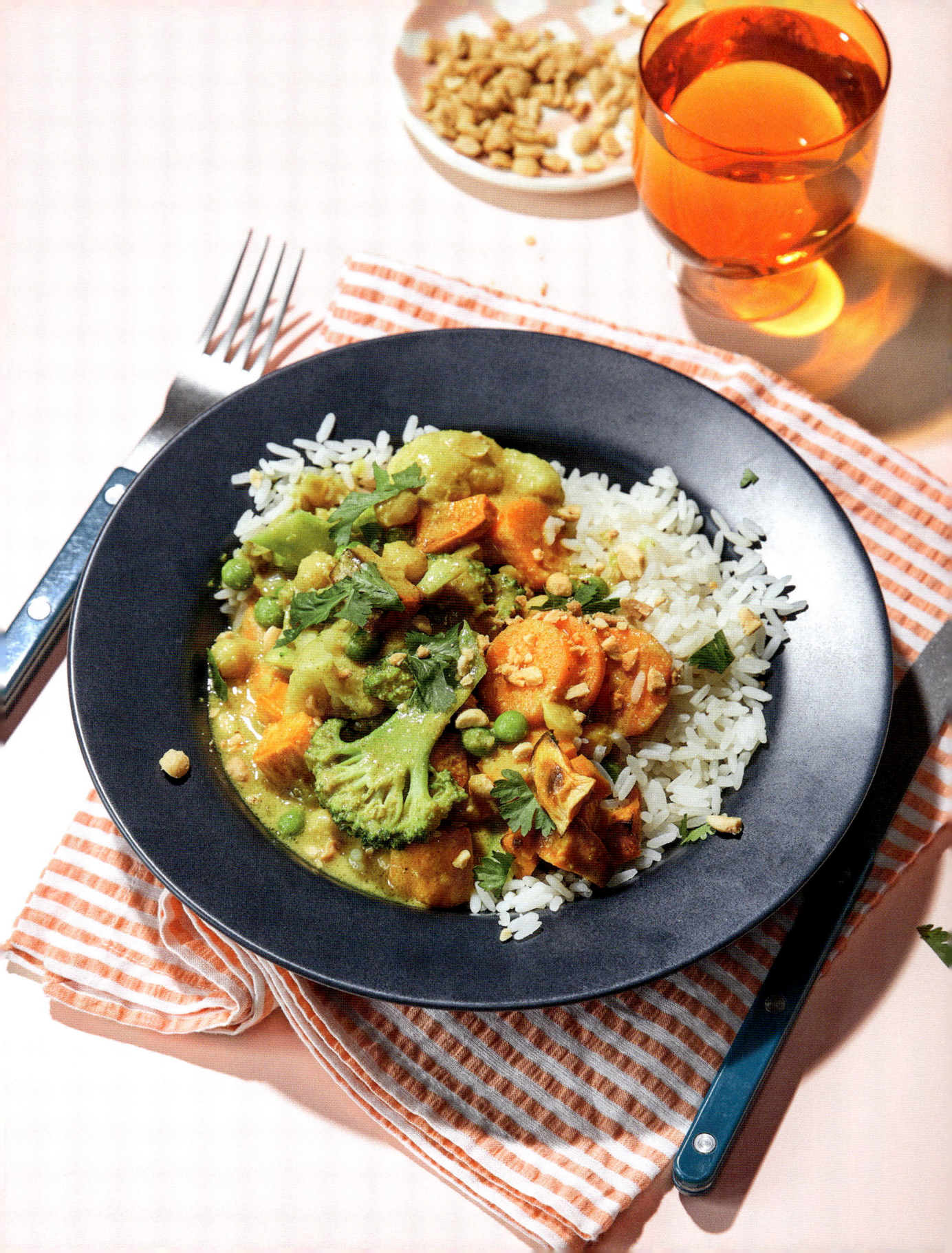

PEANUT BUTTER CURRY

This coconut and peanut butter vegetable curry is a firm favourite in our house, with that sweet and crispy sweet potato being an extremely gratifying pairing. This recipe is a great one for using up any leftover veg, though in the absence of that, I just use frozen mixed veg, which is not only affordable but already pre-chopped and prepped! Serve with long-grain rice.

Serves 6–8

Prep 10 mins

Hob + Oven 1 hour or
Slow Cooker + Air Fryer
6–7 hours

DF LF V VE

❄ See freezing and defrosting guidance for soups, stews and curries on page 28.

- Vegetable oil spray
- 150g (5½oz) frozen chopped onion **or** ½ large leek, finely chopped
- 30g (1oz) jarred jalapeños, chopped
- 2 tsp garlic paste (optional)
- 1 tbsp ginger paste
- 3 tbsp mild curry powder
- 1 x 400g (14oz) can of coconut milk

- 1 litre (generous 4 cups) gluten-free vegetable stock
- 2 x 400g (14oz) cans of chickpeas, drained
- 250g (generous 1 cup) peanut butter (smooth or crunchy)
- 500g (1lb 2oz) frozen mixed veg (carrots, cauliflower, green beans, peas)

- 250g (9oz) frozen broccoli florets
- 750g (1lb 10oz) sweet potatoes, cut into 1.5cm (⅔in) cubes
- Salt and pepper

To serve

- Handful of roasted salted peanuts, crushed
- Small handful of coriander (cilantro) leaves, chopped (optional)

To cook using the hob and oven, spray the base of a large pot that has a lid with oil and place over a medium heat. Once hot, add the onion or leek and fry until the onion is browned or the leek has softened. Add the jalapeños, garlic paste, if using, ginger paste, curry powder, 1 teaspoon of salt and ½ teaspoon of pepper, then fry until fragrant.

Add half the coconut milk and bring to the boil. Allow it to bubble for 4–5 minutes before adding the rest of the coconut milk, the stock, chickpeas and peanut butter. Stir well and bring to the boil, then reduce the heat to low and simmer for 45–50 minutes until thickened. Add the frozen mixed veg and broccoli 15 minutes before it's finished.

Meanwhile, preheat the oven to 200°C fan/220°C (425°F) and spray a large baking tray with oil. Spread the sweet potatoes out on the baking tray, spray with a little more oil and season with 2 pinches each of salt and pepper. Roast in the oven for 30–35 minutes or until lightly browned all over, turning them over halfway.

Once the curry has reduced and thickened, take it off the heat and allow to cool for 10 minutes; it will thicken more as it cools. Stir in the roasted sweet potato just before serving, with the crushed peanuts and coriander sprinkled on top, if using.

To cook in a slow cooker and air fryer, spray the base of the slow cooker with oil, then add everything except the sweet potato, season with 1 teaspoon of salt and ½ teaspoon of pepper, then pop the lid on and cook on low for 6–7 hours or high for 3½ hours.

Heat the air fryer to 200°C (400°F).

Place the sweet potato in a large bowl, spray well with oil and season with 2 pinches each of salt and pepper. Stir until evenly coated. Add the sweet potato cubes to the air fryer, making sure they're touching as little as possible, and air fry for 20 minutes until browned at the edges, turning over half way or shaking 3–4 times if particularly piled up. Stir into the curry as directed above, and serve with the crushed peanuts and coriander sprinkled on top, if using.

BARGAIN BAKES

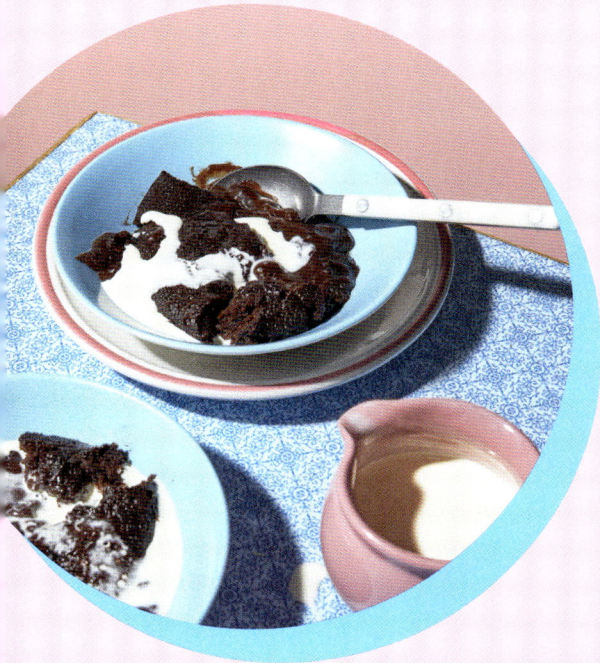

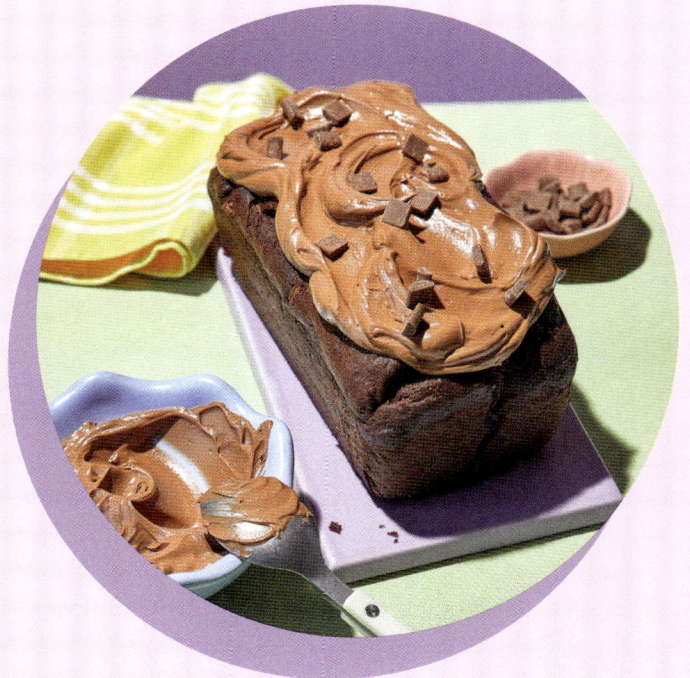

While gluten-free and 'free-from' aisles seem to be jam-packed with different cakes, biscuits and desserts these days, there's no denying that practicality, convenience and their free-from credentials are what you're getting: notice that value isn't usually present in that list!

Without a doubt, the most affordable and cost-effective way of enjoying all your past and present favourite bakes is to recreate them at home. And whether you're looking for a small sweet treat, an 'emergency' option for when nobody's catered for you, a big celebration cake that won't break the bank, or a dessert that both gluten-free folks and gluten eaters will love, this chapter covers all those eventualities and more.

There's everything from big batch bakes like my lemon drizzle traybake or slow-cooker chocolate fudge pudding, as well as budget-friendly biscuits and cookies, such as my party rings, oat and raisin/chocolate bakery-style cookies, and the ever-attractive 50:50 cookies. Of course, who could forget about dessert too? There's tons to choose from for all occasions and nobody would have any idea that they're gluten-free and all budget-friendly bakes too.

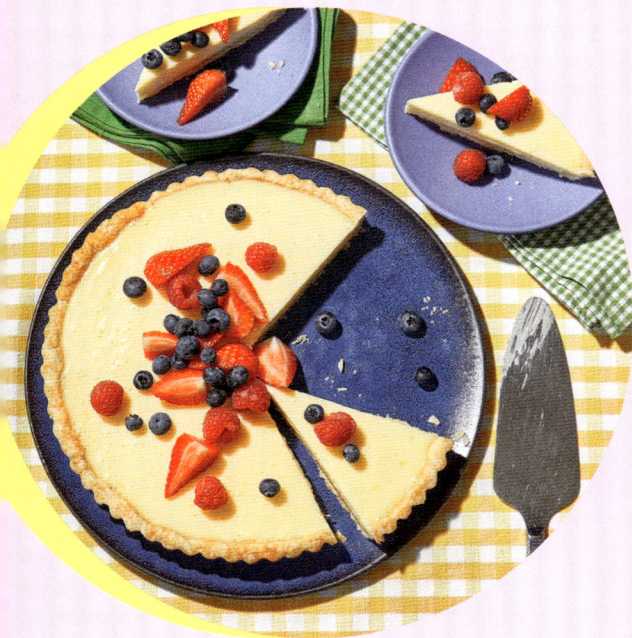

3-INGREDIENT CHOCOLATE HAZELNUT MUG CAKE

Serves 1
Prep 1 min
Microwave 1 min

V

DF Use a dairy-free alternative to chocolate hazelnut spread.

LF See dairy-free advice.

F See dairy-free advice.

It's scary to know that you're only ever a dollop of chocolate hazelnut spread, an egg, 2 tablespoons of gluten-free flour and 1 minute away from a steamed-pudding-like choc hazelnut sponge that's perfect with vanilla ice cream. However, I'm told a little fear is a good thing, and I can most definitely say that this recipe is a very good thing indeed.

- 80g (3oz) chocolate hazelnut spread
- 1 medium egg
- 2 tbsp gluten-free self-raising flour

Add the chocolate spread to a large mug, crack in the egg and beat together with a fork until well combined. If the spread clumps to the fork, just scrape it back into the mixture with a spoon and mix in.

Add the flour and mix once more until the batter is smooth and glossy, without lumps or pockets of flour; the mixture should reach halfway up the mug, giving it lots of space to rise.

Microwave at full power (mine is set to 1000W) for 1 minute – timing may vary depending on your microwave. It should rise up just above the mug, then sink back down into the mug once the microwave is done. Keep an eye on it as it cooks to ensure it doesn't rise too far out of the mug!

Allow to stand for 1 minute then serve with vanilla ice cream on top, straight from the mug.

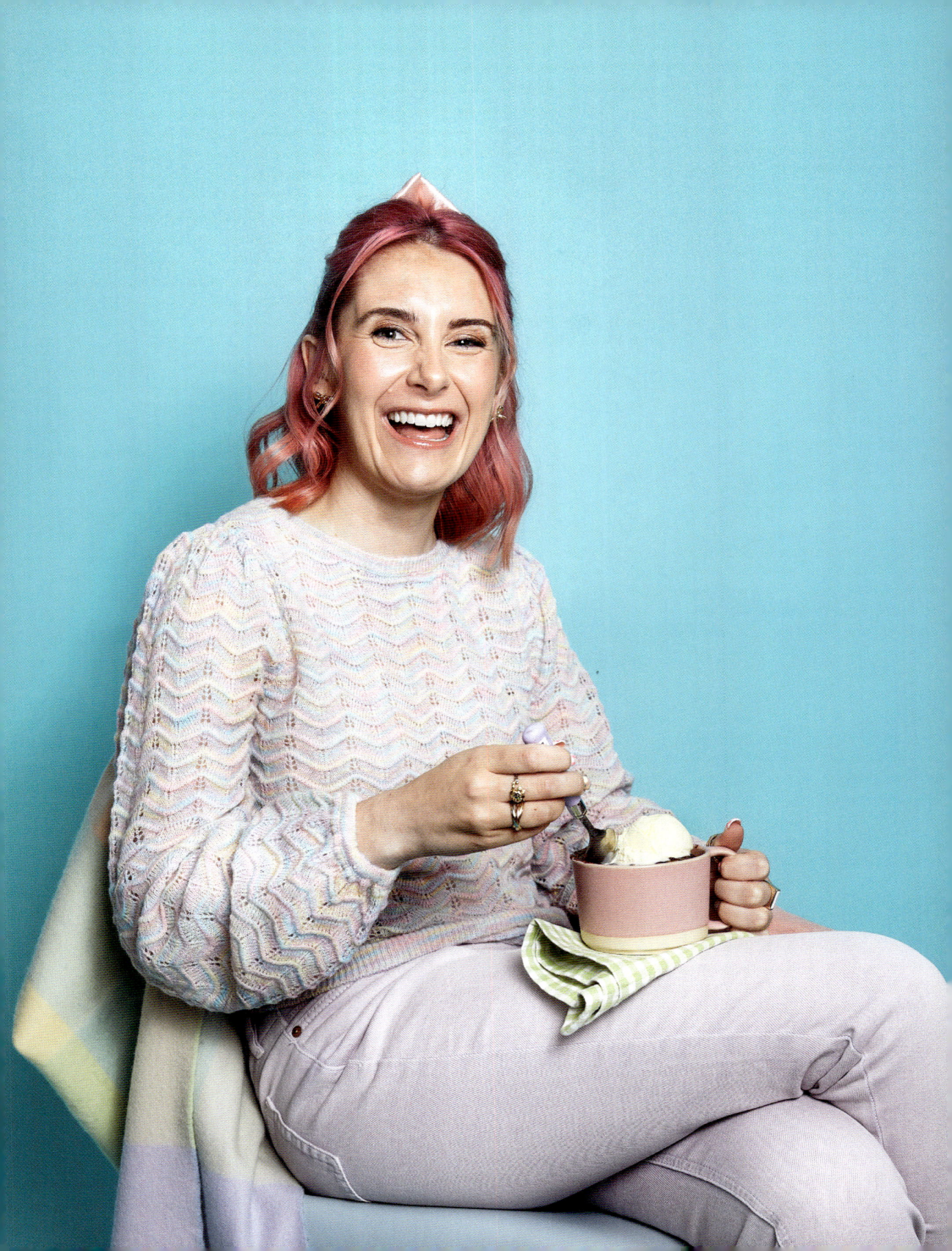

3-INGREDIENT LEMONADE SCONES

Makes 6–8

Prep 15 mins

Oven 15 mins or
Air Fryer 10 mins

If you asked me what you'd get if you mixed together gluten-free flour, lemonade and cream, I'd have probably thought you were teeing up a rib-tickling joke before I ever guessed correctly. Of course, the correct answer is: proper tea-room-style scones (biscuits) with a light and fluffy texture in the middle. Pass the jam!

V

DF Use a dairy-free alternative to cream.

LF Use lactose-free cream.

F See lactose-free advice.

VE See dairy-free advice and brush with maple syrup instead of egg.

❄ Once cooled, freeze for up to 2–3 months in an airtight container. Allow to defrost on a wire rack at room temperature for 2–3 hours. To reheat, air fry at 200°C (400°F) for 5–6 minutes.

- 325g (2½ cups minus 1½ tbsp) gluten-free self-raising flour, plus extra for dusting
- 165ml (⅓ pint plus 2 tsp) lemonade
- 155ml (⅓ pint) double (heavy) cream
- 1 egg, beaten

To make these in the oven, preheat the oven to 200°C fan/220°C (425°F). Line a large baking tray with non-stick baking parchment.

Add the flour to a large bowl, then add the lemonade and cream. Mix together using a spatula until it forms a soft dough; do not overmix.

Lightly dust your work surface and hands with a little flour. Tip the dough out of the bowl and fold it over a few times to bring it together. Then use your hands to bring the dough into a rounded shape about 4cm (1½in) thick. The taller, the better!

Using a 5cm (2in) round or fluted biscuit (cookie) cutter, push down into the dough and bring out the scones with the cutter. Gently push them out of the cutter and put to one side until you have used up all the dough. Instead of re-rolling the dough, keep re-rounding the dough back into a ball, and continue to cut out the scones.

Brush the tops of the scones with beaten egg, transfer to the lined baking tray and bake in the oven for 12–15 minutes until golden on top.

To make these in an air fryer, heat or preheat the air fryer to 180°C (350°F). Make the scones as opposite and brush with egg, then place them on individual squares of baking parchment. Air fry for around 10 minutes until golden on top.

Allow to cool briefly before enjoying warm, or allow to cool completely and serve with clotted cream and jam or lemon curd.

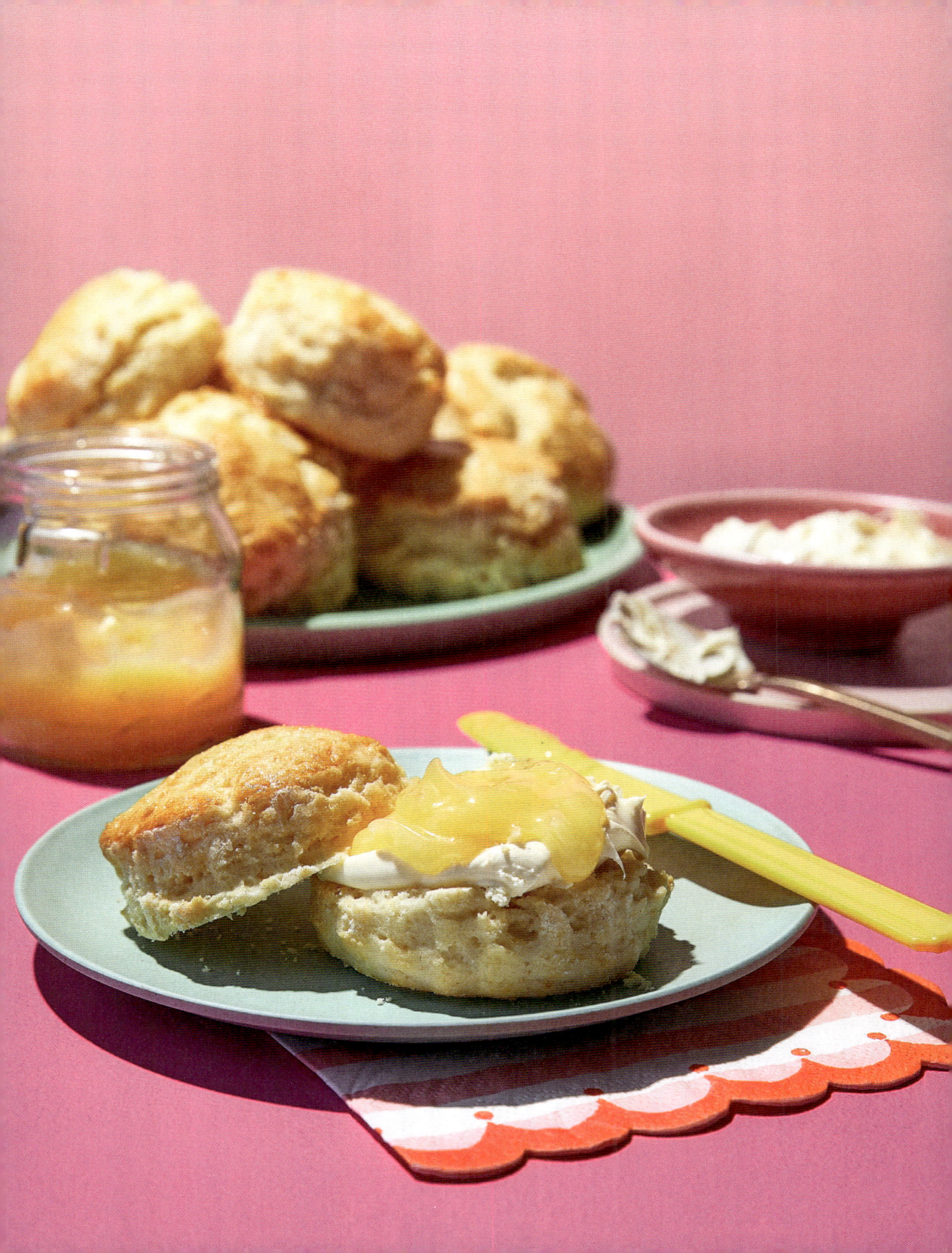

JAFFA CAKES

If you've missed these absolute classics (I won't be a part of arguing whether they're classified as biscuits or tiny cakes! Surely the answer is in the name? I've said too much already!) or been underwhelmed by supermarket versions, then trust me: this recipe is here to restore your faith and remind you of what the 'real deal' is supposed to taste like! This recipe is dedicated to one of my followers, Amy, who has been regularly asking me to make these for years... this one's for you!

Makes 12
Prep 25 mins + setting
Oven 10 mins

DF Use a (hard) dairy-free alternative to butter, and dairy-free dark chocolate.

LL Use lactose-free dark chocolate.

V Use veggie-friendly jelly.

F See low lactose advice.

❄ See freezing and defrosting guidance for biscuits and cookies on page 28.

TIP

To make cutting the circles of jelly effortless and simple, I simply use either a very small round biscuit (cookie) cutter or the wide end of a large piping nozzle. Once you've cut the circles out you'll have the remaining off-cuts of jelly leftover, but I'm sure you'll figure out what to do with it (eat it!).

- Butter, softened, for greasing
- 2 large eggs
- 50g (¼ cup) caster (superfine) sugar
- ½ tsp vanilla extract
- 50g (6 tbsp) gluten-free self-raising flour, sifted
- Pinch of xanthan gum
- 150g (5½oz) dark (bittersweet) chocolate, melted and cooled

For the jelly
- 135g (4¾oz) orange jelly (jello) cubes
- 1 tbsp orange marmalade
- 150ml (⅝ cup) boiling water

Preheat the oven to 160°C fan/180°C (350°F). Grease the holes of a 12-hole cupcake tray with a little softened butter.

For the jelly, place the jelly cubes in a jug (pitcher) with the marmalade and pour the boiling water over the top of it. Stir until the cubes dissolve completely and then pour into a 23cm (9in) square tin (I line my tin with cling film/plastic wrap as I find it easier to lift the jelly out). Refrigerate to fully set (1–2 hours).

Meanwhile, make the sponges. Crack the eggs into a medium bowl, add the sugar and vanilla and whisk together using a electric hand mixer for about 5 minutes until light and fluffy. Sift in the flour and xanthan gum and carefully fold it in (sifting the flour is very important to reduce the chance of getting any lumps).

Pour or spoon the mixture evenly between the 12 greased holes and bake in the oven for 8–10 minutes until cooked through. Remove from the oven and allow to cool briefly before removing from the tin and transferring to a wire rack to finish cooling.

Once the sponges are cooled and the jelly set, cut out circles of the jelly very slightly smaller than the sponges and place a circle on top of each sponge.

Spoon the melted chocolate over each of the cakes so the jelly circle is completely covered, all the way to the edges. Use the back of a fork to create a pattern in the melted chocolate, then allow it to fully set.

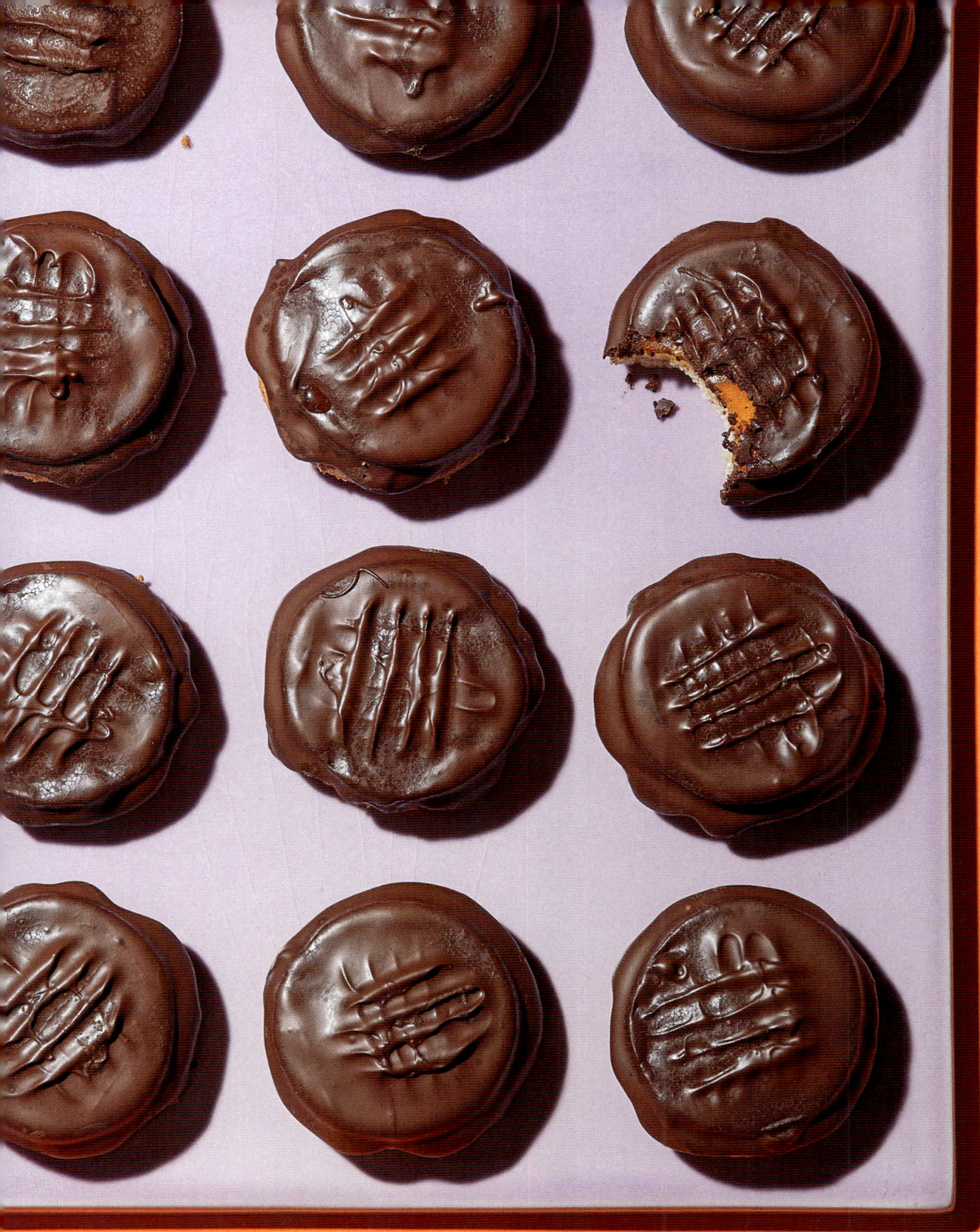

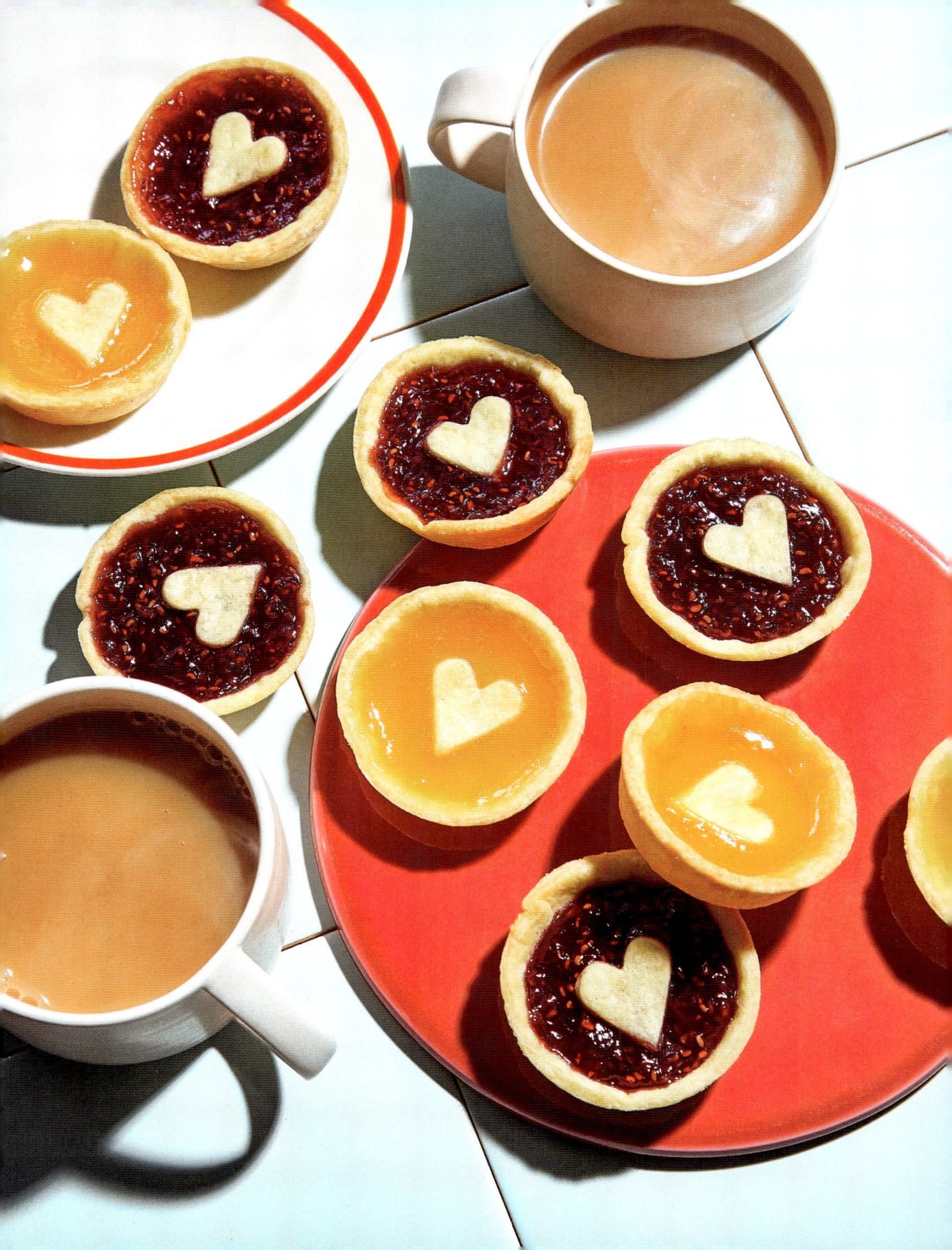

JAM OR LEMON CURD TARTS

I never thought I'd put out a recipe for something that I've always thought of as so simple, but I *always* get requests for jam tarts and it's a good reminder of my super-simple ultimate shortcrust pastry recipe, which can also be used for everything from pies, to quiches, tarts and loads more.

Makes 12
Prep 20 mins
Oven 15 mins

LL **F** **V**

DF Use a (hard) dairy-free alternative to butter.

❄ Once cooled, freeze in an airtight container. Allow to defrost fully at room temperature on a wire rack for 1 hour.

For the pastry
- 150g (1 cup plus 2 tbsp) gluten-free plain (all-purpose) flour, plus extra for dusting
- ¾ tsp xanthan gum
- 75g (⅓ cup) very cold butter, cubed, plus extra, softened, for greasing
- 1½ tbsp caster (superfine) sugar
- 1 large egg, beaten

For the fillings
- Any flavour jam
- Lemon curd

TIPS

If the pastry dough is quite firm after being chilled in the fridge, leaving it out at room temperature ahead of time is definitely advised. Simply remove it from the fridge and place it to one side until you're able to easily roll it out.

If you have a shallow cupcake tray (rather than a conventional, deeper one) then this recipe presents a perfect opportunity to put it to good use!

Though tempting, please don't overfill your tarts with jam or curd! When spooning it in, you might feel like you haven't added enough; however, adding too much will cause it to bubble up and overflow out of the pastry cases when baked, leaving you with very little left. There's a moral to be learned from that, I'm sure!

In a large bowl, mix together the flour and xanthan gum. Make sure the butter is really cold; if not, put it in the fridge or freezer until nicely chilled. Add the cubes to the bowl and mix them into the flour. Using your fingertips, rub the butter into the flour to form a breadcrumb-like consistency. Make sure your hands are cool, as we want to avoid the butter getting warm! (You can also achieve the same result by using a food processor to blitz the ingredients together.)

Next, stir in the sugar, then add in the beaten egg. Use a knife to carefully cut it into the mixture until it comes together. It should form a ball and not be crumbly; it will be a little sticky to touch but not unmanageable. Wrap in cling film (plastic wrap) and leave to chill in the fridge for around 1 hour before using.

Preheat the oven 180°C fan/200°C (400°F). Lightly grease a 12-hole cupcake tray.

If the chilled pastry dough is quite firm, remove it from the fridge and place to one side to soften (see **TIPS**, left).

Remember not to excessively handle the dough from this point onwards as this will warm it up and make it stickier.

On a sheet of non-stick baking parchment, roll out the dough to a large rectangle around 3mm (⅛in) thick. Use a round or fluted biscuit (cookie) cutter about 8cm (3¼in) in diameter to cut out 12 circles for the base of the tarts. Carefully ease them into the holes of the greased cupcake tray, pressing them in gently.

Spoon around 2 teaspoons of either jam or lemon curd into each hole and, optionally, use any spare pastry to cut out mini heart shapes to place on top of the jam or curd.

Bake in the oven for 12–15 minutes until the pastry is slightly golden. Allow to cool in the tin before removing.

You might have a small amount of pastry left over which could make 3–4 extra jam tarts. Just allow the tin to cool before using again.

LEMON DRIZZLE TRAYBAKE

Serves 12–16
Prep 15 mins
Oven 55 mins

LL **F** **V**

DF Use a (hard) dairy-free alternative to butter.

❄ See freezing and defrosting guidance for sponge cakes on page 28.

This classic cake is super-versatile, budget-friendly, easily serves a crowd and works for absolutely any occasion. Yet even ignoring all that, with a golden cake crumb that's extra zesty thanks to the drizzle, topped with a sweet and sharp glacé icing (frosting), you don't really even need any extra reasons to make this!

For the sponge
- 400g (1¾ cups) butter, softened
- 350g (1¾ cups) caster (superfine) sugar
- Grated zest of 4 lemons and 2 tsp juice
- 6 medium eggs
- 395g (2⅔ cups) gluten-free self-raising flour
- ¼ tsp xanthan gum

For the drizzle
- 175g (scant ¾ cup) granulated sugar
- Juice of 2 lemons (use the lemons from the zest in the cake)

For the icing (frosting)
- 100g (scant ¾ cup) icing (confectioners') sugar
- 2–3 tsp lemon juice
- Grated lemon zest, to finish

Preheat your oven to 160°C fan/180°C (350°F). Line a 23 x 33cm (9 x 13in) rectangular baking tin with non-stick baking parchment.

In a large bowl, cream together the butter and sugar until light and fluffy (I prefer to use an electric hand mixer for this). Add the lemon zest and juice, then beat once more. Crack in the eggs, one at a time, mixing in between each one until well combined. Don't worry if it curdles a little; once the flour is added it will all come together. Sift in your flour and xanthan gum and fold it in.

Spoon the mixture into your prepared tin and bake for 50–55 minutes until golden. If the cake is browning too much on top, cover with foil (shiny side up) for the final 5–10 minutes. Check that it's cooked by sticking a skewer into the centre – if it comes out clean, it's done.

Meanwhile, for the drizzle, grab a small bowl. Add the sugar and lemon juice and mix until well combined.

When the cake is out of the oven and still hot, use a skewer to poke lots of holes all over the top, then gradually pour over all of the drizzle. Allow to cool in the tin for a good 20–30 minutes before carefully lifting onto a wire rack to finish cooling.

For the icing, add the icing sugar and lemon juice to a medium bowl and mix until it reaches a smooth, slightly thick, yet still pourable consistency. Once the cake has fully cooled, drizzle the icing all over the top of the cake, then sprinkle on a little lemon zest and slice into squares.

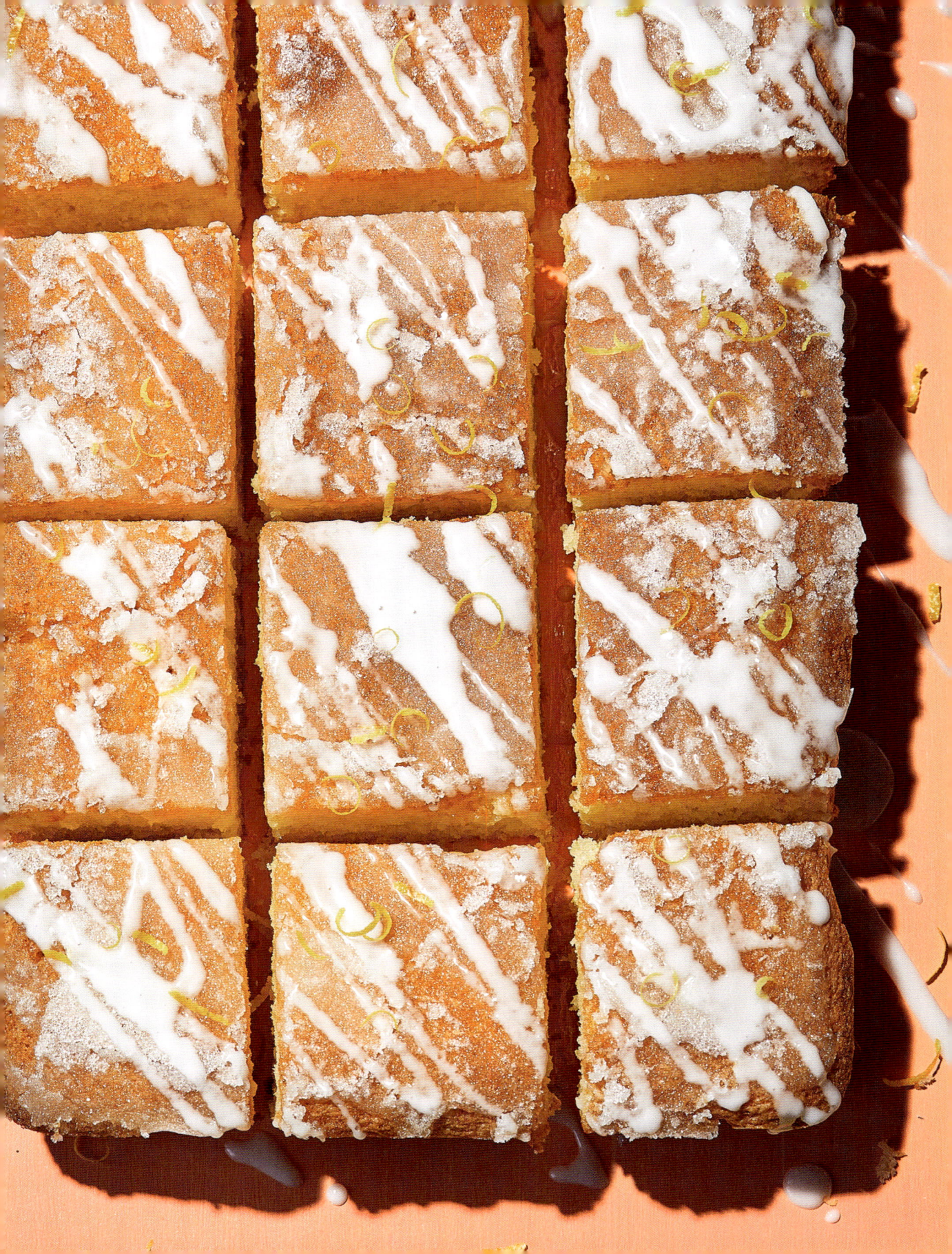

CHOCOLATE BANANA BREAD

Serves 8–10

Prep 20 mins

Oven 60 mins or
Air Fryer 50 mins

V

DF

Use a (hard) dairy-free alternative to butter, dairy-free chocolate chips and dairy-free dark chocolate. Use dairy-free milk, if needed.

LL

Use lactose-free chocolate chips and lactose-free dark chocolate. Use lactose-free milk, if needed.

❄

See freezing and defrosting guidance for sponge cakes on page 28.

Letting those overripe bananas go to waste wouldn't be anything less than a crime while this recipe exists: they're exactly what you need for the ultimate, indulgent banana bread loaf. With a velvety smooth chocolate frosting and fluffy banana bread loaded with chocolate chips, this is a loaf that all will love.

For the cake
- 115g (½ cup) butter, softened
- 115g (½ cup plus 1¼ tbsp) light brown sugar
- 2 medium eggs, beaten
- 400–500g (14–17oz) ripe bananas, mashed (peeled weight; about 4 bananas)

- 210g (1½ cups) gluten-free plain (all-purpose) flour
- 40g (½ cup minus 1½ tbsp) unsweetened cocoa powder, sifted
- ¼ tsp xanthan gum
- 1 tsp bicarbonate of soda (baking soda)
- 150g (5½oz) chocolate chips, plus an extra handful to finish (optional)

For the frosting
- 55g (2oz) dark (bittersweet) or milk chocolate
- 125g (generous ½ cup) butter, softened
- 90g (⅔ cup) icing (confectioners') sugar
- 25g (¼ cup) unsweetened cocoa powder

To make this in the oven, preheat the oven to 160°C fan/180°C (350°F). Line a 900g (2lb) loaf tin (pan) with non-stick baking parchment.

In a large bowl, cream together the butter and sugar until light and fluffy (I prefer to use an electric hand mixer for this). Add the beaten eggs and mashed banana and mix until well combined.

Sift in the flour, cocoa powder, xanthan gum and bicarbonate of soda and mix briefly until no dry flour can be seen. Lastly, add the chocolate chips, if using, and mix once more.

Spoon the mixture into the prepared tin and bake in the oven for about 1 hour. Check that it's cooked by sticking a skewer into the centre – if it comes out clean, then it's done. Allow to cool in the tin briefly, then carefully lift onto a wire rack to cool.

To make this in an air fryer, heat or preheat the air fryer to 150°C (300°F). Make and spoon the mixture into the prepared tin as opposite and air fry for 40–50 minutes – check with a skewer as opposite to ensure it's done.

Meanwhile, to make the frosting, melt the chocolate (I do this in the microwave, stirring between short bursts until melted), then allow to cool slightly.

Place the butter in a large bowl and mix for 5 minutes with an electric hand mixer until the butter is fluffy and pale. Add the icing sugar and start mixing slowly to avoid creating a mini icing sugar explosion, but then increase the speed as it starts to combine. Sift in the cocoa powder then mix again.

Add the slightly cooled, melted chocolate to the bowl and mix until fully incorporated. If it seems too thick, add a teaspoon of milk to loosen it up.

Spread over the top of the cooled banana cake and finish with extra chocolate chips, if you like.

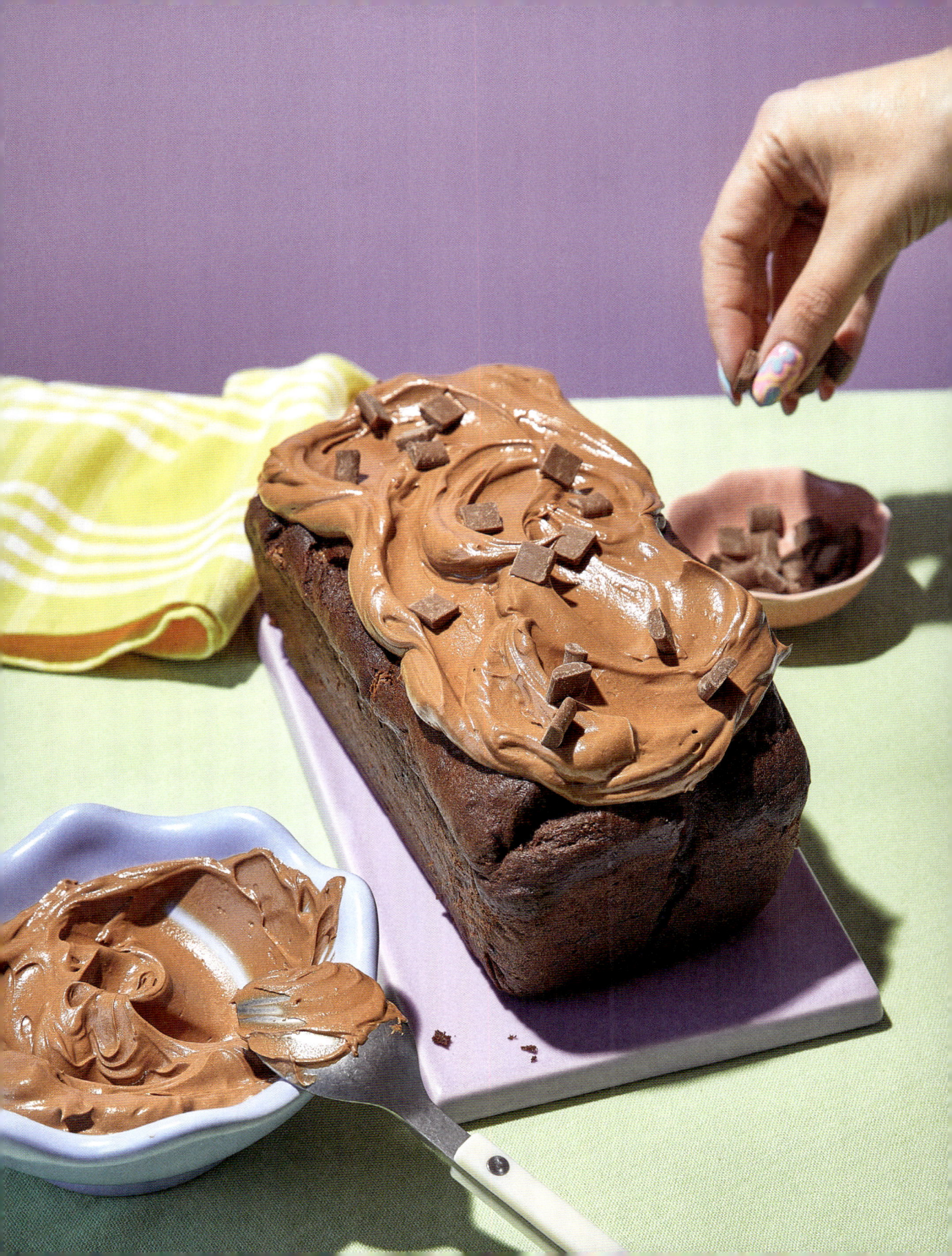

VANILLA RAINBOW CUPCAKES

Makes 12–16

Prep 20 mins

Oven 22 mins or
Air Fryer 15 mins

Nothing says 'it's party time' quite like a batch of these rainbow cupcakes! The rainbow colours are actually super simple to achieve: just ensure you have enough bowls handy. These go down so well at parties that, quite often, you'll find you won't even need the whole 'one big cake' as a centrepiece.

V

DF Use a (hard) dairy-free alternative to butter and dairy-free milk, if needed.

LL Use lactose-free milk, if needed.

F See low lactose advice.

❄ Once cooked, cooled and iced, freeze on a tray for 1–2 hours. When the buttercream is solid, transfer to airtight containers and freeze for up to 3 months. Defrost at room temperature.

- 225g (1 cup) butter, softened
- 225g (1 cup plus 2 tbsp) caster (superfine) sugar
- 225g (1¾ cups) gluten-free self-raising flour
- 4 eggs
- 1 tsp vanilla extract

- 1 tsp gluten-free baking powder
- ¼ tsp xanthan gum
- 4–5 different colours of concentrated food colouring gels

For the buttercream
- 200g (generous ¾ cup) butter, softened
- 400g (2¾ cups) icing (confectioners') sugar
- 1 tsp vanilla extract
- 1–2 tsp milk (if needed)
- Colourful gluten-free sweets and sprinkles

TIP

Though the method instructs you to make 12 cupcakes, depending on the size of your cupcake cases, you might end up with leftover batter. If that's the case, once all 12 cupcake cases are filled, simply use the remaining batter to fill additional cupcake cases. Bake these using a second cupcake tray in the oven (placed in at the same time as the main batch on a separate shelf) or in the air fryer after the first 12 cupcakes are done.

To make these in the oven, preheat the oven to 160°C fan/180°C (350°F). Line a 12-hole cupcake tray with cupcake cases. I like to sprinkle a few grains of uncooked rice beneath each case as it helps to absorb unwanted moisture.

In a large bowl, cream together the butter and sugar until light and fluffy (I prefer to use an electric hand mixer for this). Add the flour, eggs, vanilla, baking powder and xanthan gum and mix until well combined.

Separate the mixture into 4–5 separate bowls and add a tiny amount of food colouring to each bowl. Mix through carefully but thoroughly so you don't have any bits of vanilla mixture visible.

Spoon small amounts of each coloured mixture, one at a time, into each cupcake case, carefully spreading out the different colours if need be. Do this evenly between all the cupcake cases, then bake in the oven for around 22 minutes until fully cooked. Check that they're cooked by sticking a skewer into the centre of a cupcake – if it comes out clean, then they're done.

To make these in an air fryer, heat or preheat the air fryer to 160°C (320°F). Line two 6-hole silicone cupcake trays with cupcake cases. Make the cupcake batter and fill the cases as opposite, then air fry for 12–15 minutes.

Allow to cool in the cupcake tray for a couple of minutes before transferring to a wire rack to cool completely.

Meanwhile, to make the buttercream, mix the butter in a stand mixer on a medium speed or in a large bowl with an electric hand mixer for about 5 minutes or until pale. Add the icing sugar in 2 stages, beating for about 3 minutes between each addition. Add the vanilla and mix once more – it should be a perfect pipeable consistency. If it's too thick, add a small amount of milk; if it's too thin, add a little extra icing sugar.

Spoon the buttercream into a piping (pastry) bag with a large star nozzle attached, then pipe the buttercream on top. If you don't want to pipe it, you can always just spoon it on top! Finish with some colourful gluten-free sweets (candy) and sprinkles.

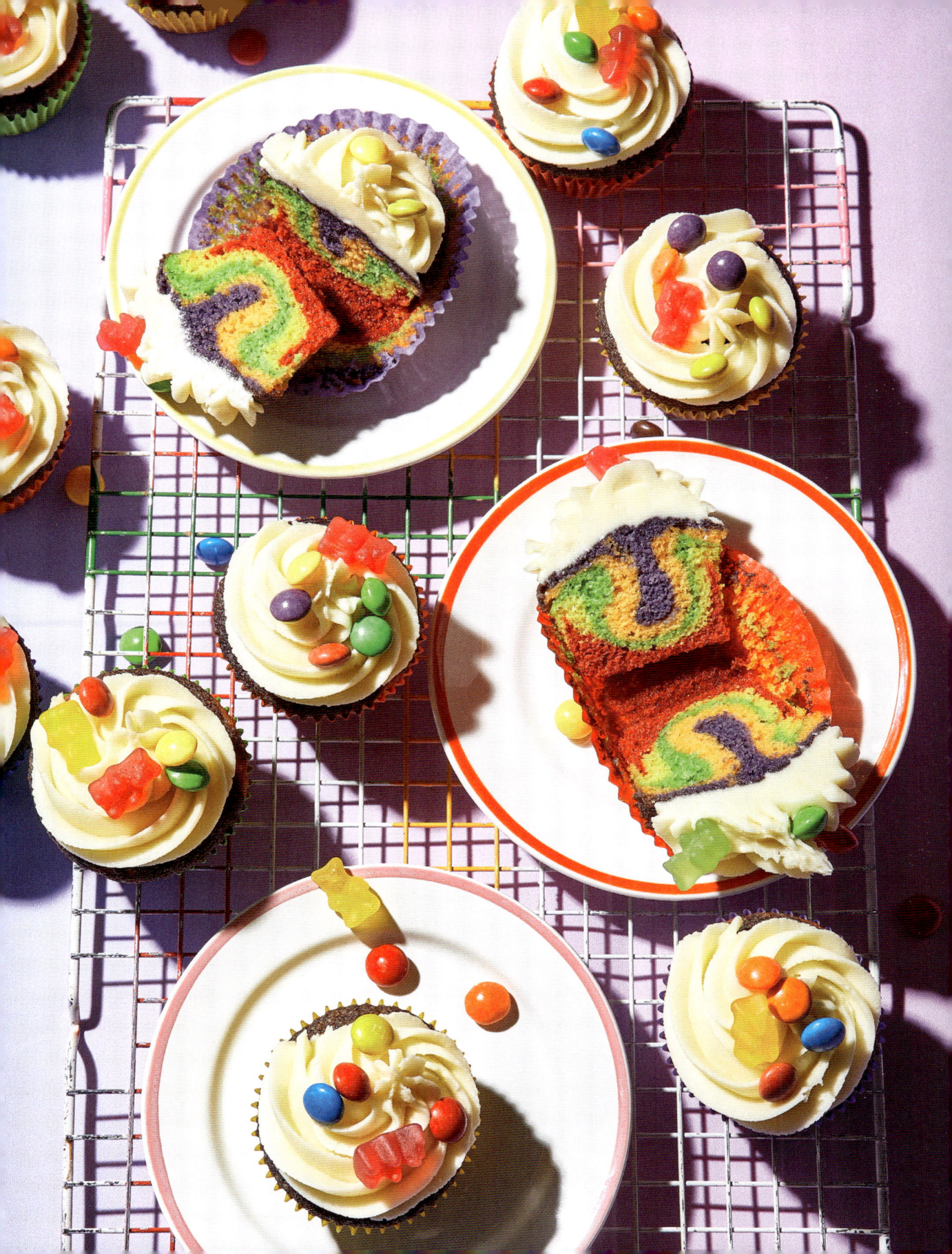

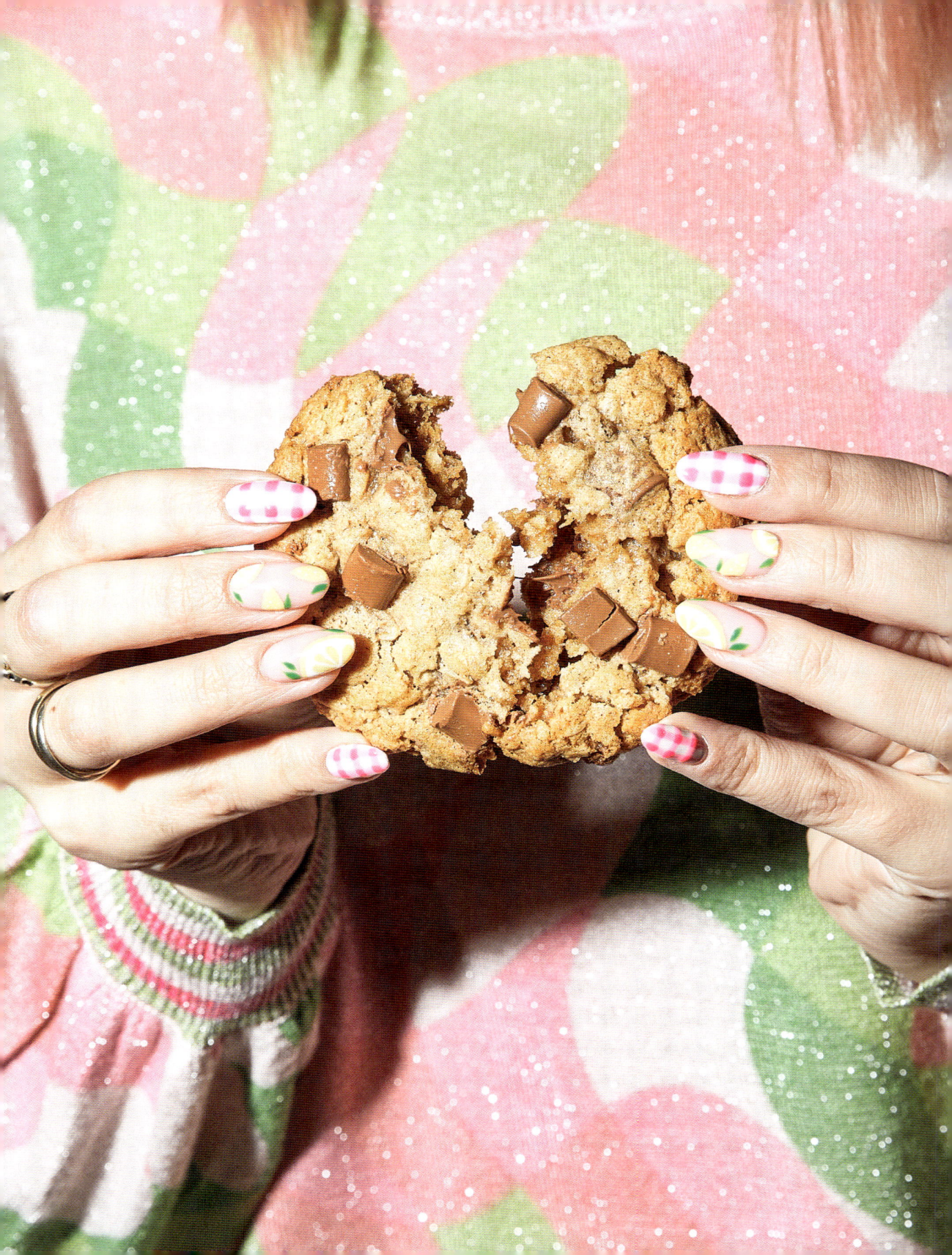

OAT + RAISIN
OR OAT + CHOC CHIP
COOKIES

It wasn't until I couldn't eat these anymore that I realized how much I'd missed them. While in the past I'd always go for a classic chocolate chip cookie, I can no longer deny how great the addition of oats (along with either raisins or chocolate chips) is to these soft, bakery-style cookies. Give them a try and tell me I'm wrong!

Makes 12

Prep 10 mins + 20 mins chilling

Oven 12 mins or
Air Fryer 12 mins

- 125g (½ cup plus 1 tbsp) butter, softened
- 150g (¾ cup) light brown sugar
- 1 medium egg

- 1 tsp vanilla extract
- 150g (1 cup plus 2 tbsp) gluten-free self-raising flour
- ½ tsp bicarbonate of soda (baking soda)

- 1 tsp ground mixed spice or ground cinnamon
- 150g (1½ cups) gluten-free oats
- 100g (3½oz) raisins or chocolate chips

V

DF Use a (hard) dairy-free alternative to butter and dairy-free chocolate chips, if using.

LL Use lactose-free chocolate chips, if using.

F See low lactose advice. If making raisin cookies, one cookie is a safe low FODMAP serving size.

❄ See freezing and defrosting guidance for biscuits and cookies on page 28.

TIP

Once the cookie dough is rolled into balls, you can freeze them for another day and bake them straight from frozen. Simply bake the frozen cookie dough balls in the oven or air fry for an extra 2–4 minutes on top of the timings given in the method.

In a large bowl, cream together the butter and sugar until light and fluffy (I prefer to use an electric hand mixer for this). Crack in the egg and add the vanilla, then mix in.

Add the flour, bicarbonate of soda and mixed spice or cinnamon, mix well, then add the oats and mix once more. Finally, stir in the raisins or chocolate chips.

Using your hands, roll the cookie dough into balls that weigh around 60g (2¼oz) each and place into the freezer for around 20 minutes or in the fridge for around an hour, to firm up. This step is important as it prevents them from spreading too much in the oven while baking.

To make these in the oven, preheat the oven to 180°C fan/200°C (400°F). Line 2 large baking trays with non-stick baking parchment.

Place the chilled cookie balls on the lined baking trays, leaving plenty of space for them to spread in the oven. Bake for 11–12 minutes until lightly golden; they should still be soft at this stage and they will firm up as they cool.

Allow to cool for 10 minutes on the trays before transferring to a wire rack to cool completely.

To make these in an air fryer, heat or preheat the air fryer to 160°C (320°F). Make the cookies as opposite and, once chilled, place the cookie balls on individual 12cm (4¾in) squares of baking parchment. Air fry for 10–12 minutes until lightly golden.

Allow to cool for 5 minutes with the air fryer drawer open before moving them to a wire rack to cool completely.

FRUIT TEA LOAF

Sometimes only a proper classic will do and that's exactly what my fruit tea loaf is. With slices of tea-infused, moist, cinnamon-tinged sponge packed with sweet and softened dried fruit, this budget bake is surprisingly quick to throw together and will disappear just as fast!

Serves 8–10

Prep 15 mins + 1 hour soaking

Oven 1 hour 10 mins or
Air Fryer 50 mins

DF **LF** **V**

❄ See freezing and defrosting guidance for sponge cakes on page 28.

- 3 tea bags
- 175ml (¾ cup) boiling water
- 225g (8oz) mixed sultanas, raisins, prunes, dates, apricots (larger fruit chopped)
- 200g (1½ cups) gluten-free plain (all-purpose) flour
- 2 tsp gluten-free baking powder
- ¼ tsp xanthan gum
- 1 tsp ground cinnamon
- 110g (½ cup plus 2½ tbsp) light brown sugar
- 2 medium eggs
- 3½ tbsp vegetable oil

Put the tea bags in a jug (pitcher) and pour the boiling water over them. Allow to brew for 5 minutes or so before adding the mixed dried fruit to the jug too – leave the tea bags in at this stage. Ensure the fruit is fully submerged, and leave to soak for a minimum of 1 hour.

To make this in the oven, preheat the oven to 160°C fan/180°C (350°F). Line a 900g (2lb) loaf tin (pan) with non-stick baking parchment.

Add the flour, baking powder, xanthan gum, cinnamon and sugar to a large bowl and mix. Add the eggs and oil and mix to combine, then tip in the dried fruit and remaining tea, but remove the tea bags. Mix together to fully combine (all of this can be done with a spatula).

Spoon the mixture into the prepared tin and bake in the oven for about 70 minutes until well risen, golden and cooked through. Check that it's cooked by sticking a skewer into the centre – if it comes out clean, then it's done.

To make this in an air fryer, heat or preheat the air fryer to 150°C (300°F). Make and spoon the mixture into the prepared tin as opposite and air fry for 40–50 minutes – check with a skewer as above to ensure it's done.

Allow to cool in the tin for about 20 minutes then carefully lift onto a wire rack to finish cooling.

Slice and enjoy warm or cold spread with butter.

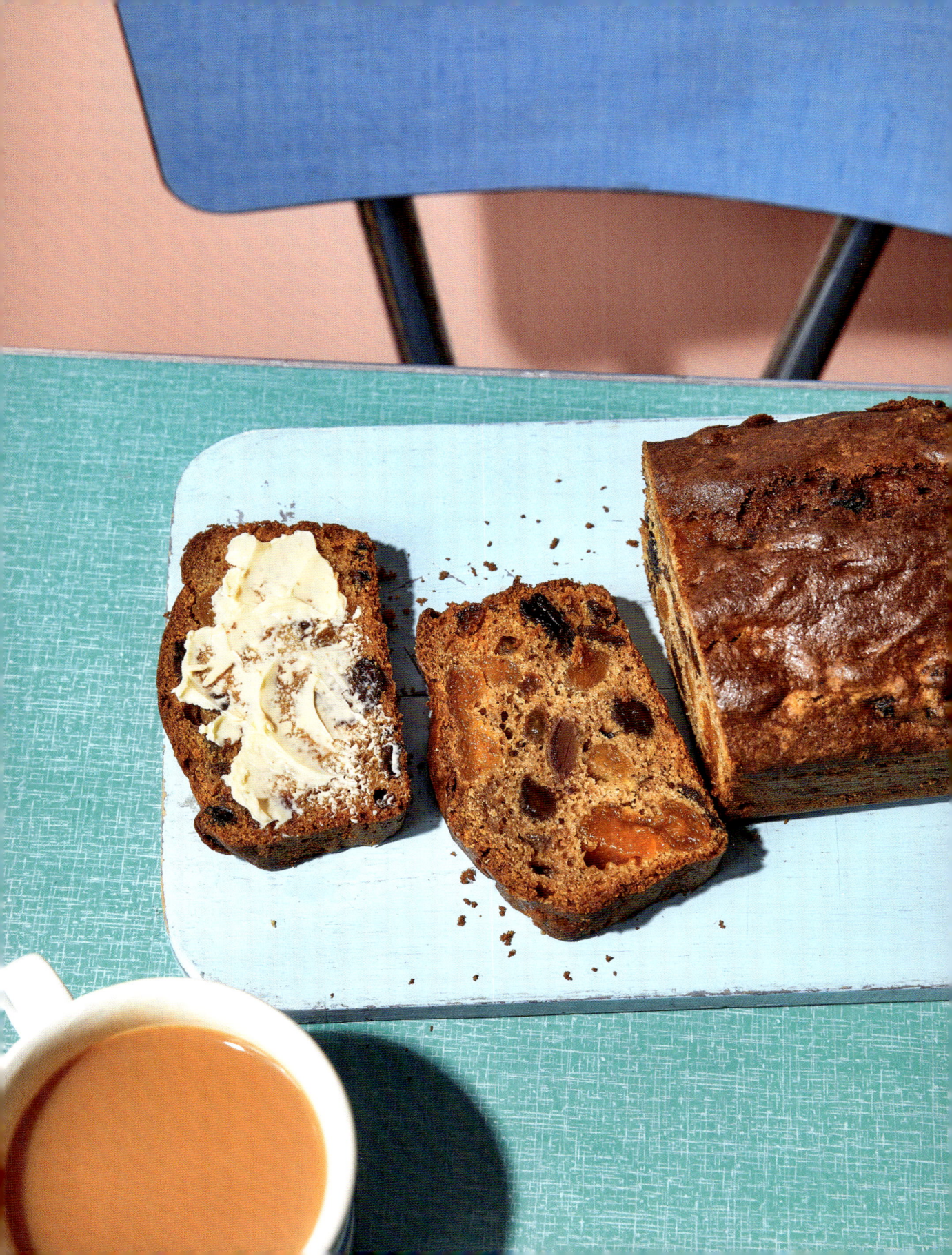

PARTY RINGS

Though I've had a party rings recipe on the blog for a decade, this is an improved version using my foolproof vanilla biscuit recipe. What's best about it is that the dough doesn't spread in the oven – that I can guarantee! Whether it's been 10 minutes or 10 years since you last ate one of these, my gluten-free party rings will never fail to put a smile on your face.

Makes about 15
Prep 25 mins + setting
Oven 10 mins or
Air Fryer 10 mins

LL **F** **V**

DF Use a (hard) dairy-free alternative to butter.

❄ See freezing and defrosting guidance for biscuits and cookies on page 28. Ideally freeze the biscuits without icing for the best results, then make the icing once defrosted.

- 100g (½ cup minus 1 tbsp) butter, softened
- 100g (½ cup) caster (superfine) sugar
- 1 large egg, beaten
- 1½ tsp vanilla extract

- 270g (2 cups) gluten-free plain (all-purpose) flour, plus extra for dusting
- ½ tsp xanthan gum

For the icing (frosting)
- 300g (generous 2 cups) icing (confectioners') sugar
- Concentrated food colouring gels

To make these in the oven, preheat the oven to 170°C fan/190°C (375°F). Line a large baking tray with non-stick baking parchment.

In a large bowl, cream together the butter and sugar until light and fluffy (I prefer to use an electric hand mixer for this). Add the beaten egg and vanilla and briefly mix in. Add the flour and xanthan gum and mix until all the flour is combined and it starts to come together as a dough.

Lightly flour a large sheet of non-stick baking parchment (and a rolling pin) and roll out the dough to a 6mm (¼in) thickness. Cut out circles using a 7cm (2¾in) cookie cutter then cut out a hole in the middle of the dough using a smaller 1–2cm (½–¾in) cookie cutter (or a rounded piping/pastry nozzle).

Transfer the circles to the lined tray, ideally using a small palette knife, then bake in the oven for 8–10 minutes until the edges are very, very slightly golden. Allow to cool briefly on the tray before transferring to a wire rack to cool completely.

To make these in an air fryer, heat or preheat the air fryer to 160°C (320°F). Make and cut out the biscuit dough as above and place onto individual 10cm (4in) squares of baking parchment. Air fry for 8–10 minutes until the edges are very, very slightly golden. Allow to cool briefly before lifting out of the air fryer using the baking parchment and transferring to a wire rack to cool completely.

For the icing, place the icing sugar in a small bowl and add water gradually until you have a thick, smooth, spreadable icing. You basically want it thick enough so that it won't drip off the biscuits, but not too thick!

Spoon the icing into a few separate bowls and add a tiny amount of different concentrated food colouring to each bowl. Steal a small amount of the different-coloured icings and spoon them into separate piping (pastry) bags fitted with very small round nozzles (or no nozzle at all – just snip off the end – or alternatively skip the piping bags and use a spoon to carefully drizzle).

Using the icing in the bowls, either spread one colour onto each cooled biscuit or dip the biscuits into them.

Pipe or drizzle thin lines of a contrasting colour icing on top of the biscuits and then, using a clean cocktail stick, pull through the lines to create a feathered pattern (switch up the colours so you have different colour combinations across the biscuits). Leave to fully set.

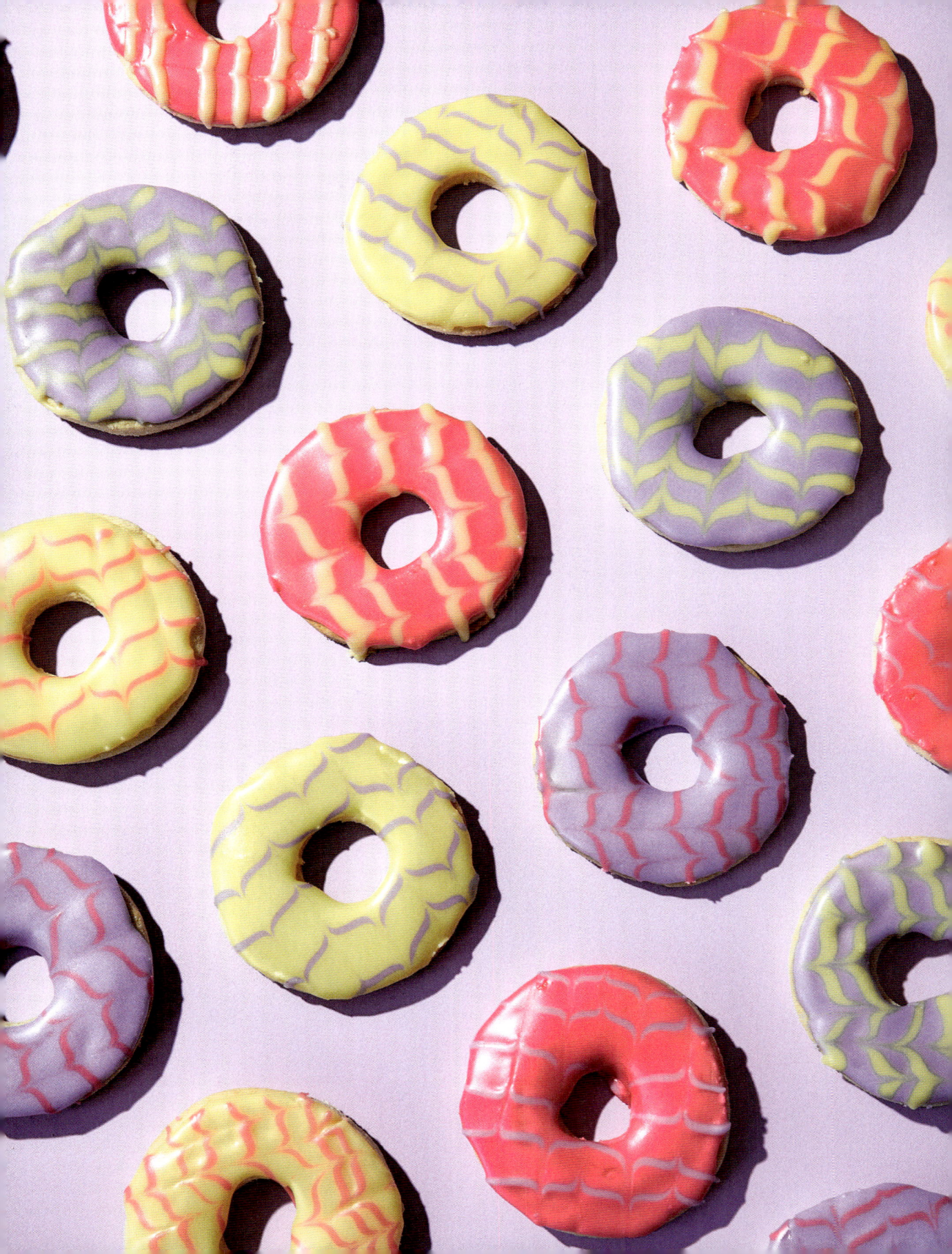

GOLDEN SYRUP PUDDING CAKE

This absolute classic is one of Mark and his dad Steve's favourite desserts, so I end up making this quite often! Fortunately, the ingredients are all mostly super-simple store-cupboard essentials, so there's certainly no need to break the bank for this one. Clearly it can be enjoyed and loved by all ages, so pour on the custard and serve this one up for dessert next!

Serves 9
Prep 5 mins
Oven 50 mins

V

DF Use a (hard) dairy-free alternative to butter and dairy-free milk.

LL Use lactose-free milk.

❄ See freezing and defrosting guidance for sponge cakes on page 28.

- 115g (½ cup) butter
- 115g (½ cup plus 1¼ tbsp) light brown sugar
- 225ml (scant 1 cup) golden syrup, plus 3 tbsp to finish
- 225g (1¾ cups) gluten-free self-raising flour, sifted
- ¼ tsp xanthan gum
- 1 large egg
- 150ml (⅝ cup) milk

Preheat the oven to 140°C fan/ 160°C (320°F). Lightly butter a 23cm (9in) square baking tin (pan) or ovenproof dish.

Put the butter, sugar and golden syrup in a medium pan and melt over a low heat, stirring occasionally. Pour it into a large bowl and leave to cool briefly.

Add the flour and xanthan gum to the bowl and mix to fully combine using an electric hand mixer. Beat together the egg and milk in a jug (pitcher), then gradually pour it in, mixing as you do until you have a smooth mixture.

Pour the mixture into the prepared baking tin and bake in the oven for 45–50 minutes until golden and cooked through.

Remove from the oven and, after a few minutes, prick the top all over and drizzle on the extra golden syrup, using a hot spoon so it drizzles fairly evenly.

Allow to cool and enjoy as a cake, in slices, or serve the ultimate way: hot with custard!

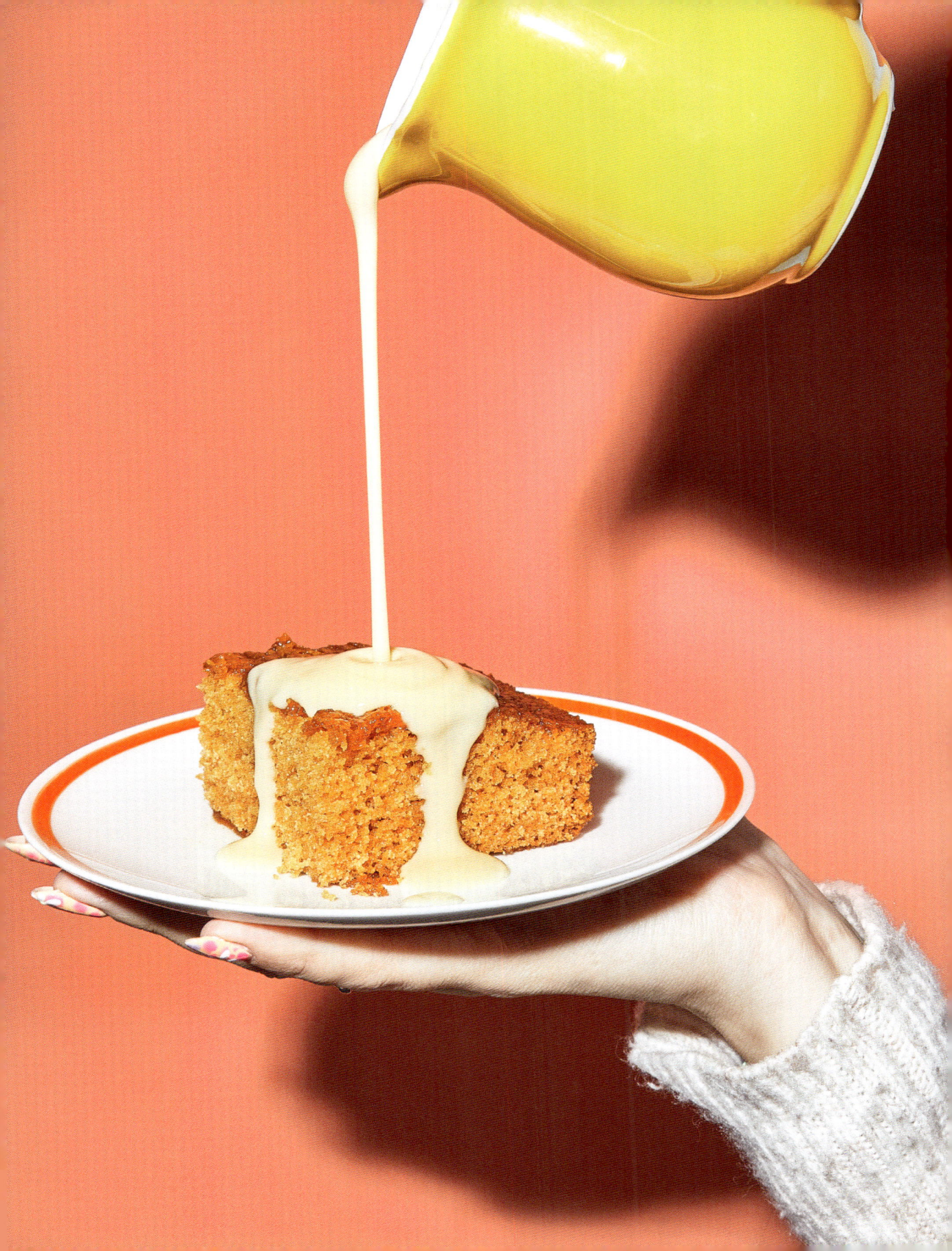

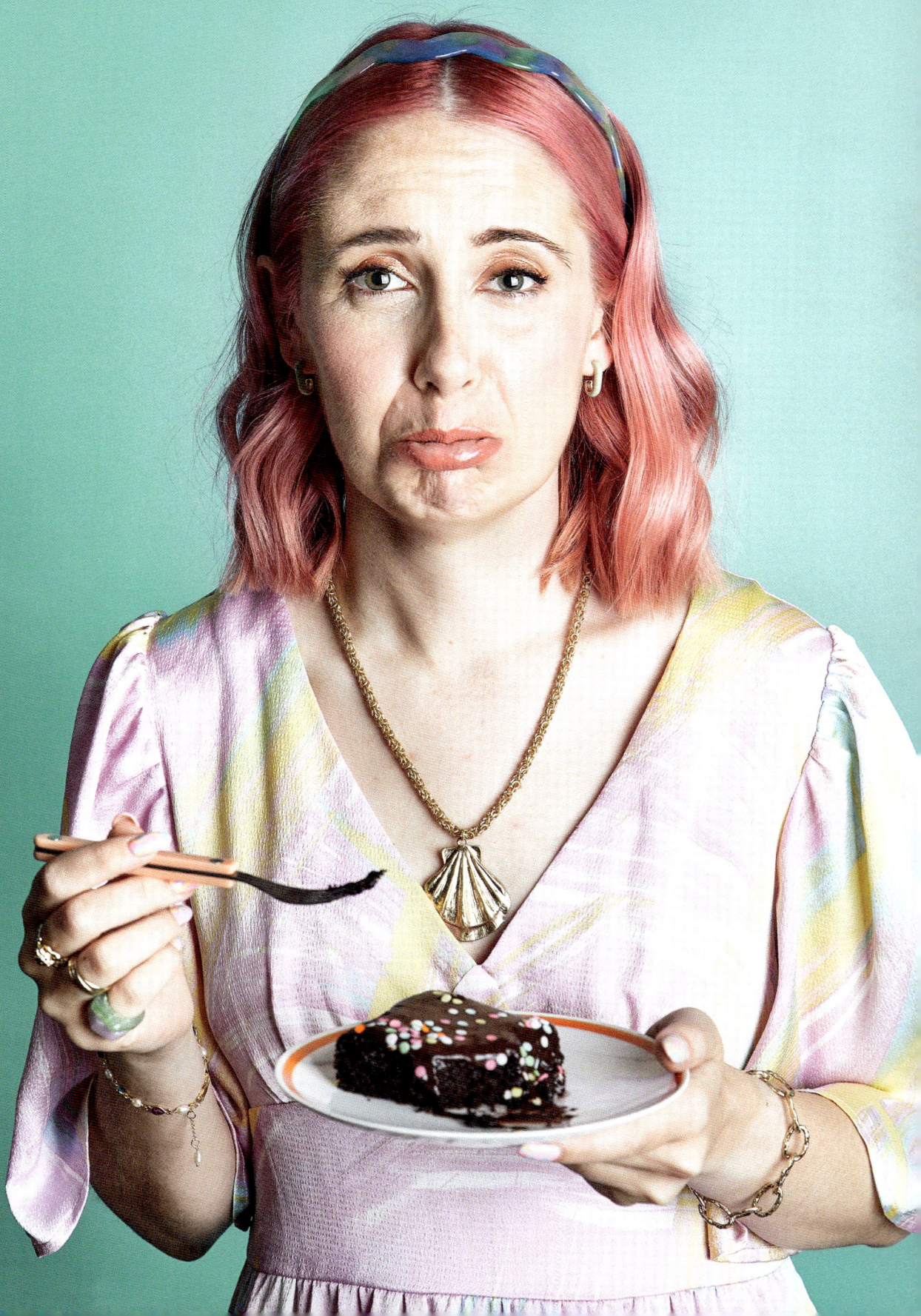

CHOCOLATE DEPRESSION CAKE

Named not because it'll make you depressed, but because it's the style of sponge cake made during the Great Depression. It contains no milk, butter or eggs because these ingredients were hard to obtain; and even when using gluten-free flour, it remains extremely budget-friendly. Don't think that all of the above makes this infinitely moist and chocolatey cake with a chocolate glacé icing any less appealing, though – there's a reason it's still being made today!

DF LF F V VE

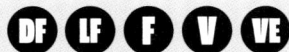

❄ See freezing and defrosting guidance for sponge cakes on page 28.

- 180g (1⅓ cups) gluten-free plain (all-purpose) flour
- 200g (1 cup) caster (superfine) sugar
- 1 tsp bicarbonate of soda (baking soda)
- ½ tsp salt
- ¼ tsp xanthan gum

- 30g (⅓ cup) unsweetened cocoa powder
- 80ml (⅓ cup) vegetable oil
- 250ml (1 cup) water
- 1 tsp vanilla extract
- 1 tbsp gluten-free vinegar

For the icing (frosting)
- 170g (1¼ cups) icing (confectioners') sugar
- 25g (¼ cup) unsweetened cocoa powder
- 50ml (3½ tbsp) water
- 1 tsp vanilla extract
- 3 tbsp gluten-free sprinkles

Preheat the oven to 160°C fan/180°C (350°F). Line a 23cm (9in) square baking tin (pan) with non-stick baking parchment.

Add the flour, sugar, bicarb, salt, xanthan gum and cocoa powder to a large bowl and mix.

Pour in the oil, water, vanilla and vinegar and mix to combine to form a smooth batter.

Pour into the prepared tin and bake for about 30 minutes. Check that it's cooked by sticking a skewer into the centre – if it comes out clean, then it's done. Allow to cool in the tin before lifting it out using the parchment.

For the icing, mix together the icing sugar, cocoa powder, water and vanilla until smooth and glossy. Spread all over the cooled cake and then top with the colourful sprinkles. Slice into 9 squares to serve.

BAKERY-STYLE 50:50 COOKIES

When you can't decide between a classic choc chip cookie or a double chocolate cookie, why even bother coming to a conclusion when you can just have both in one cookie? And that's exactly what these are: a golden choc chip cookie on one side and a chocolate cookie on the other. And yes, they taste every bit as good as they look!

Makes about 18

Prep 20 mins + 1 hour chilling

Oven 12 mins or
Air Fryer 12 mins

V

DF Use a (hard) dairy-free alternative to butter and use dairy-free chocolate chips.

LL Use lactose-free chocolate chips.

F Use lactose-free chocolate chips.

❄ See freezing and defrosting guidance for biscuits and cookies on page 28.

TIPS

If you are wondering how to halve an egg, it's simple: crack an egg into a dish, beat it so that it's all combined, weigh it and pour half into another dish!

See the tip on page 221 for advice on freezing the cookie dough balls and baking/air frying from frozen.

For the chocolate chip cookie dough

- 60g (¼ cup) butter, softened
- 50g (¼ cup) caster (superfine) sugar
- 50g (¼ cup) light brown sugar
- ½ medium egg, beaten
- ½ tsp vanilla extract
- 125g (1 cup minus 1 tbsp) gluten-free self-raising flour
- ¼ tsp bicarbonate of soda (baking soda)
- 80g (3oz) milk chocolate chips

For the double chocolate chip cookie dough

- 60g (¼ cup) butter, softened
- 50g (¼ cup) caster (superfine) sugar
- 50g (¼ cup) light brown sugar
- ½ medium egg, beaten
- ½ tsp vanilla extract
- 100g (¾ cup) gluten-free self-raising flour
- 25g (¼ cup) unsweetened cocoa powder
- ¼ tsp bicarbonate of soda (baking soda)
- 80g (3oz) white chocolate chips

For the chocolate chip cookie dough, in a large mixing bowl, cream together the butter and sugars until light and fluffy. Then add in the half egg (see **TIP** below) and the vanilla, and mix until combined. Add in the flour and bicarbonate of soda, mixing well to ensure there are no pockets of flour, then mix in the chocolate chips, reserving a small handful for the tops.

Do the same for the double chocolate chip cookie dough (this time adding cocoa powder with the flour), then cover both doughs and chill in the fridge for about 1–2 hours.

To make these in the oven, towards the end of the chilling process, preheat the oven to 180°C fan/200°C (400°F). Line 2 large baking trays with non-stick baking parchment.

Take the chilled doughs out of the fridge. Take 20g (¾oz) of each dough and roll them together so you have a 40g (1½oz) cookie dough ball that looks half and half. Repeat until you've used up all the dough. Press the reserved chocolate chips into the tops of the cookie dough balls so they're more visible once baked.

Place the balls on the prepared baking trays, leaving plenty of space between them to allow for spreading. Bake for 11–12 minutes until slightly golden; they should still be soft at this stage and they will firm up as they cool. Allow to cool for 10 minutes on the tray before transferring them to a wire rack to cool completely.

To make these in an air fryer, heat or preheat the air fryer to 160°C (320°F). Make the cookies as opposite and, once chilled and rolled into balls, place them onto individual 12cm (4¾in) squares of baking parchment. Air fry for 10–12 minutes until slightly golden. Allow to cool for 5 minutes with the air fryer drawer open before transferring them to a wire rack to cool completely.

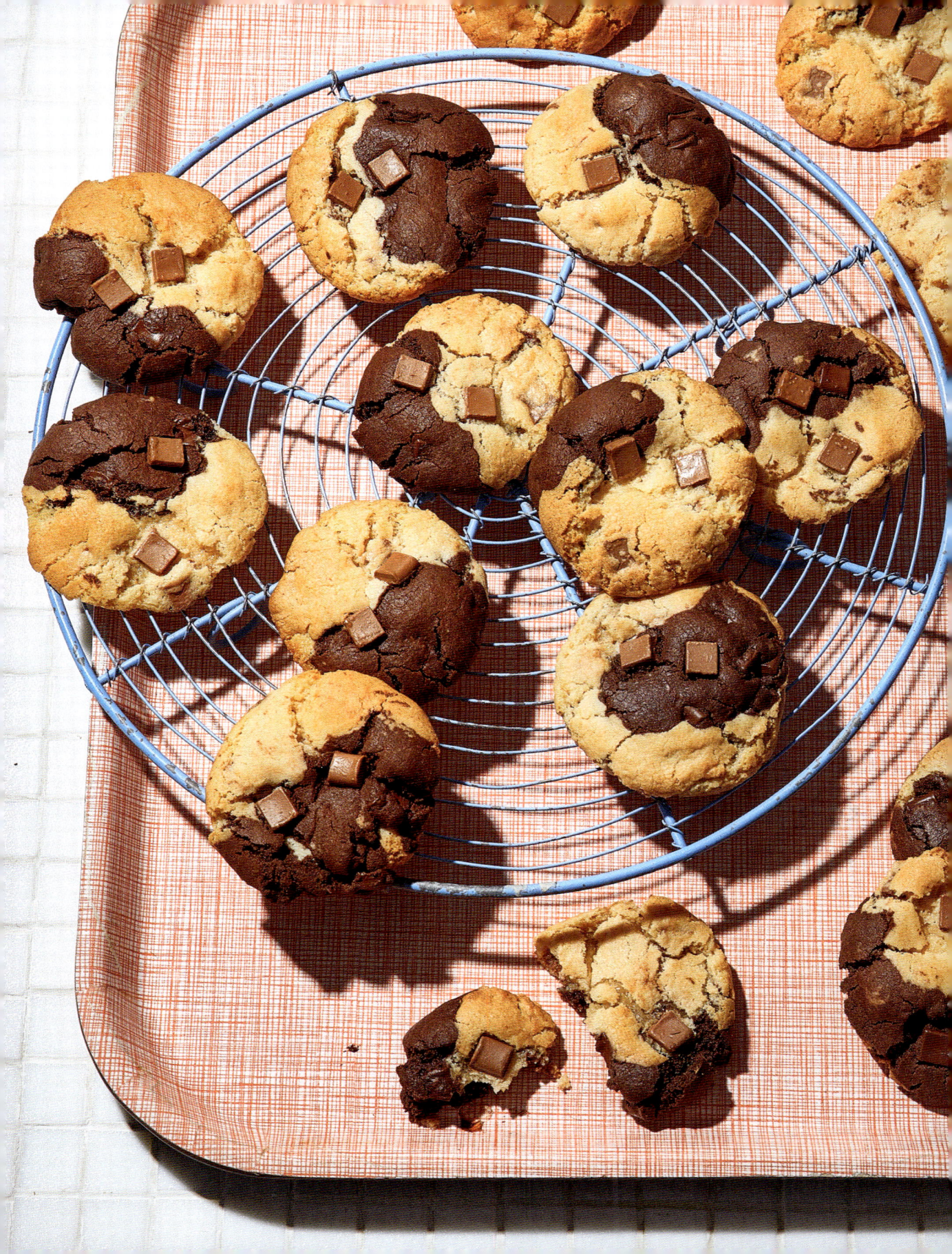

30-MINUTE PEACH ALMONDINE

This is one of my favourite quick, easy and super-simple desserts to throw together at short notice as there's a very good chance that I already have everything I need in the cupboard! Using canned peach slices is a convenient and cost-effective way of transforming this super-moist Bakewell-like sponge into a dessert to remember.

Serves 8

Prep 5 mins

Oven 30 mins or
Air Fryer 30 mins

LL **V**

DF Use a (hard) dairy-free alternative to butter.

❄ See freezing and defrosting guidance for sponge cakes on page 28.

TIP
Feel free to try this recipe with other canned fruit too – canned pear halves work especially well.

- 130g (½ cup plus 1 tbsp) butter, softened, plus extra for greasing
- 130g (⅔ cup) caster (superfine) sugar
- 130g (1⅓ cups) ground almonds
- 1½ tsp gluten-free plain (all-purpose) flour or cornflour (cornstarch)
- 1 tsp vanilla or almond extract
- 1 large egg
- 1 x 125g (4½oz) can of peach slices in juice (or use half a larger can)
- Handful of flaked (slivered) almonds
- 1 tbsp icing (confectioners') sugar, for dusting

To make this in the oven, preheat the oven to 160°C fan/180°C (350°F). Lightly grease a round (not loose-bottomed) 20cm (8in) baking tin (pan) or ovenproof dish with butter.

In a large bowl, cream together the butter and sugar until light and fluffy (I prefer to use an electric hand mixer for this).

Mix in the ground almonds, flour, vanilla or almond extract and egg until well combined.

Spread the mixture evenly in the prepared tin, then arrange the peach slices on top. Finish with a sprinkling of flaked almonds and bake in the oven for about 25–30 minutes until golden and no longer super wobbly.

To make this in an air fryer, heat or preheat the air fryer to 160°C (320°F) and ensure that the tin or dish will fit into your air fryer; if not, find the biggest size that will. Once you've prepared the mixture as opposite, transfer it to the tin and air fry for 25–30 minutes until golden and no longer super wobbly.

Serve warm or cold, dusted with icing sugar, with some vanilla ice cream or cream.

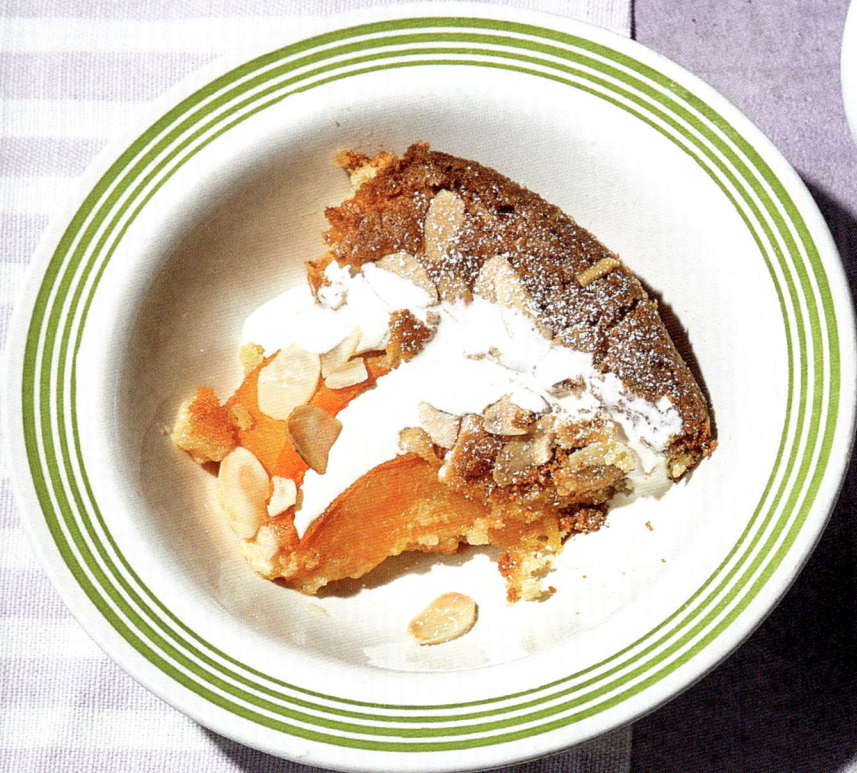

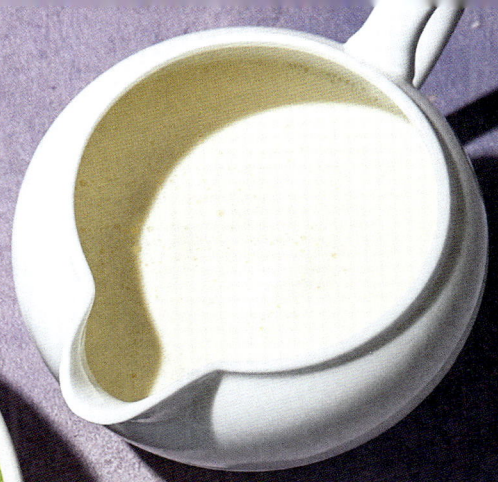

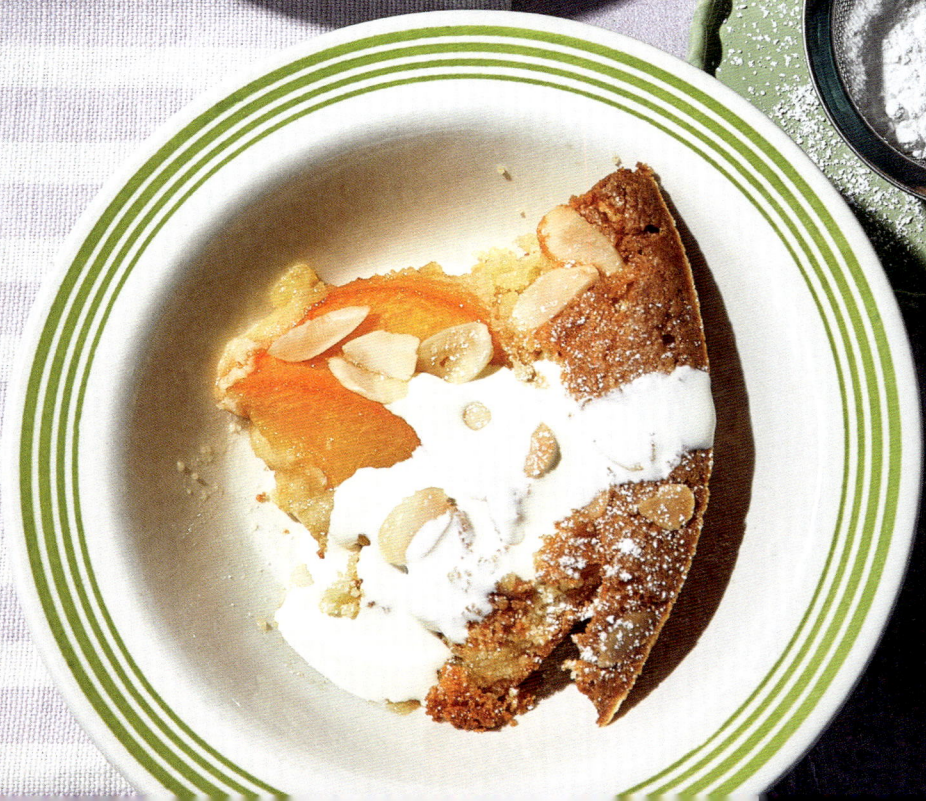

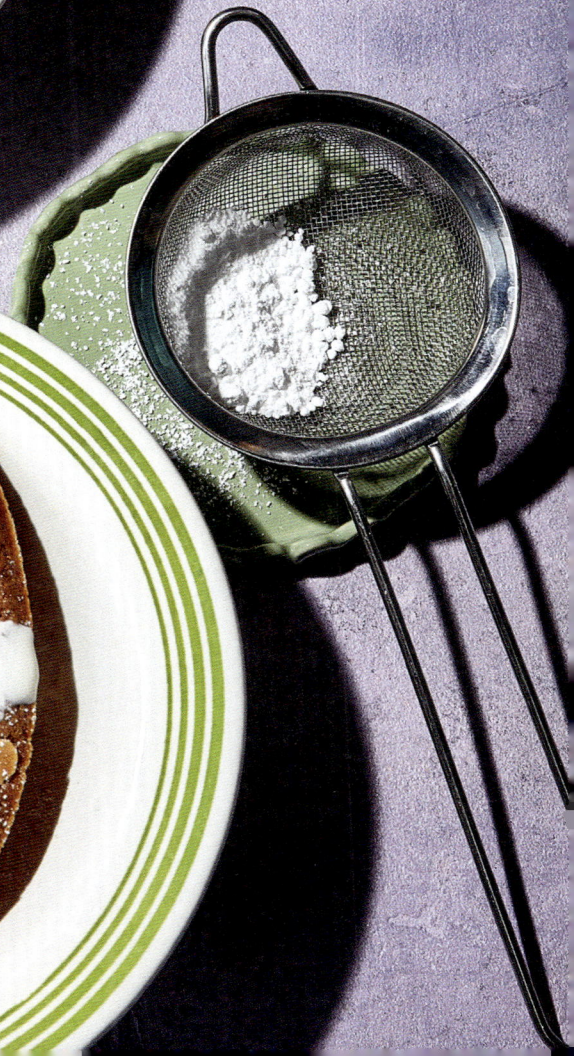

COURGETTE + LIME LOAF CAKE

Serves 8–10

Prep 15 mins

Oven 55 mins or
Air Fryer 50 mins

Now, adding courgette (zucchini) to this sweet and zesty cake isn't just a ploy to make it go further – it actually makes the cake incredibly moist without adding any unwanted flavour. Plus it's a great way to use up courgettes if you grow your own at home like we do! Gardening for baking is definitely something I didn't expect to add to my list of hobbies, but it's something I can most definitely get behind.

V

DF Use dairy-free cream cheese and a (hard) dairy-free alternative to butter.

LL Use lactose-free cream cheese.

F Use lactose-free cream cheese.

❄ See freezing and defrosting guidance for sponge cakes on page 28.

- 150ml (⅝ cup) vegetable oil
- 175g (¾ cup plus 2 tbsp) light brown sugar
- 3 medium eggs
- 200g (1½ cups) gluten-free self-raising flour
- ¼ tsp xanthan gum

- 1 tsp bicarbonate of soda (baking soda)
- 1 tsp ground cinnamon
- 175g (6¼oz) grated courgette (zucchini), weight after water squeezed out by hand
- Grated zest of 2 limes

For the cream cheese icing (frosting)
- 100g (scant ½ cup) butter, softened
- 100g (scant ¾ cup) icing (confectioners') sugar
- 200g (scant 1 cup) full-fat cream cheese
- 1 tsp vanilla extract
- Lime zest, to finish

To make this in the oven, preheat the oven to 160°C fan/180°C (350°F). Line a 900g (2lb) loaf tin (pan) with non-stick baking parchment.

Add the oil, sugar and eggs to a large bowl. Mix together, ideally using an electric hand mixer, until well combined. Add the flour, xanthan gum, bicarbonate of soda and cinnamon and mix in to combine. Ensure you've squeezed out a lot of liquid from the grated courgette, then fold that in alongside the lime zest.

Spoon the mixture into the prepared tin and bake in the oven for about 50–55 minutes. Check that it's cooked by sticking a skewer into the centre – if it comes out clean, then it's done.

To make this in an air fryer, heat or preheat the air fryer to 150°C (300°F). Make and spoon the mixture into the

prepared tin as opposite and air fry for 40–50 minutes – check with a skewer as opposite to ensure it's done.

Allow to cool in the tin briefly and then carefully lift onto a wire rack.

For the cream cheese icing, place the butter in a large bowl and mix for about 3 minutes using an electric hand mixer until it has turned a lot paler in colour. Add the icing sugar and mix for a further 3 minutes.

Before you add the cream cheese, ensure that there is no excess liquid in the tub – simply drain it if needed. Add to the bowl with the vanilla and mix for 2 more minutes until well combined, and the icing is light and fluffy, without lumps.

Spread the icing on the cooled loaf and finish with some extra lime zest.

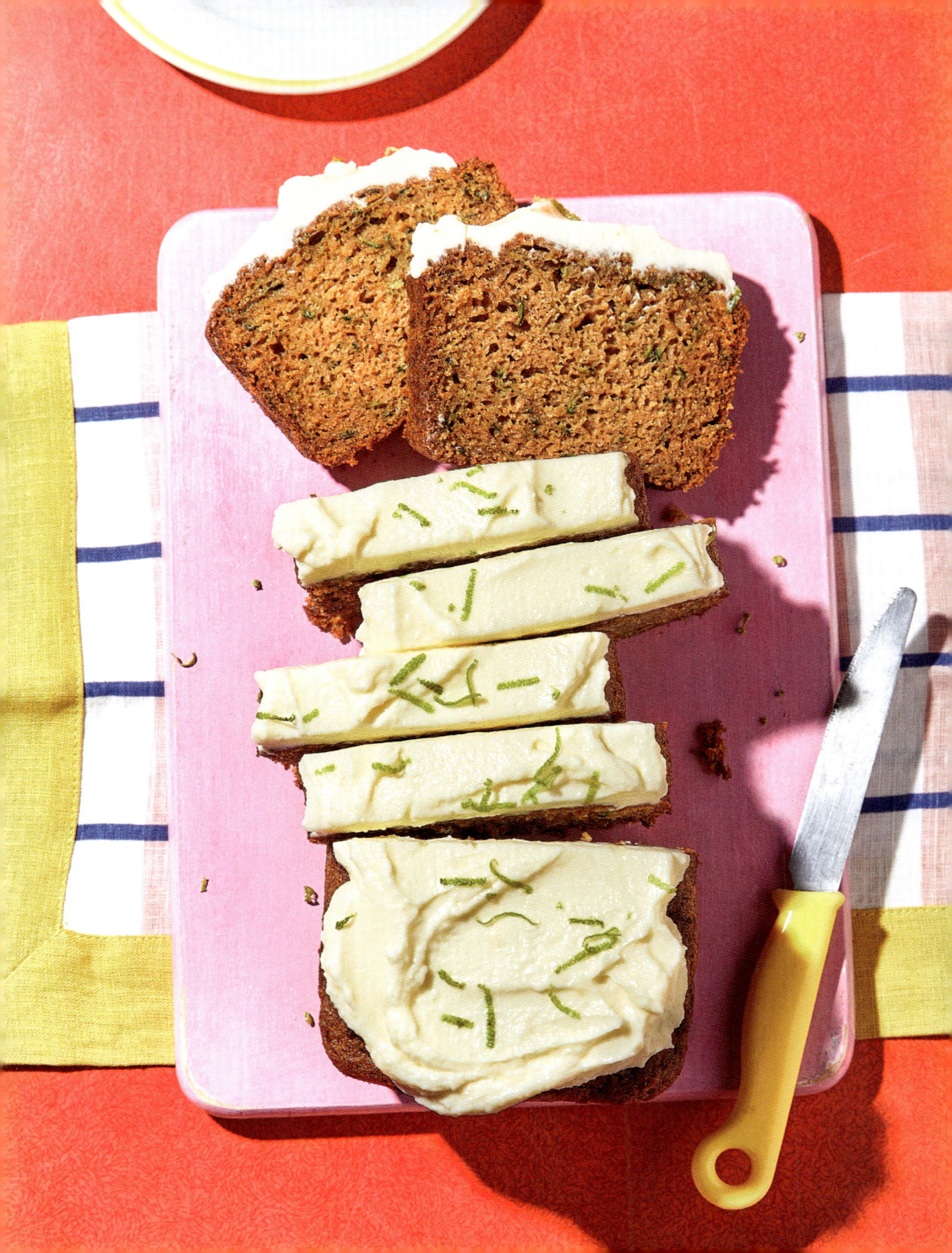

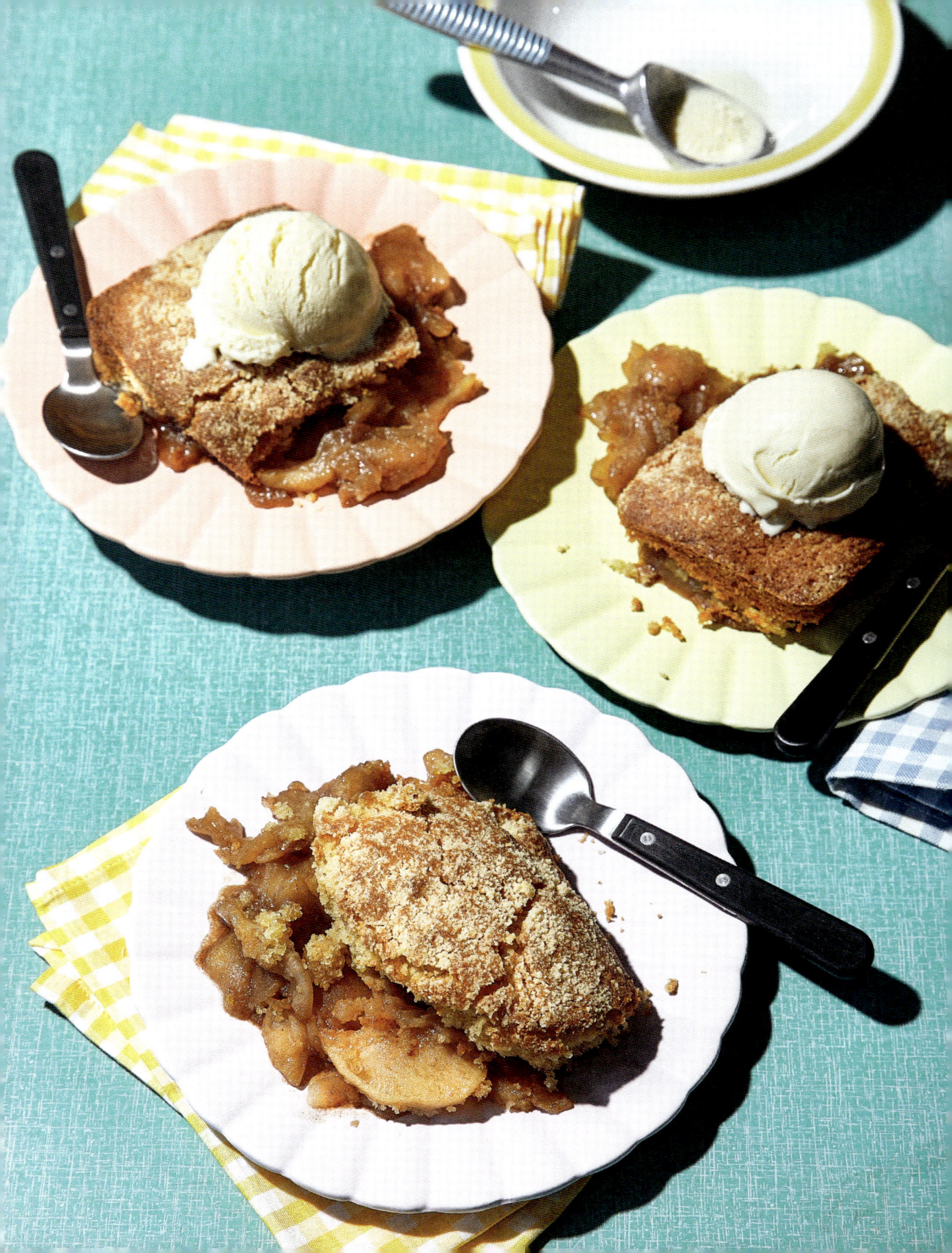

EVE'S PUDDING

This classic British apple sponge pudding is not only one of my favourite desserts when served with a catastrophic amount of gluten-free custard or ice cream, it's also a great way of using up any leftover apples that might otherwise go to waste. Traditionally you'd top this with flaked (slivered) almonds before baking, but when I'm lacking those, I often use ground almonds instead, as pictured. Feel free to use whatever you have to hand!

Serves 6

Prep 5 mins

Hob + Oven 55 mins or
Hob + Air Fryer 40 mins

LL **V**

DF Use a (hard) dairy-free alternative to butter.

❄ See freezing and defrosting guidance for sponge cakes on page 28.

For the apples
- 550g (1lb 3½oz) eating apples (about 8), peeled, cored and thinly sliced
- 2 tbsp light brown sugar
- 1 tbsp lemon juice
- 2 tbsp water
- 20g (1½oz) butter
- 1 tsp ground cinnamon

For the topping
- 125g (½ cup plus 1 tbsp) butter, softened
- 100g (½ cup) light brown sugar
- 2 medium eggs
- 1 tsp vanilla extract
- 125g (1 cup minus 1 tbsp) gluten-free self-raising flour
- ground or flaked (slivered) almonds, for sprinkling (optional)

Place all the ingredients for the apples in a large saucepan over a low–medium heat. Stir to coat the apples, then pop the lid on and allow to cook for 5–10 minutes until the apples are starting to break down, and are soft and cooked. Spoon into a rectangular ovenproof dish about 22 x 16cm (9 x 6in) and put to one side while you make the topping.

To make this in the oven, preheat the oven to 160°C fan/180°C (350°F).

In a large bowl, cream together the butter and sugar until light and fluffy. Add the eggs one at a time, beating between each addition. Mix in the vanilla before folding in the flour. Spoon the mixture on top of the apples and optionally sprinkle with some ground or flaked almonds.

Bake for 40–45 minutes, until golden and the sponge is fully cooked.

To make this in an air fryer, heat or preheat the air fryer to 150°C (300°F) and ensure that the dish or tin will fit into your air fryer; if not, find the biggest size that will. Follow the steps opposite to create the cake mixture, then arrange it along with the apples and ground or flaked almonds in the prepared tin. Air fry for 30 minutes until golden and the sponge is fully cooked.

Serve warm with custard or vanilla ice cream.

EMERGENCY BERRY SWIRL NO-BAKE CHEESECAKE POTS

Serves 4

Prep 20 mins

Fridge 1–2 hours (optional)

I know, I know, a 'dessert emergency' is probably quite low in the grand scheme of emergencies, but it's one that can happen all too often when you're gluten free. Fortunately, when you make these little sharp, sweet and creamy cheesecakes with a buttery biscuit base, the time from prepping to eating is the shortest it could possibly be when making a no-bake cheesecake. That's because the pot supports the filling so it never needs to freely stand on its own, meaning you can basically enjoy it straight away, or allow it to set in the fridge for a couple of hours if you'd prefer it to be a bit firmer. It's totally up to you!

V

DF Use a (hard) dairy-free alternative to butter, dairy-free cream cheese and a dairy-free alternative to cream.

LL Use lactose-free cream cheese and lactose-free cream.

❄ Cover and freeze the assembled cheesecakes. Make sure the glasses or ramekins you are using are freezer safe. Defrost fully in the fridge before eating.

For the berry sauce
- 200g (7oz) frozen berries
- 40g (scant ¼ cup) caster (superfine) sugar
- 50ml (3½ tbsp) water
- 1 tsp cornflour (cornstarch)

For the biscuit base
- 100g (3½oz) gluten-free digestive biscuits (graham crackers)
- 35g (2½ tbsp) butter, melted

For the filling
- 250g (generous 1 cup) full-fat cream cheese
- 55g (6 tbsp) icing (confectioners') sugar
- 150ml (⅝ cup) double (heavy) cream
- ½ tsp vanilla extract

TIP
The leftover berries that remain in the sieve (strainer) can be either enjoyed on top of the cheesecakes or even stirred through plain yoghurt as a snack. So definitely don't get rid of them!

For the berry sauce, place a medium saucepan over a low heat, then add the frozen berries, sugar and water. Simmer for 10 minutes or until the sugar has dissolved and the berries have softened, then break them down with the back of a wooden spoon. Sieve (strain) the mixture into a small bowl (keep the berries – see **TIP**) and pour the liquid back into the saucepan. Stir in the cornflour and continue to simmer until the mixture thickens, then set aside to cool.

Meanwhile, for the base, use a food processor to blitz the biscuits to a crumb-like texture – not into a fine dust! Alternatively, pop the biscuits into a zip-lock bag and bash them with a rolling pin. Add to a large bowl, pour in the melted butter and mix well. Spoon the mixture evenly between

4 ramekins, compacting it down, and pop in the fridge or freezer to chill while you make the filling.

Place the cream cheese and icing sugar in a medium bowl. Mix using a spatula or with an electric hand mixer for about 10–20 seconds, then add the cream and vanilla. Mix for about a minute or until it begins to firm up.

Spoon the mixture on top of each of the bases and then swirl or feather a little of the berry sauce onto the top of each.

Optionally chill in the fridge until completely set, for 1–2 hours; I often make mine the night before I want to serve them, for ease. Feel free to enjoy them before 1–2 hours of chilling, as the ramekins will contain them completely even if not fully set.

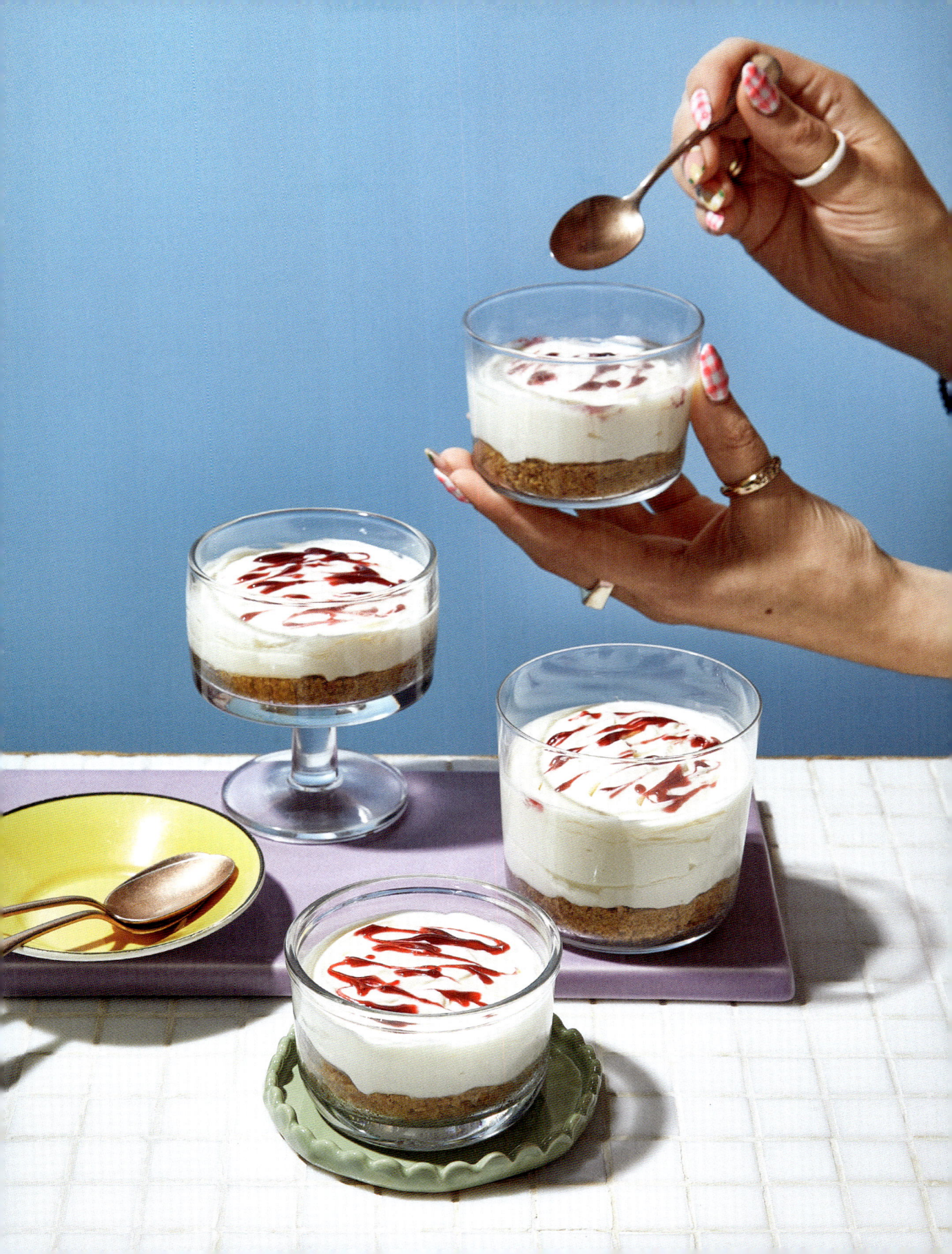

SLOW COOKER CHOCOLATE FUDGE PUDDING

Serves 8–10

Prep 5 mins

Slow Cooker 2 hours

There's absolutely no doubt that the slow cooker is an underrated, cheap-to-run, small appliance when it comes to dessert. Not only will making your dessert in it usually not get in the way of whatever you're cooking on the hob, in the oven or air fryer, but it yields an exceptionally soft, fluffy, pudding-like texture every time. And this chocolatey pudding, with a hidden, secret chocolate sauce at the bottom, is no exception! Note that I made this recipe using a 6.5l (7 quart) slow cooker. In smaller slow cookers, it can take a little longer.

V

DF Use a (hard) dairy-free alternative to butter, dairy-free milk and dairy-free chocolate chips.

LL Use lactose-free milk and lactose-free chocolate chips.

F See low lactose advice.

❄ See freezing and defrosting guidance for sponge cakes on page 28.

- 175g (1⅓ cups) gluten-free self-raising flour
- 1 tsp gluten-free baking powder
- 30g (4 tbsp) unsweetened cocoa powder
- 200g (1 cup) caster (superfine) sugar
- 2 medium eggs
- 215ml (1 cup minus 2 tbsp) milk
- 90g (½ cup minus 2 tsp) butter, melted, plus extra for greasing
- 75g (2½oz) chocolate chips of your choice

For the topping
- 185g (1 cup minus 1 tbsp) light brown sugar
- 20g (3 tbsp) unsweetened cocoa powder
- 600ml (1¼ pints) boiling water

Prepare the slow cooker dish by greasing it all over with butter.

In a large bowl, mix together the flour, baking powder, cocoa powder and caster sugar.

In a separate bowl, mix together the eggs, milk and melted butter, then add it to the dry ingredients. Mix thoroughly to ensure there are no flour lumps and it's well combined. Then fold through the chocolate chips and pour the mixture into the prepared slow cooker dish.

Mix together the light brown sugar and cocoa powder and sprinkle this over the top of the cake batter. Carefully pour the boiling water on top of that evenly.

Pop the lid on the slow cooker and cook on high for around 2 hours. As slow cookers seem to differ, I would check it after about 90 minutes, but it could take up to 2½ hours. You are looking for a firm sponge top and middle but with a degree of moisture still beneath, as this is what forms the delicious chocolate sauce.

Serve the pudding warm with lots of the chocolate sauce over the top of it. Add a little cream to serve, if you fancy.

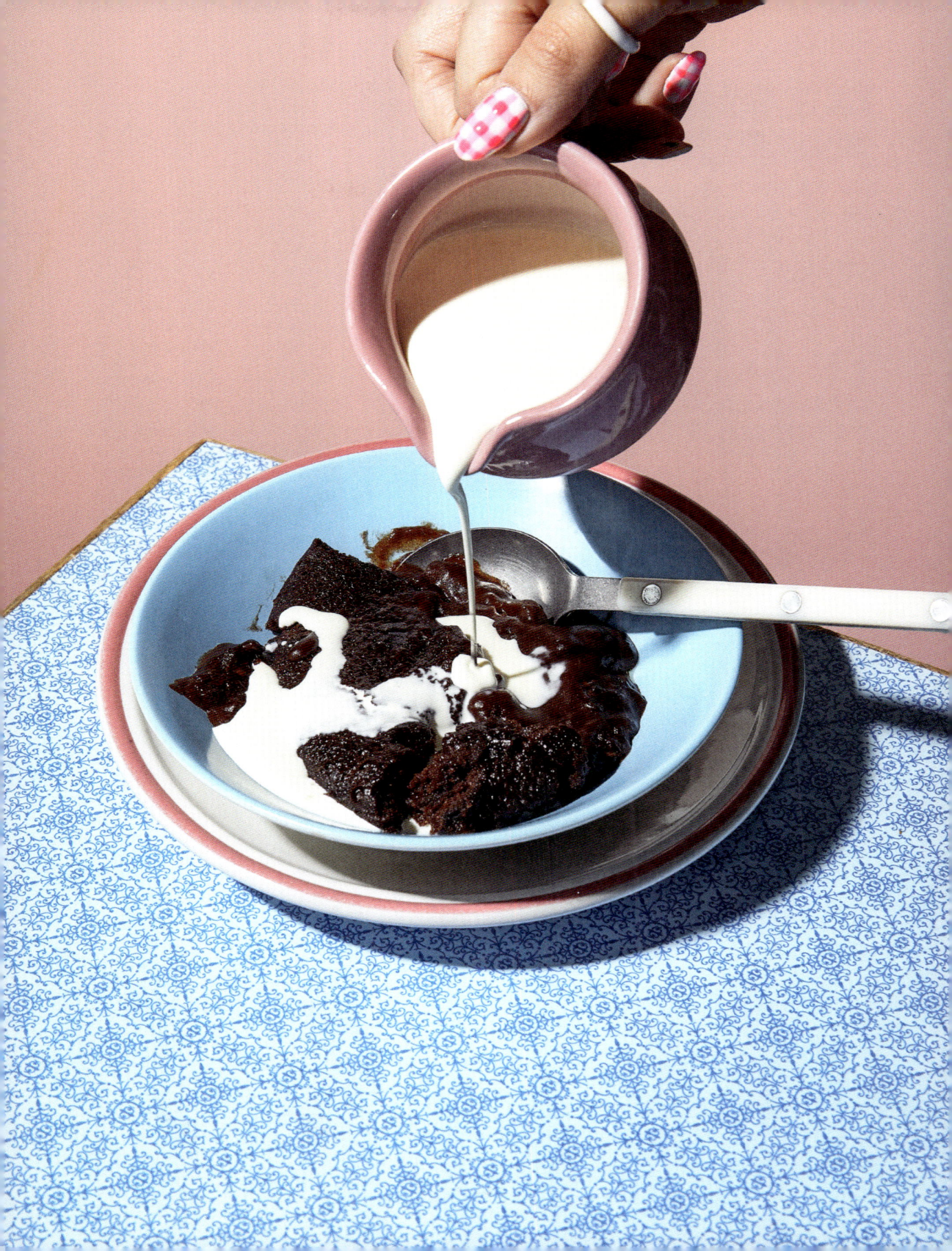

LEMON POSSET 2 WAYS

Here's a dessert to suit two situations: emergency dessert pots in a hurry, or a full-sized lemon tart centrepiece that's set to impress. Whichever you choose, you can expect the same, creamy, zesty and sweet lemon crowd-pleaser!

Makes 6–8 possets or 8–12 slices of tart

Posset Prep 5 mins + 3 hours chilling

Tart Prep 20 mins + 3–4 hours chilling

Oven (tart only) 22 mins

V

❄ Both the posset and the tart can be frozen. Make sure the glasses or ramekins you are using are freezer safe. Defrost fully in the fridge before eating.

TIPS

If the pastry dough is quite firm after being chilled in the fridge, leaving it out at room temperature ahead of time is definitely advised. Simply remove it from the fridge and place it to one side until you're able to easily roll it out. Remember not to excessively handle the dough from that point onwards, as this will warm it up and make it stickier.

Any excess pastry can be wrapped well and frozen for 2–3 months or kept in the fridge for 2–3 days. You can always easily use it up by following the method in my jam tarts recipe over on page 213.

For the filling (posset or tart)

- 600ml (2½ cups) double (heavy) cream
- 200g (1 cup) caster (superfine) sugar
- Grated zest of 3 lemons, plus 75ml (5 tbsp) juice

For the pastry (tart only)

- 300g (2¼ cups) gluten-free plain (all-purpose) flour, plus extra for dusting
- 1½ tsp xanthan gum
- 145g (⅔ cup) very cold butter, cubed
- 3 tbsp caster (superfine) sugar
- 2 large eggs, beaten

To make the lemon possets, place the cream and sugar in a saucepan over a low heat and stir until the sugar has dissolved. Increase the heat a little to bring the mixture to a simmer. Allow to simmer for 1–2 minutes before taking off the heat. Stir through the lemon zest and juice and pour the mixture evenly between 6–8 serving glasses or ramekins, then chill in the fridge for 3–4 hours or overnight, until fully set.

To make a lemon posset tart, first make the pastry. In a large bowl, combine the flour and xanthan gum. Add the very cold butter to the bowl and, using your fingertips, rub it into the flour to form a breadcrumb-like consistency. (You can also achieve the same result by using a food processor.)

Stir in the sugar, then add the beaten egg and, using a knife, carefully cut it into the mixture until it comes together. It should form a ball and be a little sticky to the touch but not unmanageable. Wrap the dough in cling film (plastic wrap) and leave to chill in the fridge for at least 1 hour (see **TIP**).

Flour a rolling pin and a large sheet of non-stick baking parchment, then roll out the dough on the parchment into a circle 3mm (⅛in) thick.

Invert the pastry into a 23cm (9in) loose-bottomed fluted tart tin (pan), then peel off the parchment. Use your fingers to carefully ease the pastry into

place, so that it neatly lines the tin. Lift the overhanging pastry and, using your thumb, squash 2mm (1⁄16in) of pastry back into the tin. This will result in slightly thicker sides, which will prevent the pastry from shrinking when baked. Allow the rest of the overhang to do its thing – we'll trim it after chilling. Lightly prick the base of the pastry case several times with a fork, then chill in the fridge for 15 minutes.

Preheat the oven to 180°C fan/ 200°C (400°F).

Remove the pastry case from the fridge and use a rolling pin to roll over the top of the tin, removing the overhang and flattening the pastry rim. Loosely line the base with a piece of scrunched baking parchment and fill with baking beans (or uncooked rice if you don't have any). Place on a baking tray in the oven and bake for 15 minutes, then remove the parchment and baking beans and bake for a further 5–7 minutes. Allow to completely cool.

Follow the instructions opposite for making the lemon possets, but pour the mixture into the pastry case instead. Leave to chill in the fridge for about 3–4 hours, or overnight, until set.

Serve both the possets and the tart simply as they are, or optionally adorn with fresh or frozen and defrosted berries – the berry sauce on page 238 also goes well with the tart.

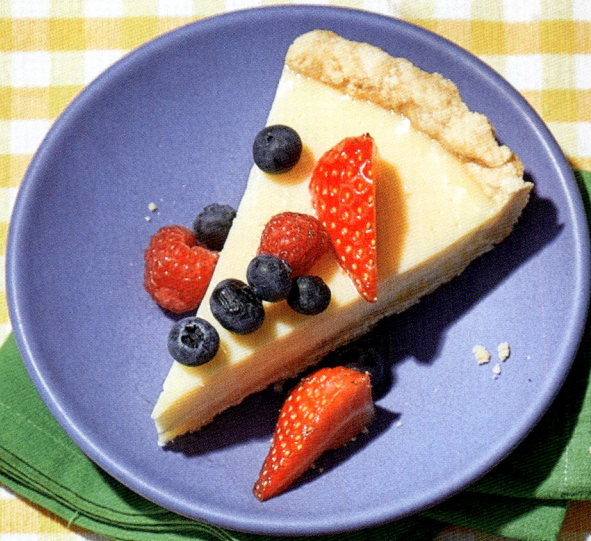

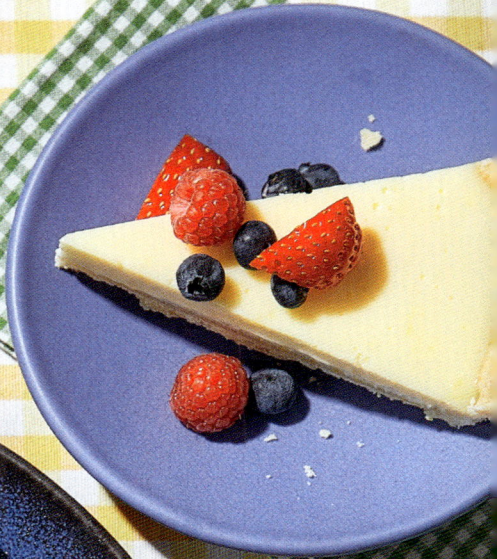

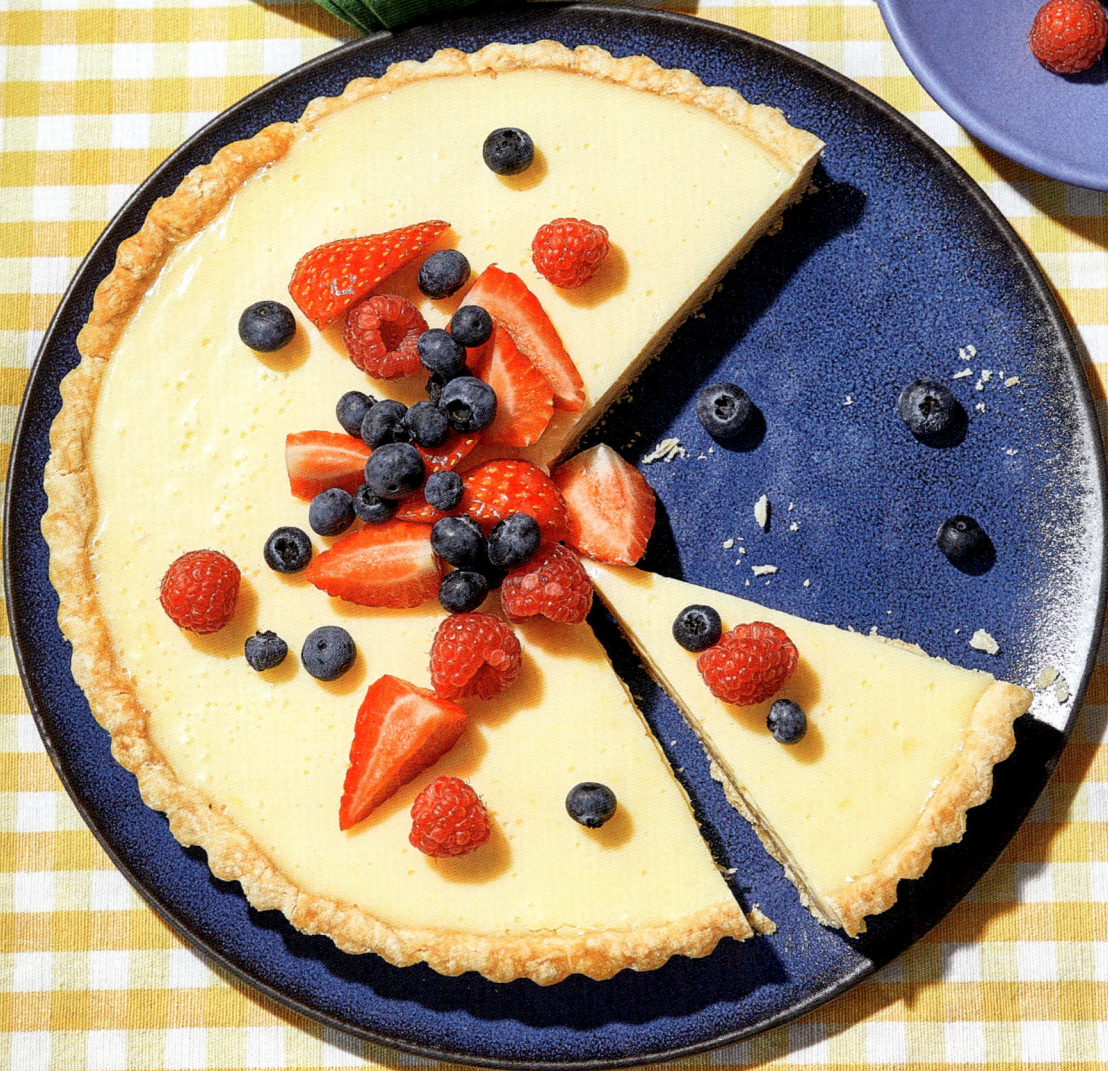

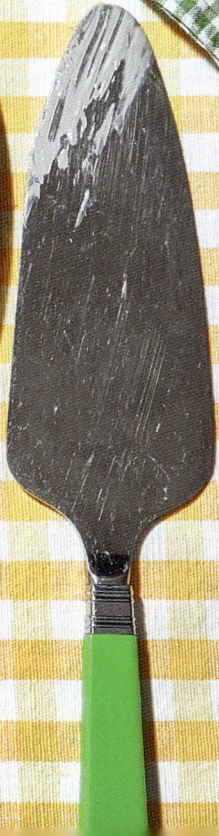

MICROWAVE SPOTTED DICK

Serves 4

Prep 5 mins

Microwave 5 mins or less

V

DF Use a dairy-free 'buttery' margarine for greasing and use dairy-free milk.

LL Use lactose-free milk.

F Use lactose-free milk and use no more than 52g (1¾oz) dried currants.

❄ See freezing and defrosting guidance for sponge cakes on page 28.

TIP

Some supermarkets in the UK sell gluten-free vegetarian suet at a very reasonable price – you'll usually find it down the baking aisle. However, most suet products aren't gluten-free, so always check the ingredients and labelling on the packaging first.

If you're not from the UK, then I should probably first start this by apologizing for the title. If you are from the UK, then you'll already know that this super-traditional dessert is a soft and fluffy sponge with a hint of lemon that sets off the sweet little currants perfectly. All you need is some custard to serve, and you're set. Apparently the 'spotted' part of the name refers to the appearance of the currants and the 'dick' part came from a shortening of the word 'pudding' to 'ding', which somehow became... well, I'm not typing it again!

- Butter, softened, for greasing
- 100g (¾ cup) gluten-free self-raising flour
- 75g (2½oz) gluten-free vegetarian suet
- 75g (6 tbsp) caster (superfine) sugar
- Grated zest of ½ lemon
- 1 large egg
- 125ml (½ cup plus 1 tsp) milk
- 75g (2½oz) currants

Prepare either one 1-litre (2-pint) pudding basin or 4 individual microwave-safe pudding moulds by greasing them with a little softened butter.

In a medium bowl, stir together the flour, suet, sugar and lemon zest. Mix in the egg and milk so it is well combined, then fold through the currants. This can all be done with a spatula.

Spoon the mixture into the larger pudding basin or divide equally between the small pudding moulds. Microwave at full power (mine is set to 1000W) for 4½ minutes for the larger pudding or around 1 minute 20 seconds for the smaller puddings.

Carefully remove from the microwave and use a palette knife to loosen around the edges. Use a plate (or plates) to invert the pudding(s) and carefully lift the basin/moulds off to reveal the perfect spotted dick.

Serve straight away, with custard.

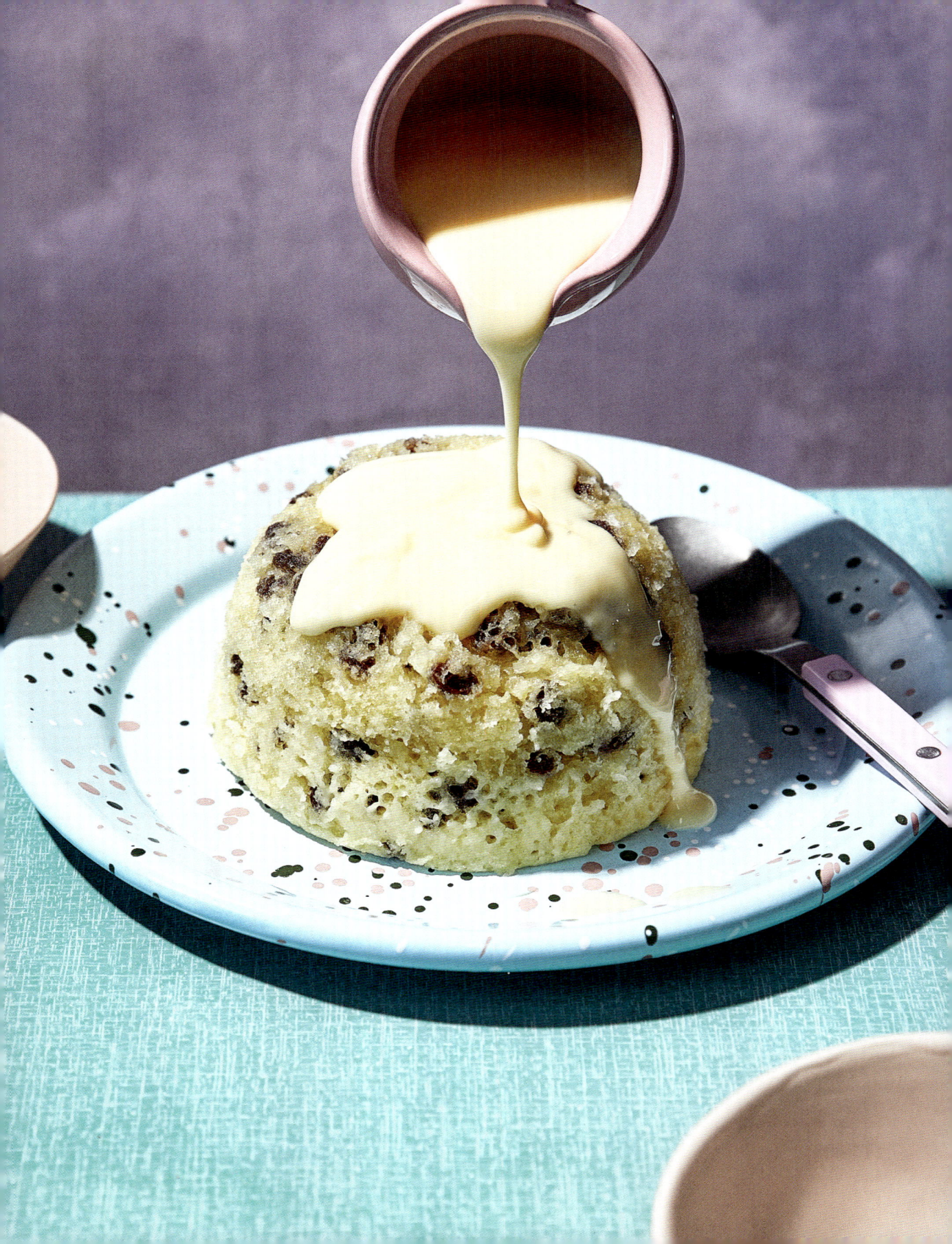

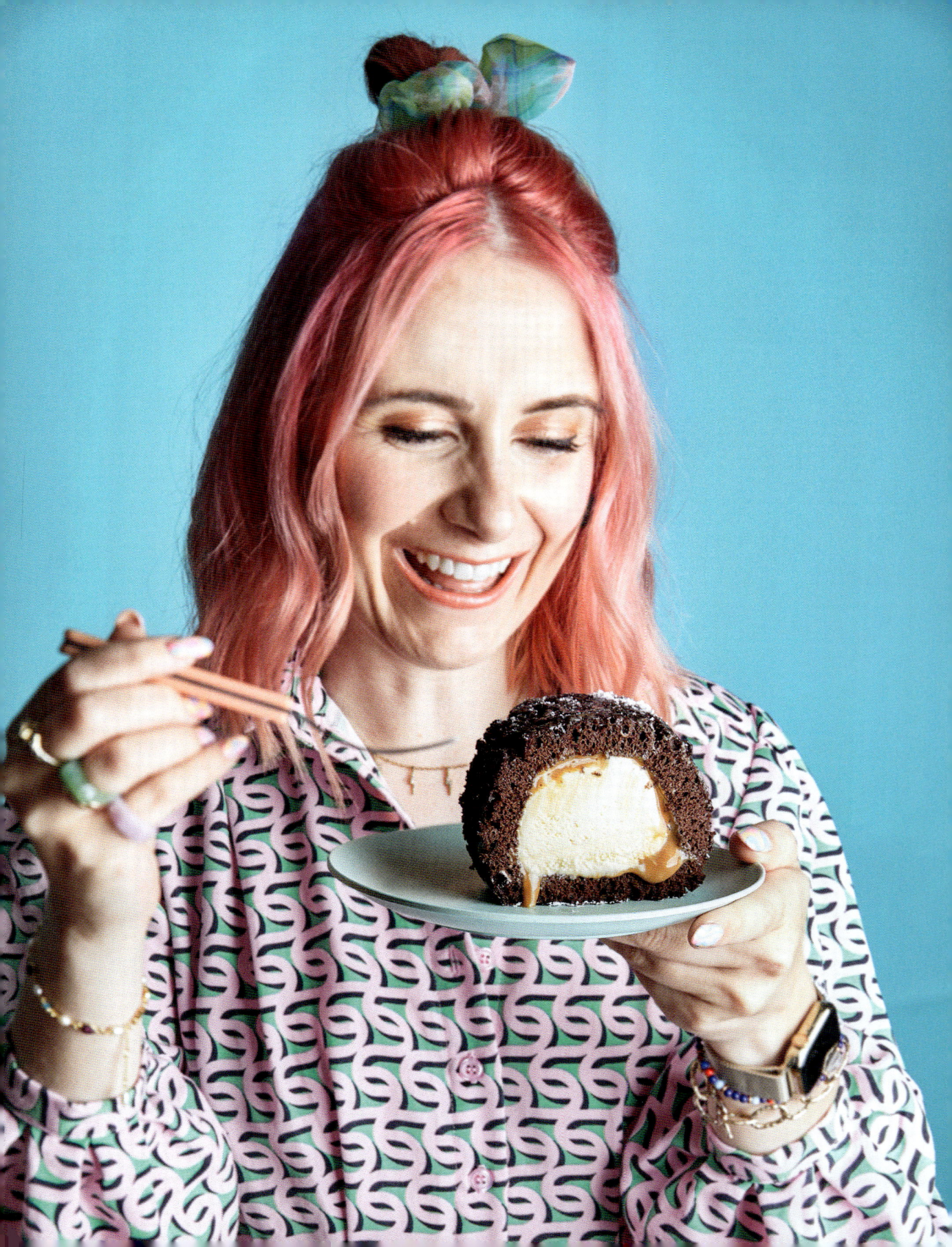

CHOCOLATE + CARAMEL ARCTIC ROLL

Serves 8–10

Prep 25 mins

Oven 9 mins

Freezer 2 hours

V

DF Use dairy-free ice cream and dairy-free caramel.

LL Use low lactose ice cream and lactose-free caramel.

F See low lactose advice.

❄ Store in airtight containers (ideally sliced) for up to 2–3 months.

Ice cream in the world's lightest chocolate Swiss-roll-style sponge with lashings of caramel sauce? Gluten free? Oh sorry, I must be dreaming. No actually, it's definitely real, because I just made and enjoyed many slices of this! This chocolate, caramel and vanilla take on a classic dessert might be too good to believe, but as I always say, eating is believing.

- 100g (½ cup) caster (superfine) sugar
- 4 large eggs
- 65g (½ cup) gluten-free self-raising flour
- ¼ tsp xanthan gum
- 40g (½ cup minus 1 tbsp) unsweetened cocoa powder
- Icing (confectioners') sugar, for dusting

For the filling
- 900g (2lb) vanilla or caramel vanilla ice cream
- 200g (7oz) caramel

Remove the ice cream from the freezer and, on a large sheet of cling film (plastic wrap), larger than a 30 x 23cm (12 x 9in) Swiss roll tin (pan), form a long sausage-like shape of ice cream that's roughly 3.5cm (1¼in) in diameter. Roll it up tightly in the cling film, then carefully place in the freezer to firm up again.

Preheat the oven to 180°C fan/200°C (400°F). Line a Swiss roll tin with non-stick baking parchment. Make sure the baking parchment fits well, as you'll need the full shape of the tin.

In a large bowl, whisk together the sugar and eggs until light and a little frothy. It should only take a few minutes (I prefer to use an electric hand mixer for this). Sift in the flour, xanthan gum and cocoa powder, then fold into the mixture carefully until fully combined.

Pour the mixture into the tin and spread it right to the edges. Try your best to get it nice and even, as it will rise more consistently in the oven.

Bake in the oven for about 9 minutes. The sponge should have come away a little bit from the sides of the tin and be slightly risen.

Remove from the oven and very carefully invert the sponge onto another piece of baking parchment that's lightly dusted with icing sugar. Carefully peel off the parchment that was on the bottom of it in the oven.

Now, while the sponge is still warm, roll it up with the parchment inside it as you roll – ensure a long side of the sponge is closest to you before you roll. Place the rolled-up sponge to one side and leave it to cool completely while rolled up. I usually put something heavy against it to ensure it stays fairly tight and doesn't unroll itself.

Once completely cooled, carefully unroll the sponge and remove the parchment. Spread the caramel all over the inside of the unrolled sponge, then remove the ice cream from the freezer. Remove the cling film and place the ice cream 'sausage' along a long side of the sponge, about 2cm (¾in) in from the edge, and carefully roll the sponge up around the ice cream. Re-wrap in cling film and place back in the freezer for a couple of hours to firm up.

To serve, remove from the freezer and allow to sit for about 5 minutes, then dust with icing sugar and slice.

INDEX

THANK YOU

I'm always told I write too much here... so I'm going to again as this book would not exist without a lot of incredible people!

Firstly, thank you to my super-star editor Harriet Webster. We've somehow worked on seven books together now and I just want to say thank you for putting up with me, I don't know how you do it!

Thanks always to Sarah Lavelle for her continued belief in me and my books and for taking a punt on me in the first place all those years ago! Thanks a million to Stacey Cleworth for your valued input and for always being at the end of an e-mail whenever I need help.

Huge thanks to my literary agent, Emily Sweet, who always seems to have all the answers when I have none! I infinitely appreciate your honesty and input.

Thank you once again to my copy editor, Sally Somers, for your knowledgeable and insightful edits as always.

Thanks to the talented designer of this book, Emily Lapworth, for making *Budget Gluten Free* as vibrant, fun and even more visually appealing than I could have ever imagined. I don't know how you do it, but you are the best in the business!

Thank you to Hannah Hughes for all the truly mind-blowing food photography – we'd expect no less! Shout out to photography assistant Sasha Burdian too.

Thank you to Amy Stephenson (and baby Annie – food stylist in the making!) for your flawless food-styling yet again, as well as food stylist assistant Áine Pretty-McGrath. Huge thanks to prop stylist Max Robinson for yet another stunning curation of all things props.

I'm once again super grateful to Cat Parnell for her hair and make-up magic on set! Thanks to Nicky for the flawless cut and colour of my hair and thank you to Amy for your amazing nail art skills as always.

Thanks to Laura Eldridge and Alice Hill, as well as Ruth Tewkesbury, Iman Khabl and Di Kojik, for flying the flag for my books. You all continue to help gluten-free people find my books and for that, I am forever grateful.

And of course, thank you to the entire 'Quad Squad' at Quadrille Publishing for their persistent enthusiasm, care and making the process of publishing a book so seamless from start to finish.

A massive thank you to Ros Dundas for not just helping to get the book out there and seen, but myself too!

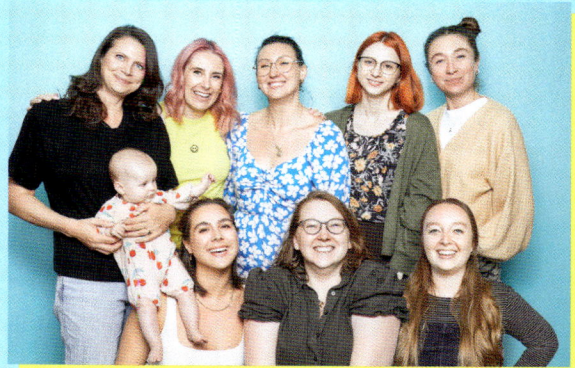

(Most) of the photoshoot crew!

Big thanks to Robyn Tyrer and the team at M&C Saatchi Merlin, I'm so happy to be working together now – the sky's the limit!

The BIGGEST thank you to my boyfriend, recipe tester and proofreader, Mark, who still did all of that even after a late night trip to A&E and several months of being one-handed! I genuinely couldn't do this without you. Thanks to my dog and mini mascot, Peggy, who probably thinks I spend way too much time at home, in the kitchen. She's asleep on my lap as I type this!

Thank you sincerely to my Mum and Dad for always supporting me and believing in me – if you're reading this, then you will have to come over and let us make you dinner!

Thanks again to my brother Charlie and his fiance Gemma, my Auntie Carol, as well as Mark's mum, dad and sister, Lisa, and her partner Michael (as well as Micah and Evelyn!) for all the constant support, recipe testing and positivity.

A huge thank you to my Facebook group moderators past and present including Kirstie, Lizzie, Sharon, Amanda, Bindu and Debbie. Your help in managing the group has not only been invaluable, but just chatting to you all about life in general means a lot to me. You rock!

And finally, thanks to YOU and all of my dedicated followers/readers (especially those of you in the Facebook group!) for the unyielding support and enthusiasm across all of my books and everything I do. There absolutely wouldn't be a seventh book without you and I sincerely hope that together, we can continue to improve the lives of gluten-free people and achieve a greater understanding from others.

ABOUT THE AUTHOR

Becky Excell is a best-selling author and gluten-free food writer with a following of over 1 million on her social media channels and over 1 million monthly views on her award-winning blog.

She won the *Observer Food Monthly*'s Best Food Personality award in 2022, the BCreator Award's Food Creator of the Year 2022 and BBC Food and Farming's Digital Creator of the Year Award 2023.

She's been eating gluten-free for 16 years and writes recipes for numerous print and online publications. She has made various TV appearances, most recently on ITV's *This Morning*, raising awareness and showing the nation how easy it is to make delicious gluten-free food, as well as cooking and baking at events including the Good Food Show, The Big Feastival, Carfest and Pub in the Park.

She gave up a career working in PR and marketing to focus on food full-time, with an aim to develop recipes which reunite her and her followers with the foods they can no longer eat. Her previous six best-selling cookbooks, *How to Make Anything Gluten Free*, *How to Bake Anything Gluten Free*, *How to Plan Anything Gluten Free*, *Quick and Easy Gluten Free*, *Gluten Free Christmas* and *Gluten Free Air Fryer* were published by Quadrille. She lives in Essex, UK.

You can find more of Becky's delicious and fuss-free gluten-free recipes on her website **glutenfreecuppatea.co.uk**, on Instagram **@beckyexcell**, or on her Facebook page **Becky Excell Gluten Free**.

RECIPE NOTES

MEAT TEMPERATURE GUIDE

As I said in the 'Not Mandatory but Super Handy' part of the Essential Equipment section on page 21, a digital food thermometer can not only be incredibly handy at telling you when your food is sufficiently cooked or reheated, but they can also be surprisingly affordable. →

EGG CONVERSION GUIDE

Did you know that egg sizes are different in various parts of the world? Me neither! That's why I thought I'd pop in a handy egg conversion guide in the back of this book to help make things simple. I've used UK egg sizes in all my recipes, so just convert from there. ↓

UK	USA + CANADA	AUSTRALIA
Small	Medium	Large
Medium	Large	Extra-large
Large	Extra-large	Jumbo

FOOD	TYPE	MINIMUM INTERNAL TEMPERATURE
Beef, lamb, pork and goat	Steaks, roasts and chops	63°C (145°F) Rest time: 3 minutes
	Mince (ground) meat and sausages	71°C (160°F)
Chicken, duck, turkey and other poultry	All: whole bird, breasts, legs, thighs, wings, mince (ground meat), etc.	74°C (165°F)
Seafood	All fish (whole or fillet)	50–60°C (120–140°F)
	Prawns (shrimp), lobster, crab, shellfish	63°C (145°F) Or at your own discretion

Quadrille, Penguin Random House UK,
One Embassy Gardens,
8 Viaduct Gardens, London
SW11 7BW

Quadrille Publishing Limited is part of the Penguin Random House group of companies whose addresses can be found at global.penguinrandomhouse.com

Penguin
Random House
UK

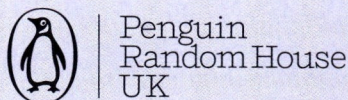

Published by Quadrille in 2025

www.penguin.co.uk

A CIP catalogue record for this book is available from the British Library

ISBN 978-1-83783-245-3
10 9 8 7 6 5 4 3 2 1

Managing Director Sarah Lavelle

Senior Commissioning Editor Stacey Cleworth

Project Editor Harriet Webster

Design and Art Direction Emily Lapworth

Designer Sarah Fisher

Photographer Hannah Hughes

Props Stylist Max Robinson

Food Stylist Amy Stephenson

Makeup and Hair Stylist Cat Parnell

Production Manager Sabeena Atchia

Head of Production Stephen Lang

Colour reproduction by F1

Printed and bound in Germany by Mohn Media

The authorised representative in the EEA is Penguin Random House Ireland, Morrison Chambers, 32 Nassau Street, Dublin D02 YH68.

Penguin Random House is committed to a sustainable future for our business, our readers and our planet. This book is made from Forest Stewardship Council® certified paper.

FSC
www.fsc.org

MIX
Paper | Supporting responsible forestry
FSC® C018179

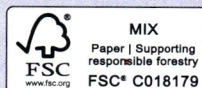

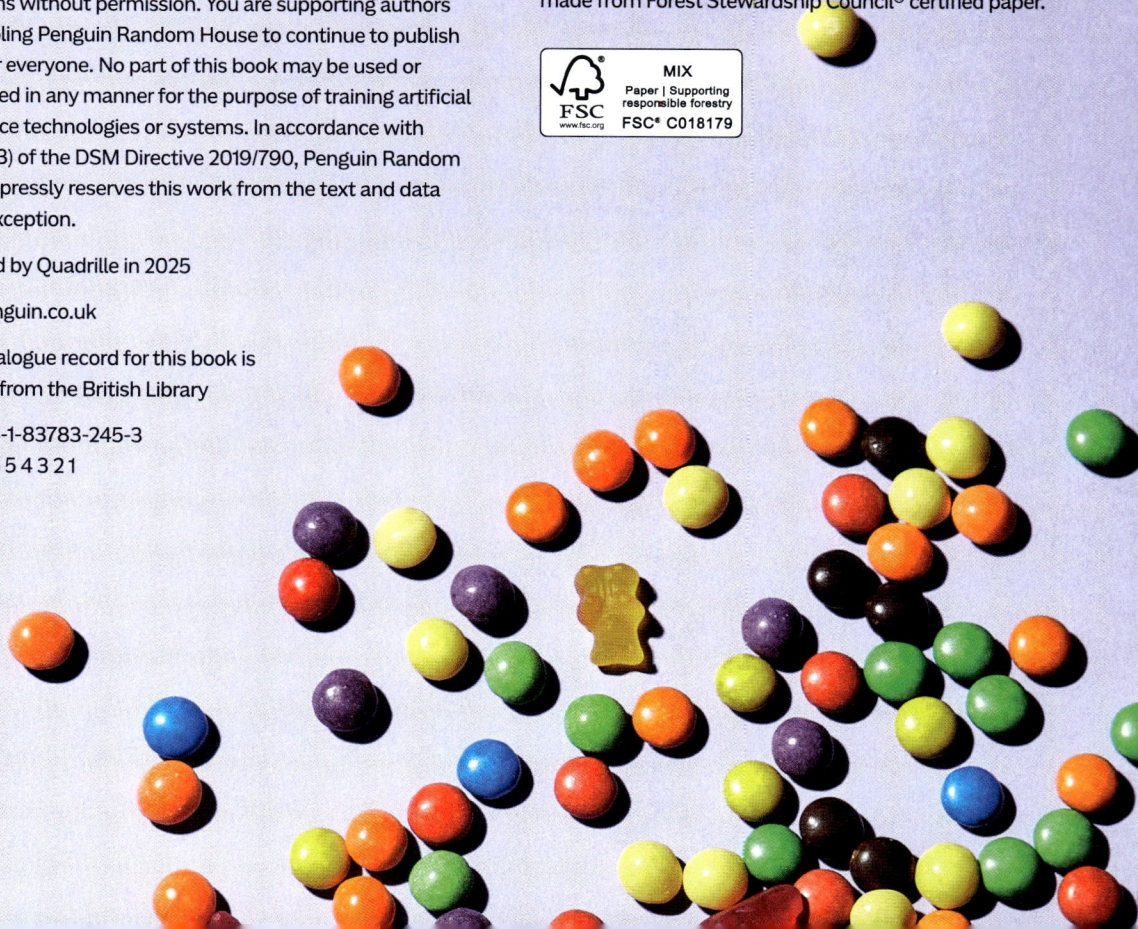

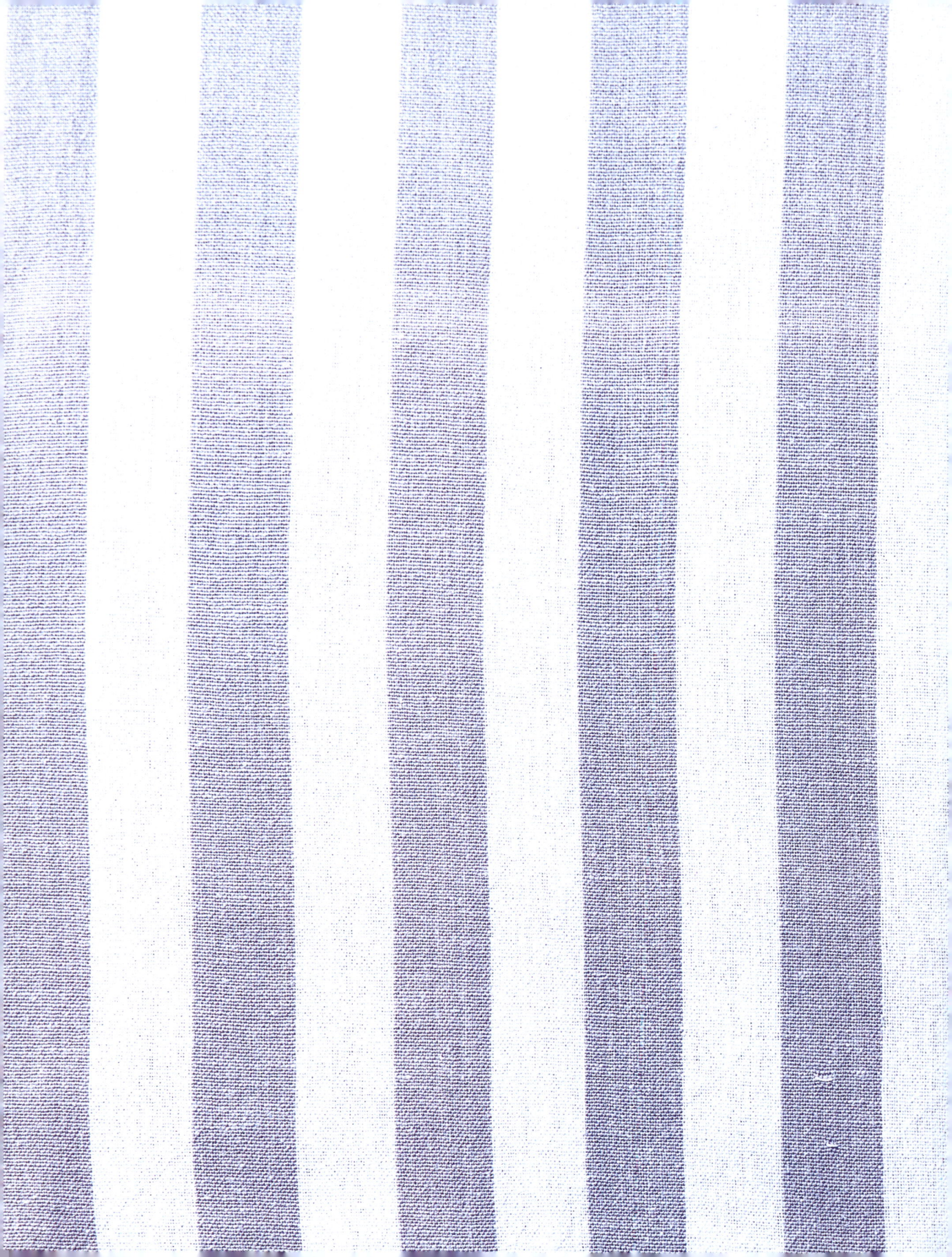